Therapeutic Footwear

A Comprehensive Guide

For Elsevier

Commissioning Editor: Robert Edwards
Development Editor: Nicola Lally
Project Manager: Sukanthi Sukumar
Designer/Design Direction: Charles Gray
Illustration Manager: Merlyn Harvey
Illustrator: Antbits

Therapeutic Footwear A Comprehensive Guide

Wendy Tyrrell MEd, FHEA, DPodM, MChS, FCPodMed
Principal Lecturer, University of Wales Institute Cardiff

Gwenda Carter MChS, FCPodMed, MSSF, City & Guilds A&FE
Orthopaedic Footwear Consultant, Founder of The Footwear Centre,
Mile End Hospital

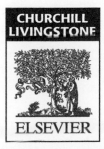

CHURCHILL
LIVINGSTONE

ELSEVIER

EDINBURGH LONDON NEW YORK OXFORD PHILADELPHIA ST LOUIS SYDNEY TORONTO 2009

CHURCHILL
LIVINGSTONE
ELSEVIER

© 2009, Elsevier Limited. All rights reserved.

ISBN: 978-0-443-06883-6

British Library Cataloguing in Publication Data
A catalogue record for this book is available from the British Library

Library of Congress Cataloging in Publication Data
A catalog record for this book is available from the Library of Congress

Notice

Knowledge and best practice in this field are constantly changing. As new research and experience broaden our knowledge, changes in practice, treatment and drug therapy may become necessary or appropriate. Readers are advised to check the most current information provided (i) on procedures featured or (ii) by the manufacturer of each product to be administered, to verify the recommended dose or formula, the method and duration of administration, and contraindications. It is the responsibility of the practitioner, relying on their own experience and knowledge of the patient, to make diagnoses, to determine dosages and the best treatment for each individual patient, and to take all appropriate safety precautions. To the fullest extent of the law, neither the Publisher nor the Authors assumes any liability for any injury and/or damage to persons or property arising out or related to any use of the material contained in this book.

Neither the Publisher nor the Authors assume any responsibility for any loss or injury and/or damage to persons or property arising out of or related to any use of the material contained in this book. It is the responsibility of the treating practitioner, relying on independent expertise and knowledge of the patient, to determine the best treatment and method of application for the patient.

The Publisher

ELSEVIER your source for books, journals and multimedia in the health sciences
www.elsevierhealth.com

Working together to grow
libraries in developing countries

www.elsevier.com | www.bookaid.org | www.sabre.org

ELSEVIER BOOK AID International Sabre Foundation

The Publisher's policy is to use **paper manufactured from sustainable forests**

Printed and bound by CPI Group (UK) Ltd, Croydon, CR0 4YY

Transferred to Digital Print 2011

Contents

Contents

Preface

Until recently footwear was largely ignored as a therapeutic strategy, even though many of the disciplines associated with medicine have long been aware of the damage it can cause to foot health. Sometimes footwear was low down the list of priorities that the healthcare practitioner wanted to discuss with their patient. All too frequently footwear was blamed for a condition and the patient told to change their footwear. The big questions were what should they change to and where could they find this ideal footwear. If they found it could they afford to buy it, would they like it and would they wear it? Sometimes it was far simpler for them to attend clinics at regular intervals for treatment of their problem and to continue to wear the shoes that they liked, even though the shoes were implicated in the causal pathway which led to foot lesion formation and to foot pain.

Orthotists in Britain and pedorthists in the US have done a valiant job in providing footwear for patients with severe foot conditions, but they can only act on the patients referred to them from other practitioners – usually orthopaedic surgeons. Practitioners such as physiotherapists, occupational therapists, podiatrists, and nurses who treat foot problems often have little knowledge of what suitable footwear might be available, how to evaluate footwear needs, how to advise patients, and how to prescribe for them.

It seems now that the range of patients who would benefit from therapeutic footwear has increased partly due to the explosion in the incidence of diabetes and the foot complications that accompany it. In the United States this became acknowledged when the Therapeutic Shoe Bill became part of the Medicare program in 1993. But it is not only in diabetes that therapeutic footwear has a role. Patients with conditions such as rheumatoid disease, other connective tissue disorders, spina bifida, post polio syndrome, and those with local foot pathologies such as hallux valgus syndrome, pes cavus and toe deformities may be among those who would benefit considerably from therapeutic footwear.

New developments in manufacturing techniques and materials technology have led to the production of footwear which contains materials with a variety of properties making it suitable for use in numerous pathological conditions. Retail footwear can be used successfully in a large number of patients if the practitioner knows what features are important, which footwear contains those features and how to obtain it. When retail footwear is outside the range of suitability for a patient, therapeutic footwear is the only option. This is available in several ranges: stock orthopaedic footwear made on special lasts, but available off-the-shelf from a range of manufacturers; modular orthopaedic footwear where a minor modification to an existing stock footwear last would meet the patient's needs; and fully bespoke footwear for unusual foot shapes where a unique last is made for the patient and footwear is constructed around that last.

Designs in therapeutic footwear have improved and frequently they cannot be differentiated from footwear bought on the high street. This is a far cry from the days not so long ago when like the Ford cars of the 1920's the patient could have an orthopaedic footwear in any colour, provided it was black, when footwear was available generally as a boot and then only with a deep toe box. These shoes were rarely clinically perfect and were very unattractive. After all which patient wants a shoe that marks them as handicapped or physically challenged.

At a very few centres in Britain skills in therapeutic footwear prescription have been fostered but there is a notable dearth of literature in this area. Not since the 1950's has any definitive text book been written and those using this text will note that the references included are quite dated. There was a danger that the knowledge base which previously existed would be lost, hence the need for this book. There also seems to be little relevant published research and perhaps some practitioners will now be stimulated to develop the subject further and investigate specific aspects of footwear therapy.

Wendy Tyrrell and Gwenda Carter have been at the forefront of this development in prescribing and using footwear therapy. They have designed and developed courses for practitioners wishing to learn to prescribe therapeutic footwear and their clinical experience, gained over many years of practice, and the development of therapeutic footwear as a Master's level academic discipline has made the need for a dedicated text more urgent.

This text is designed to support practitioners who wish to prescribe, fit and assess the effectiveness of therapeutic footwear. It is intended to provide a base for clinical practice, an instructional guide and an aid to problem solving. The book takes the reader through the various stages in assessing patients' footwear needs and identifies the types of footwear available. It examines both the various materials

suitable for use in footwear manufacture and also the footwear construction methods available. It provides useful guides to assessing fit and takes an in-depth look at prescribing orthotics and footwear, enabling the practitioner to ensure that these function as a single entity. Perhaps the most challenging aspect of therapeutic footwear is the successful prescription of bespoke footwear and several chapters in the book focus on this topic. These sections lead the practitioner through an evaluation of the patient's needs, describe how to use the British Standard measurement system, and suggest the means of solving specific footwear fitting problems.

Throughout the text the authors emphasise the need for patient concordance. All too often in the past, orthopaedic footwear has found a permanent home in the patient's wardrobe rather than on their feet. The high value of well prescribed and well fitting therapeutic footwear is seen by the increased mobility, freedom from pain and improved quality of life that it provides for patients. It's really not 'just a pair of shoes'.

Biography

Wendy Tyrrell MEd, FHEA, DPodM, MChS, FCPodMed

Wendy qualified in 1977 and worked for many years in the health service and in private practice before being appointed lecturer at the Wales Centre for Podiatric Studies (then the Cardiff School of Chiropody). She taught undergraduates for many years and footwear was one of the areas in which she specialised.

Whilst her academic career progressed Wendy was determined to further develop her professional skills and in 1992 began to work with the Wales College of Medicine Wound Healing Research Unit in treating diabetes related foot wounds. This led to the introduction of several specialist clinics in NHS Trusts where treatment focussed on plantar pressure off-loading techniques. Her previous expertise in footwear led to the development of a specialist therapeutic footwear service. The effectiveness of the clinical strategies provided by this service was evaluated via a research project funded by the Wales Office of Development for Health and Social Care and the positive findings of this work were disseminated nationally and internationally. Her broad research portfolio has also included an EU Funded international collaborative project for the development of effective off-loading footwear devices to improve healing of foot wounds.

She has worked widely in collaboration with other academic bodies, with footwear manufacturers throughout Europe and with colleagues in a variety of health related professions to further the understanding of the therapeutic benefits of footwear, its component parts, footwear technology and construction techniques when applied to the spectrum of foot pathologies. On the basis of this expertise she developed various CPD programmes and introduced the first Post Graduate Certificate in Therapeutic Footwear. This was validated by the University of Wales and accredited by both the Society of Chiropodists and Podiatrists and by the British Association of Orthotists and Prosthetists.

Wendy has published widely on a variety of podiatry related topics and has presented at many national and international conferences. Until September 2008 Wendy was Principal Lecturer and Director of Research and Enterprise for the Cardiff School of Health Sciences at University of Wales Institute Cardiff. She now undertakes consultancy work specialising in footwear.

Gwenda Carter MChS, FCPodMed, MSSF, City & Guilds A&FE Tutor, Orthopaedic Footwear Consultant

Gwenda trained at the Chelsea School of Chiropody qualifying in 1973. She gained experience in both the private sector and NHS service over a period of 36 years. Gwenda joined a partnership in private practice for ten years, where a footwear service, offered to the patients, gave her a growing interest in this area. In 1993, an unusual post was offered at the Mile End Hospital for a Health Professional to start up a Specialist Footwear Service, Gwenda was appointed, and dedicated the next fifteen years developing and expanding this highly specialised department into a beacon centre of excellence.

By developing a CPD training day Gwenda has also been responsible for the re-introduction of footwear training to the Profession. She also introduced her own orthopaedic footwear course which was unique in its conception and as a result was awarded the Silver Medal by City & Guilds. It went on to be very successful in attracting and developing more specialised clinicians.

During her career she has continually promoted the benefits of all types of footwear training and has encouraged a number of colleagues to specialise and go on to start up other specialised footwear services. This has lead to the formation of the special Interest group in footwear being set up by some of these colleagues.

She is also a very active member of the Society of Shoe Fitters and has contributed to the rewrite of their unique retail fitting qualification and has been involved on their council and liaised between SSF and the SCP professions. Gwenda's contribution to the Podiatry profession has been recognised by receiving a Citation in 2006 and recently she was awarded a fellowship status.

Gwenda has recently taken early retirement from the NHS and now concentrates on writing on the subject of footwear.

Acknowledgments

The authors wish to express their sincere appreciation to the many orthopaedic footwear manufacturers who have willingly and patiently spent time explaining and demonstrating the numerous skills that are needed to manufacture and fit bespoke footwear well. The support and co-operation they offered over many years in allowing us to spend time in their factories and clinics gave us the opportunity to develop our expertise.

In particular we wish to thank County Footwear, Gilbert and Mellish, Jane Saunders and Manning, Ken Hall, Klaveness UK, Reed Medical and Tay Care.

It's not 'just a pair of shoes'

There is little doubt that footwear can be a mechanical and sometimes a chemical irritant to feet, but it can also be used as a therapy to reduce morbidity, and to improve foot health, mobility and quality of life. The footwear worn by patients with foot pathologies is often criticized and condemned as the cause of many foot lesions, but maybe consideration should be given to the reason why individual patients are wearing the shoes they have chosen. It is important that their footwear choices are carefully evaluated, that the criteria identified by patients as being of significance in their choice of footwear are assessed and consideration is given to previous experience that has affected their footwear selections. This information should form the basis on which footwear advice or prescription is founded. Without it, the likelihood of success in finding footwear which meets the needs of patients in terms of acceptability, style and improvement in foot health is much reduced.

In considering the prescription of therapeutic footwear, the underlying foot pathology and foot shape will determine the type of footwear required – be it advising on retail footwear which the patient may purchase, stock surgical footwear, modular surgical footwear or the fully bespoke footwear option. If patients' needs can be addressed by the retail option, they will have control over the purchase. This option of course represents a cost saving for the NHS or for medical insurance companies. For patients who require more specialized footwear, the options are many. The variety of companies supplying footwear made on different lasts and in different styles and colours means that the choice available to patients has greatly increased in recent years.

Most people today have a footwear wardrobe with shoes for various activities and occasions. It is quite important that the footwear worn is appropriate for the activity being undertaken. In addition to hobbies, the needs of the workplace need to be considered. In general, men can wear classic laced-up style shoes, but ladies are expected to wear a very different style for many occupations. The favourite for them is probably the court shoe and this may be the culprit causing many foot lesions and deformities. The fact that it is slipped onto the foot means that it has to be tightly wedged in order for it to stay on the foot during the swing phase of the gait cycle, when the foot is off the ground and is non-weight-bearing. Its elevated heel means that weight is thrown forward and the toes are compressed into the toe box. The generally slim, elevated heel gives a small ground contact point which may lead to instability and an increased incidence of ankle sprains. The heel height can also cause knee, hip and lower back problems. When ladies wear this shoe style throughout the day during their working life, the end result can be deformed toes, and painful superficial lesions on the toes, the plantar surface of the metatarso-phalangeal joints and on the medial and lateral borders of the forefoot. This shoe style is often the one of choice for many social and dancing activities, both of which make heavy demands on foot function, and so, because of its popularity, the opportunities for damage from this type of footwear are many.

Those doing heavy industrial work will need to wear footwear which protects their feet from possible injury. These are often boots with steel toe caps contained within them to protect from direct impact injuries. Such footwear often has rigid rocker soles with deeply patterned soling to provide grip on a variety of surfaces. There may be issues around obtaining adequate fit when patients need to wear industrial footwear. It is often made without any width choice and, as the footwear is so rigid, patients often develop lesions as a result of it. Many industrial companies tend to link with a single supplier of industrial footwear, hence their workforce has no choice of fitting. If requested to do so, companies may allow their employees to obtain footwear from alternative suppliers whose footwear may be made on lasts which more closely approximate the particular wearer's foot shape (see also Ch. 6).

Why we wear shoes

Why do people wear shoes? The classic answer is 'protection'. When underfoot conditions were unfavourable, it seems that even primitive man covered his foot to make ground contact more comfortable and protect his feet from external trauma. It is thought that very early footwear was made of vegetable fibres which of course have decomposed without trace in archaeological deposits. Spanish rock paintings from about 15000 years ago provide images of footwear, and in the Fort Rock caves in Oregon, USA, sandals made of sagebrush bark dating from 9000 BC to 7000 BC

have actually been found. As man developed tools and manufacturing capability, he used the spoils of his hunting and harvesting prowess. He manufactured tools made of stone, horn or animal bones to pierce animal skins, used bone needles for sewing and used stone blades to remove flesh and fat from skins, and he would have fashioned a protective covering for his feet from those skins. The mummified remains of prehistoric man from the quaternary period (3300 BC) found on a glacier at Alto Adige in Italy was wearing rough footwear, with rawhide bearskin soles and deerskin uppers strengthened with strings of woven grass and stuffed with hay to insulate the foot from the cold (www.vannacalzature.it).

The evidence provided by statues, tomb paintings, papyruses and parchments show that the ancient Egyptians who were members of high classes wore footwear, while lower classes walked unshod. Here we see footwear used as a sign of social distinction. The office of 'bearer of sandals' to the Pharaoh and to other noblemen is known to have existed, signifying that shoes were indeed a valued possession. A variety of materials was used by the Egyptians for footwear. Some sandals had wooden soles, but leather, papyrus, reeds or palm leaves were also woven to form soles (Fig. 1.1). The sandals were often secured onto the foot with a thong from the upper attached to the sole between the first and second toes. The shoes of the wealthy were embellished with jewels. It is interesting to note that Egyptians were able to tan skins and used vegetable oils extracted from acacia pods, and so had a way of preserving leather.

From displays in the British Museum, the Assyrians and Babylonians are seen to have worn leather boots for riding and for driving chariots. Such foot and leg coverings would provide protection for those activities. The first time we see the development of styling in shoes rather than sandals seems to be in Turkish history, where ankle boots made of soft leather with extended and turned up toes are seen dating from about 865 BC. The Phoenicians were the first known to have perfected leather dying, so that coloured footwear became available, but in Turkey during the reign of Mahomet II (1451–1481 AD), shoe making had become an established craft, with shoemakers organized into a corporation with state controls in place to ensure quality standards. Here also we see the colour of footwear used to denote class, rank, religious belief and ethnicity.

Figure 1.1 Examples of natural fibre sandals (Yukka) (left) and wood (right) 2500 BC. (Courtesy of Bata Shoe Museum.)

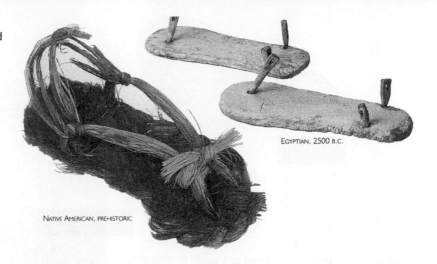

EGYPTIAN, 2500 B.C.

NATIVE AMERICAN, PREHISTORIC

We know that the Greeks and Romans wore similar kinds of open sandals and boots and that this footwear was used as class and rank indicators.

On the other side of the world, in central America, from 5000 BC, people are seen depicted as wearing manufactured footwear – in other words, not rough animal skins, but crafted shoes made from cutting and stitching together pieces of animal hide. In South America, it is interesting to note that Patagonia derived its name from 'Patagones' which actually means 'big feet'. It seems that the native inhabitants wrapped their feet in hides to protect them from the cold, and when the invading Spanish saw their footprints in the snow they deduced that they were gigantic men with big feet.

In North America, the native Americans wore moccasins made from animal hide tanned using animal fat combined with bark, sewn together with strips of leather or animal tendons using bone needles or thorns. The Inuit population tanned hides using smoke and used different footwear according to the time of year. Winter boots had soles made of caribou with the fur side outwards next to the ground to give a grip on the ice and snow. Summer footwear needed to be waterproof and was made with very dense stitching to minimize the penetration of water through the seams. Inuits from coastal regions used sealskin, and the skins of hares and other small animals were also used for footwear.

In medieval Europe, footwear styling developed under the influence of fashion. Shoes with pointed toes became popular. These points extended in length and sometimes were so long that they had to be strapped to the leg around the calf to allow the wearer to walk safely. This became such an issue that, during the fourteenth century, laws were passed in some European countries fixing the length of the point that was allowed to be worn by noblemen, by the middle classes and by commoners.

Pointed shoes were succeeded by round and square toe styles and medieval women wore ankle shoes with laced fastenings.

The development of high-heeled shoes was noted in Florence in the thirteenth century, when they are thought to have developed from shoes with both elevated soles and heels which were worn to raise the wearer above the level of the waste material which clogged the streets. In Britain and elsewhere in Europe, pattens were often worn over delicate footwear to prevent the feet of the wearer contacting the filth in the street (Grew et al 2004). These were mainly wooden sole and heel units with a band over the forefoot into which the shod foot was placed, similar in appearance to a wooden clog. The fashion then developed into footwear called 'chopines' where their shape and height became exaggerated and reached extremes of heel height and shape.

In Elizabethan England, shoes became heavily decorated, with embroidered satin as the material of choice for the upper, and by the end of the reign of Elizabeth I, heels had become as high as 7 centimetres.

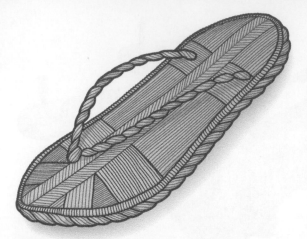

Figure 1.2 The 'flip-flop' started as a sandal in 2000 BC made from woven vegetable fibre. (Reproduced with permission from Peacock 2005.)

All footwear was made straight so that a shoe would fit both left and right feet. During the reign of Charles I, flamboyant knee boots made of leather became popular. Later centuries have seen shoe shapes change from pointed to round, to square and back again, with both men and women wearing court style shoes, boots and mules.

It is very interesting to compare styles from history with more familiar present day ones. The Egyptian worker's sandal of 2000 BC and the Solea from Roman times are of very simple construction and were often made from local grasses or papyrus. They were the first style of crafted footwear to follow on from primitive foot wrapping (O'Keeffe 1996). These are minimalist thong strap sandals which are still popular today as a rubber flip-flop, or a classy leather sandal (Fig. 1.2).

A patten from the fourteenth and fifteenth centuries, usually made from wood, was designed as a platform to raise the wearer high off the ground. It had leather straps to fasten it to the sole of the foot and was a very practical item to protect the feet from the mud and dirt of the unmade roads of the day. This has reinvented itself around the world over the centuries as a fifteenth century Venetian chopine which reached heights of up to 30 inches high, and the Italian chopine of the sixteenth century which was nearer to 7–8 inches high. A stilted early twentieth century sandal was also found in parts of Turkey

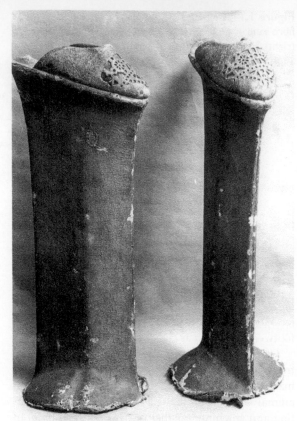

Figure 1.3 Example of sixteenth century Venetian chopines approximately 20 inches (51 cm) tall. Platforms made from wood or cork and often covered in fabric or calfskin. (Reproduced with permission from Correr Museum, Venice.)

and of Syria. It was carved in wood and inlaid with mother of pearl. A few 'platform' shoes appeared in the mid 1940s, mostly in America, which were quite modest in height, but then, in the 1960s, platform shoes became very popular and once again reached several inches in height (Figs 1.3 and 1.4).

'The clog is one of civilisation's most successful examples of design' (McDowell 1994). Clogs were first invented by peasants as working footwear on farms and date back to the middle ages. Clogs were worn throughout Europe and were a simple hard-wearing solution to the problem of footwear for the poor and hardworking populace. They were made by carving out a solid piece of wood, shaping and honing it to fit the individual's feet, often by the worker for himself. Later, a variation of design included a

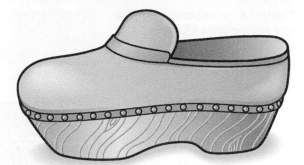

Figure 1.5 Typical working clog made from leather and wood.

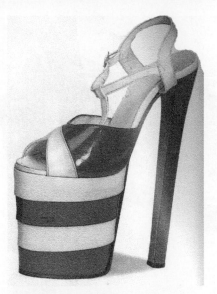

Figure 1.4 Example of 1970s platform shoe. (Reproduced with permission from Northampton Museum and Art Gallery.)

separate top piece which formed the upper, made from a variety of materials such as leather, plaited raffia or a fabric, nailed around the sides to the wood base. Clogs were very hard wearing and protective, warm and comfortable and could be considered a forerunner of safety footwear. The casual clog is still very popular today, made from modern materials such as plastic, cork and fabric, and it has also been adapted for the modern workplace, for example static-free moulded shoes for the operating theatre. Heat-resistant plastic and industrial rubber and metal have also been incorporated into industrial clogs. The current trend for Crocs is also another reinvention of this style (Figs 1.5 and 1.6).

Many of the early shoes were made from soft fabrics like velvet and silk rather than calf leather. These did not wear particularly well and yet they were very attractive, often highly decorated with embroidery and beads and even jewels. In the sixteenth century, the pantoffe became a notable style, being very soft and flat with a large spacious toe shape. These soft shoes are similar to today's slipper although the shape has changed dramatically. Mules derive their origins from the soft slip-on idea, but are more open with the toe piece removed. Their style has changed slightly and has gradually changed from flat soles to being a wedge shape. The beautiful yet highly

impractical fabrics suggest a life of wealth rather than poverty, inactivity compared to manual work and one where the ladies of the times were almost always transported to wherever they wished to go rather than having to walk or ride on horseback (Fig. 1.7).

The original 'court shoe' dates from the seventeenth and eighteenth centuries when it was worn in the courts of the palaces by the ladies in waiting. They were very simple flat silk pumps hidden under the magnificent dresses of the time which allowed the ladies to walk about very sedately and quietly on the flag stone floors of the day. Court shoes with higher heels were also worn by men at court and were particularly fashionable in France at the time of Louis XIV. Today the court shoe has taken on a completely different identity, as a very neat, tight fitting high-heeled shoe, first made popular by the designer Dior in 1952. He introduced a very pointed stiletto heel which emphasized the shape of the calf, and as skirt lengths gradually became shorter, more leg could be admired. There are very few ladies today who do not have a 'court shoe' in their footwear collection as it has never lost its appeal (Fig. 1.8).

Boots have featured throughout the centuries with the earliest being about 1000 BC (Peacock 2005). Roman soldiers wore boots with specific designs to denote rank, while the lower ranks wore sandals. Many of the boot and sandal designs are still recognizable today. Boots have featured in every century in some way, some as bootees, mostly made from soft hide and fastened with a simple lace system up the side. They have been a consistent part of army uniform throughout the world. For centuries, boots were

Figure 1.6 A clog-based style now very popular called a 'Croc'.

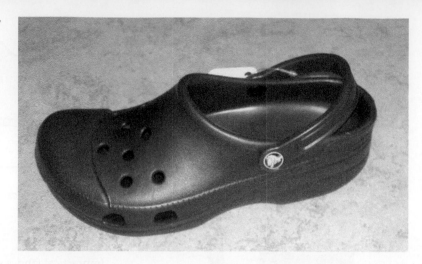

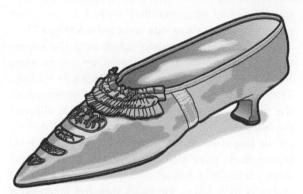

Figure 1.7 A French silk slipper dated 1785. (Reproduced with permission from O'Keefe 1996.)

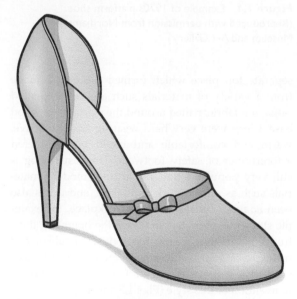

Figure 1.8 Classical 1950s stiletto style. (Reproduced with permission from Peacock 2005.)

worn more by men than ladies, often as a class distinction denoting wealth and property. Interestingly, men travelled mainly by horseback until the mid nineteenth century and therefore heels on their boots or shoes were essential to keep the foot in the stirrup. Heels were simply a practical solution for riding, but were limited in height as higher heels made walking difficult and tapered ones tended to break off (McDowell 1994). At this time, ladies were most often transported around in a sedan chair, or later by carriage, arriving without having to step out into the dirty tracks, hence their footwear was kept clean. By the same token, higher heels became very attractive to ladies as they needed only to walk indoors. By the 1800s, women also adopted the boot as a valuable part of their wardrobe, and have continuously

worn boots high and low, fabric and leather, plain and highly decorated ever since (Fig. 1.9).

The 'Mary Jane' shoe dates back to 1902, named from a character in the 'Buster Brown' comic strip which appeared first in the *New York Herald* (O'Keeffe 1996). This basic and simple style has changed little over the years and keeps reappearing in many variations as footwear fashion. This style has been around for centuries, and examples of the simple

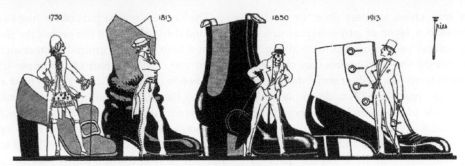

Figure 1.9 An early twentieth century advertisement for Barthman Schuhe. (Reproduced with permission from McDowell 1994.)

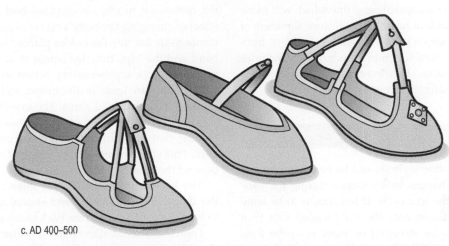

c. AD 400–500

Figure 1.10 Examples of the Mary Jane style dating back to the Byzantine period. (Reproduced with permission from Peacock 2005.)

strap design can be found as early as the Byzantine period, 400–1100 AD (Peacock 2005) (Fig. 1.10). It is a classic children's style which has also been popular with adults.

While shoe styles and shapes have changed with fashion through the centuries, it is only in latter years that developments in manufacturing techniques and shoe materials – particularly soling materials – have advanced. From vegetable matter through to raw animal skins and tanned leather, technology has now provided the means of developing a range of natural and synthetic soling materials which are available to provide rigidity, flexibility, durability, shock absorption, grip or pure decoration as required.

Looking at the modern day scenario, it is clear that wearing footwear in inclement conditions provides a protection against the cold and wet. In rough terrain, soling will minimize trauma and the risk of damaging the integrity of skin. However, even when conditions are fair, and underfoot surfaces are non-traumatic, for example indoors, we wear shoes. Maybe still today the major influences are not only climatic and not solely related to underfoot surfaces but also to the influences of fashion, peer pressure and habit. In warmer climates, particularly in the Mediterranean regions, fishermen may be seen comfortably walking barefoot during the day, without sustaining damage to their feet, but then during the evening they may chose to wear shoes or sandals. Their feet develop a layer of physiological callous to provide a natural protection against walking on firm surfaces, but the shoes or sandals they choose to wear out of work form part of their social dress code.

This dress code has often been down-played in considering the role of footwear, but we should consider the part that footwear style and colour play in body image for all our patients and pay due account to the effect that this will have on the patients' acceptance of any footwear recommendation we may make to them. The eventual footwear prescription derived in consultation with the patient may well be a compromise, but it will be a compromise that the patient will find acceptable and one which will minimize damage to foot health. This historical picture of footwear provides a profile of its development from a purely protective function to one which includes fashion and status. However, using footwear as a therapy is a relatively recent development.

Shoe styles

The choice of shoe style should be based on the fact that the foot changes in dimension during the various stages of the gait cycle. If the shoe is to be large enough to accommodate the fully loaded foot then it will need to be strapped or laced onto the foot, otherwise it will fall off during the swing phase of the gait cycle when the foot is unloaded and of different dimension. Slip-on or court shoes will need to be wedged onto the foot, and if they are to stay on the foot during the swing phase they will be too small for the fully loaded foot. They only stay on the foot by the gripping action of the toes. This can lead to the development of corn or callous on prominent toe joints and in some cases can lead to toe deformities through the constant clawing action. Functional straps or laces provide a mechanism for holding the foot back in the shoe and minimizing the forward slip of the foot into the toe space of the shoe causing compression of the forefoot. It is worth checking that laces are actually done up and undone to take the shoe on and off. Sometimes fashion dictates to younger adults that laces should remain undone, and older folk, perhaps because of difficulty in reaching their feet, may not undo their laces. In such cases, alternatives such as Velcro® fastening might be worth considering.

The heel is the first part of the foot to contact the ground during gait and the heel of the shoe needs to form a firm base for ground contact and for stability in gait. The heel part of the upper (the quarter) also needs to be fairly firm and to hold and contain the soft tissue surrounding the calcaneus, otherwise this tissue will be subject to tensile stress during heel contact, will splay over the edge of an open-backed sandal or mule-style shoe and will lead to the development of heel callous which may in turn become cracked, fissured and infected.

The heel height should ideally be about 2.5 cm but no more than 4 cm. The higher the heel, the greater the forward displacement of body mass onto the metatarsal heads. An elevated heel also has the effect of changing the body's centre of gravity, and to compensate for this the ankles plantarflex, the knees bend and the hips flex (De Lateur et al 1991). There may then be a compensatory action in the lumbar spine. This can lead to discomfort and to arthritic changes in the affected joints. The same basic principles apply to children's footwear with one additional feature; that of additional length for growth allowance. This should amount to a length of about 14 mm beyond the length of the longest toe.

The heel counter of the shoe should conform to the shape of the calcaneus and should grip the heel to hold the foot firmly at the back of the shoe.

Footwear should allow free movement of the toes, should be of good fit and of adequate length with quarters of adequate height and shape to grip the heel. It should have good contact with the surface of the foot, and should cradle the foot at this point. The shoe should absorb humidity, limit any increase in foot temperature and be of low weight. Brazil became the first country to develop norms for footwear comfort in 2002 and identified the following factors (World Footwear 2006):

- Mass (weight) of shoe
- Plantar pressure distribution
- Internal temperature control
- Weight-carrying capability
- Pronation angle control
- Fitting (individual perception).

Table 1.1 outlines the suitability of the major shoe styles in relation to foot shape and pathology.

Table 1.1 Foot pathology and shoe styles: a table of suitability

Foot type	Shoe styles					
	Gibson (lace style) (men & ladies)	Oxford (men & ladies)	Mary Jane (ladies only)	Boots (men & ladies)	Trainer (men & ladies)	
'Average' instep, normal range of motion (ROM)	Very suitable. 3 eyelets minimum. 4–6 eyelets creates a lower opening allowing easier entry and more adjustment.	Needs the facings to fit correctly over instep but good choice especially for men.	Position of strap is critical for comfort. A good style that many people can wear.	May limit ROM. The choice of fabric and soling affects the flexibility of boots.	Very suitable but heel to ball fit needs to be correct. Depth at counter can cause pressure on Achilles tendon. Need to be properly fitted.	
High instep and pes cavus	2–3 eyelet facings generally do not sit well on high-instep foot. 5–6 eyelets allow more ease of entry and adjustment. Look for extra depth in 'stock' (ready-made) ranges.	Poor choice for these foot types as facings cannot lay properly so foot appears to be 'bursting' out of the shoe.	Not a good choice as strap can cause extreme pressure on dorsum of foot. This may damage veins or cause swelling to occur.	Style of boot matters here as high-instep feet need an easy entry. Styles that have a side zip or front low lace are worth trying.	With careful selection, a trainer with a padded tongue should fit well.	
Low instep and pes planus	3–5 eyelet styles are good but need to be fitted properly otherwise heel slip will occur. If facings butt together, shoe is too deep in instep circumference. May be solved with an extra in-sock or looking at alternative last proportions.	Can be successful for low-instep shape as long as facings do not overlap. With careful fitting, this style can help to hold foot firmly back into counter. Search for different last proportions until you find the right one.	Depending on strap width and position, this style can work. A twin strap style is best. Check depth of vamp and instep as gaping may occur if too deep.	Most boot styles work well on low-arched feet. Plenty of choice available. Check foot is not sliding forward to end of toe puff.	Trainers with 'built in' arch support may be quite uncomfortable for a low-arched foot. Check depth as too much space allows the foot to slide forward. Laces rather than Velcro® are best for this foot type but need to be correctly fastened.	
Hallux abducto valgus (HAV) and lesser toe deformities	Extra width required for ease of entry. Lower opening facings with 4–6 eyelets are easier to get on. A very adaptable style – can have extra depth added for clawed toes or to accommodate the enlarged HAV joint.	Not suitable due to restricted entry.	This style can work if made to correct depth and has a wide strap. Look for variety of last choices as many 'stock makers' have this style in their selection.	Choice limited by boot styles that will go on easily. Low facing position. Velcro® straps or laces best. Watch weight and flexibility as these may limit ROM too much.	Not ideal as layers of stitching and seams often rub the joint or dorsum of toes. If made to order then depth can be adjusted over toes, and minimal 'design features' to simplify construction helps.	

(Continued)

Table 1.1 Continued

Foot type	Shoe styles				
	Gibson (lace style) (men & ladies)	Oxford (men & ladies)	Mary Jane (ladies only)	Boots (men & ladies)	Trainer (men & ladies)
Hyper-mobile foot	Great style that works well with control orthotics to give good support and stability.	Firm close fit of Oxford can be very successful here but search for best last proportions. Little room for orthotics.	Not suitable due to lack of instep control.	A lace-up boot style is very helpful, gives good control and plenty of space for orthotics.	Trainers are very suitable and work well with orthotics.
Limited ROM or fixed ankle position	Gibson lace style is very suitable but needs to fit firmly to hold onto foot. Addition of rocker sole may be helpful but assess gait carefully first. Plenty of choice in stock ranges to find a good fitting last. Must have heel to ball flexion accurately fitted especially if adding a rocker sole.	Oxford style OK in general but entry might be difficult with fixed ankle position. If made with leather soles, can be very helpful as less flexibility and reduced ground grip aids limited gait movement.	The Mary Jane is unsuitable for this foot type as it lacks support and is not adaptable to the change in foot position.	Boots can be helpful and supportive but entry can be difficult for limited ROM unless style is open to toe for ease of entry. Lace or Velcro® fastenings work well. Be aware of excess weight or bulk, e.g. padded collar and tongue, as these can compromise the little movement still available.	Trainers are great style especially if supplied with rocker soles and are properly fitted from heel to ball.
Oedema	4–6 eyelet styles are best or twin Velcro® straps. Add padded collar for extra comfort if swelling collects around the ankle. Extra depth may be needed and readily available in stock ranges. Keep heel height as low as possible for stability. May need extended medial heel for instep support.	Oxford is a poor choice for oedema due to limited opening and fixed base of facings. Style does not allow for swelling to increase over a few hours.	Mary Jane is often chosen but swelling can bulge out through 'key hole' opening which can look unsightly. Strap can cause major problems cutting into swelling. The style is more suited if elastic stockings are worn to control the oedema.	Boots with easily adjustable fastenings can be comfortable. However, in severe cases, boots are too cumbersome and bulky and, if oedema is variable, very difficult to fit around the ankles.	Trainers with padded tongue and collar enable this style to be very comfortable for oedema. Low opening laces are advantage for ease of adjustment.

Severe valgus deformity; Charcot-Marie-Tooth	Choose a 3–6 eyelet style which may need to be modified or bespoke version to fit the deformity. Medial facings often need to be specially cut to accommodate the foot shape. Style can also be made to accommodate cradles or orthotics. Medial heel flare or extension also very useful for control.	Oxford style is unsuitable, even if bespoke, due to limit of style over instep; does not work well when modified for a valgus foot shape.	Mary Jane is unsuitable for this foot type as lack of support in instep and problems with gaping spoil the overall appearance.	Boots are often the first choice and require a low opening for ease of entry. Very adaptable via modification or bespoke for most foot shapes. Good casts often needed and accurate measurements essential.	Trainers can be adapted to suit if chosen with minimal design features. Can accommodate moulded cradle or orthotics. Very popular as foot shape can be disguised quite successfully.
Diabetic	Gibson is an ideal style that can be modified to protect the diabetic foot with whole cut vamp and wall linings (seam free), wall toe puff (mudguard), very soft uppers. However, if the footwear is too soft there is a risk of the foot distorting the shoe and causing pressure points. By keeping a firm heel counter for control and when very carefully fitted, the diabetic foot can wear a firm shoe that does not cause any damage.	Oxford style is less suitable due to stitching and overlap at base of facings. A very difficult style to make seam free.	Mary Jane can be used for diabetic feet provided the firm heel counter remains, and a twin strap would be best choice.	Boots are frequently prescribed for diabetic feet, as they are so adaptable, accommodative and protective. Watch weight and flexion of sole. Rockers often used as ROM is reduced in this style.	Trainers are less suitable due to the number of pieces forming the upper causing extra stitching and seams. If very well designed and fitted with care this style can be used to satisfy patient compliance.

(Continued)

Table 1.1 Continued

	Shoe styles				
Foot type	**Gibson (lace style) (men & ladies)**	**Oxford (men & ladies)**	**Mary Jane (ladies only)**	**Boots (men & ladies)**	**Trainer (men & ladies)**
Rheumatoid arthritis	Very suitable style. 3 eyelets minimum. 4–6 eyelets creates a lower opening allowing easier entry and more adjustment. Extra depth required for a reasonable depth of cushioning under the foot to toe end and keep lightweight and flexible by using a thinner sole (3 mm) unit if necessary.	This style does not lend itself to be extra deep, and is also less flexible, with a leather sole, so is less likely to be a suitable choice.	This is a popular style as it is lightweight and smart. Extra depth can be added to toe and vamp and, provided the strap holds firmly, it will be comfortable.	Boots can be heavy and cumbersome so the rheumatoid foot is less likely to be very comfortable in them. If ankle support is required, keep top height as low as possible and reduce weight by using 'Bontex' midsole and lightweight outer soling.	Trainers are less suitable due to the number of pieces forming the upper causing extra stitching and seams. If very well designed and fitted with care, this style can be used to satisfy patient compliance.
Amputees: single digit or all toes back to mid-tarsal joint	Gibson style will work if the facings are cut to grip the foot as high as possible on the dorsum, as close to the front of ankle as is comfortable. Very firm fastenings required to keep shoe from slipping is vital. Partial foot filler can be placed inside shoe to compensate for short lever arm and prevent collapse of the upper and unsightly creases.	Oxford style can be very successful as it fits so well to the foot and grips on. Very careful fitting checks should be done to reduce risk of pressure.	Mary Jane is unsuitable as it lacks body and good grip over the instep.	Boots can be adapted for amputees. Allows great grip above the ankle and extra height helps to accommodate cradle or filler. Often necessary to add a rocker sole and extended shank to improve toe off.	Trainers can be used provided the lining is smooth inside to reduce any rubbing from extra seams on vamp. The ankle-high top style is more suitable combined with a padded collar and tongue.

What do patients want from footwear?

A bold headline in one of the daily newspapers states: 'One woman in ten splashes over £1000 a year on shoes' (*Daily Mail*, August 10th, 2006). Another headline states: '£80000 on shoes! Why we're all addicts' (*In The Know* magazine, August, 2006). It appears from these articles that the enjoyment of buying shoes fulfils many needs and can be a therapeutic activity. Women particularly love shoes, as these articles suggest, especially high-heeled, sexy, impractical styles that lengthen the leg, increase height, and alter their posture and make them feel good about themselves even if the shoes are very uncomfortable to wear. There are many who will spend over £100 a month on shoes, and keep them in boxes, carefully stored away only to be worn once in a while. It's the buying and owning of lovely shoes that has such appeal and any suggestion that they may be damaging their feet is treated with disdain.

As a clinician, it is important to understand patients' views of their footwear before attempting to discuss their footwear needs. Some people seem unable to relate their footwear to their foot health, disconnect footwear from any aspect of health care and regard any suggestion that footwear may be damaging their feet and other parts of the kinetic chain as an unwelcome intrusion into a somewhat fantasy world of fun and elegance.

Patients may subconsciously use a list of preferential features, which might well include:

- Does the shoe suit me?
- Do I like the look of it?
- Do I like the colour?
- Is it what I want/need?
- Is it comfortable?
- Is the price right?

Before beginning to consider the suitability of the footwear presented by the patient, the type of footwear normally worn for the large part of the day and the reasons why the particular style and material were chosen should be established. It is also advisable to identify whether patients have had any bad footwear experiences. For example, have they been persuaded to buy 'sensible' footwear only to find that it was expensive and did not improve their foot comfort or their foot health? The purpose for which the footwear is to be used is significant and we should consider whether it is essentially designed to be smart or casual, for work, for special occasion, for regular use or for a specific activity.

Part of the skill in advising someone about footwear is having a clear understanding of what style to suggest in each individual situation. The suitability of a particular style will depend on foot shape, mobility factors, medical history and the circumstances in which it is to be worn. The decision on whether or not to wear a certain style rests with the wearer. Where footwear may be damaging foot health, a change of style or heel height may be beneficial, but the advice offered needs to be clear and unambiguous about the rationale for change. It can be counterproductive to suggest that patients should use a lace-up shoe if they buy a decorative lace rather than a functional one. Guidelines and boundaries will always be stretched to the limit and clear advice is essential to avoid such misunderstandings. It is worthwhile to suggest that a patient brings new shoes to the clinic for evaluation before they are worn, especially if orthoses are involved, to ensure that the best choice has been made within the budget available.

Continuing to consider the patient's perspective, thought must be given to the way in which a patient evaluates the fit of a shoe. A patient would probably consider a well-fitting shoe to be one which doesn't hurt or slip, which seems to be long enough, feels wide enough, which doesn't cause discomfort and doesn't rub and which has a heel height which the patient likes.

This patient perspective may be summarized in the word 'comfort'. Comfort is a relative term which relates to a lack of discomfort or pain and is directly related to sensitivity levels. It appears that, in comparison with the hand, the foot has much lower sensitivity. Table 1.2 indicates the findings when monofilaments are applied to sites on the hand and foot, and the awareness of two-point discrimination at specific distances on those same sites (Goonetilleke 1998).

The footwear comfort factor is important to patients and healthcare professionals alike. But 'comfort' may mean different things to different people. Is it the right feel, causing no discomfort or pain? But when patients like particular footwear and want to wear a favourite pair of shoes, they can block the

Table 1.2 Sensitivity to Semmes–Weinstein monofilament and two-point discrimination at points in the hand and foot

Site	Touch sensitivity measured with Semmes–Weinstein monofilament (in mg)	Two point discrimination (in mm)
Middle finger	6.8	2.5
Palm	20.1	11.5
Sole	35.9	22.5
Hallux	36.7	12.0

pain sensation. Feet and shoes are different, and when we put shoes onto our feet we are generally trying to fit an irregular shaped object into a more regularly shaped piece of footwear. However if we try to replicate the actual individual foot shape into a shoe, that will also give rise to problems as the foot undergoes changes in shape on load-bearing, deformation due to temperature changes, impact, oedema and so on. For a shoe to fit, it ought to allow a certain 'feel' against the foot so that the wearer knows they have a shoe on their foot, but it should not cause any discomfort or pain or trauma. Neither should it require the foot to do any additional work in the form of gripping to make the shoe stay on the foot. The shoe should be secure at locations on the foot where deformations during gait will not be significantly large. Such positions will depend on shoe design and some possibilities include grip around the heel and waist, with the girth and height of the shoe matching that at the midfoot. Forward movement of the foot should be restricted by a secure fastening across the instep. This will prevent the foot slipping forward into the toe box of the shoe and minimize the risk of the toes impacting on the forepart or vamp of the shoe.

Many foot lesions presented by patients are footwear related. Where there is intermittent compressive stress from footwear over parts of the foot with little soft tissue covering over superficial bone, hard corns or even ulcers can develop. Where there is friction between foot and shoe, blisters or callous develop. Foot health professionals may clearly see the link between presented lesion formation and the footwear being worn by the patient, but the patient

may not be able to see that link, or may not wish to see it. Quite often, patients do not identify the footwear as contributing to their foot lesion or to the pain and discomfort associated with it. This scenario is seen quite frequently when patients change from summer footwear comprising open-toed, loose-fitting sandals into winter shoes. They expect to feel discomfort and accept it as normal. In fact, they may say that the summer sandals have 'spoilt their feet' and that the compression from winter shoes is the norm and is what should be expected from footwear.

What footwear should achieve

What then is suitable footwear for the patient? In answering that question, the activity for which the footwear is intended to be used needs to be considered first. Is it to be worn when walking distances, for shopping, for work; is it intended for occasions when smart dress is required or for casual events; is it for regular use or occasional wear, or for specific activities? Rather than being completely rigid about recommending a particular shoe style, the healthcare professional must examine the patient's lifestyle needs. It is no use insisting that a female patient wears a laced-up, low-heeled shoe continuously if she wants to go dancing. A happy compromise can be reached so that the ideal shoe for foot health is worn for the greater part of the day and footwear for selected activities is worn only when undertaking that activity.

Generally footwear should be suitable for use during the activity for which it is designed. It should be of a suitable style with appropriate heel height and shape. It needs to provide a non-irritant covering for the foot and footwear for general use should also include a functional fastening. Probably the most evident feature is that shoes should fit the feet they are intended for. The heel part of the shoe upper should grip the calcaneus and hold the foot at the back of the shoe. The shoe should flex where the foot is designed to flex – at the metatarso-phalangeal joints. The foot should have to make no effort to keep the shoe on and the outer sole should provide enough grip to prevent the foot slipping as the individual walks or runs.

Shoes should be long enough. They should be deep enough to accommodate the depth of the toes even if they are hammered or clawed, wide enough not to cause any part of the foot to be compressed and should have adequate girth throughout.

The length of the shoe should be great enough to allow the toes to function unimpeded when the foot is fully loaded with body weight and is at its maximal length. The shoe needs to accommodate the longest part of the foot, always remembering that digital formulae are not standard and that, in some patients, one or more of the lesser toes may be longer than the hallux. The shoe length should then be subdivided into the length from the heel to the first metatarso-phalangeal joint and the length from the first metatarso-phalangeal joint to the toes. The proportions of each of these measurements should match those of the foot. All feet are different and, even if the overall shoe length is correct, if the heel-to-ball length of the shoe does not correspond with the heel to metatarso-phalangeal joint measurement of the foot, foot flexion will fail to correspond with the point at which the shoe is designed to flex (the tread line). If the tread line of the shoe is too far proximal for the flexion of the foot, the shoe will acquire additional toe spring from the foot flexion point and the vamp will crease excessively. If it is too far distal, the toe spring of the shoe will be depressed by the foot and lead to cramping of the toes. Different manufacturers' shoes will have different heel-to-ball measurements and it is often worthwhile to try various shoes to ensure that heel-to-ball length is adequate for the foot which is to wear it.

Shoe width increases incrementally with length and patients with wide feet often choose shoes which are too long for them in order to obtain the width. This also means that the metatarso-phalangeal joints will be positioned proximal to the shoe tread line and shoe flexion will not correspond to foot flexion. The shoe will then acquire additional toe spring and the vamp will crease. If the shoe contains a shank, the shank may break through the outer sole as the relationship between the heel height and the tread line has been changed with the foot requiring the shoe to flex in a more proximal position than it was designed to do.

The length of the shoe is only one factor; the others include width and girth. These are two separate features, and both measurements must be taken if the shoe is to fit adequately (Fig. 1.11).

The shoe should be of correct width and girth at the metatarsal heads and of correct girth at the instep. Several other girth measurements need to be matched if the shoe is to fit properly. The long heel measurement is perhaps one of the most significant in obtaining a good fit and it dictates the positioning of the instep fastening. It is also necessary to remember that the shoe needs to change shape with the foot in gait. The time of the day when taking measurements is also important, since normal daytime changes result in a 3% increase in foot volume (Janisse et al 1995) and vigorous exercise can cause an increase in foot volume by 8% (Merriman & Tollafield 1997). The shoe should be large enough to allow for changes in dimension as the day progresses and should also allow for changes in volume required by variation in hosiery worn or dressings/padding where needed. If the patient needs to wear orthoses, accommodation for these should be available within the shoe. The shoe should be of adequate width and depth and there should be no localized tight spots. The heel of the shoe should be broad based for stability on heel contact. There should be a functional fastening to hold the foot back in the shoe and to prevent impaction of the toes against the front of the shoe. The top line of the shoe should fit snugly and should not gape. It should not irritate the malleoli nor the tendo-Achilles.

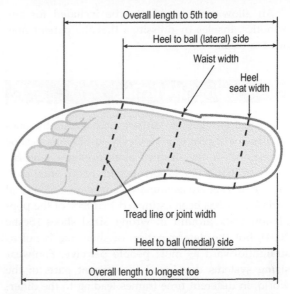

Figure 1.11 Plantar view of foot and sole to identify fitting points. (Reproduced with permission from Rossi & Tennant 1993.)

An allowance should also be included for any orthotics, insoles or dressings that the patient may need to wear.

Shoe sizing and fitting

Shoes that are likely to cause a problem are the ones that do not fit properly. However, just because a shoe corresponds to the size measured does not necessarily mean that it fits. Problems with fit are often multifactorial. Feet are asymmetric and show anatomical variation. It has been estimated that 85% of the population walk around in wrong sized shoes (Bestic 2004), but the determination of shoe size is not as straightforward as most people perceive. Footwear sizing systems developed in different parts of the world, in different time frames leading to the difference in shoe sizes that we are familiar with today. In England, shoe sizing started in the time of Edward II where sizes were equated with barleycorns. Over time, this evolved to the current measurement of one-third of an inch, equating to a shoe size. In America, Europe and Japan, sizing systems which are currently used originated at different times based on different units and hence the present variation developed (Janisse et al 1995) (see Ch. 5 for details).

Even within the same sizing system, there is little equity between the various devices which are used to measure length. A particular device from a specific manufacturer may be representative of the size required for that make of shoe but may not be representative for others. For example, the measurements taken in a Clarks shop may not match the shoe length of the same size given to a shoe in Marks and Spencer. It is therefore important that size is taken as a guide and that patients do not rigidly adhere to a given size. This is because the size given will also include a styling allowance which may not be the same even between footwear from the same manufacturer. For example, toe shape may dictate that a larger size shoe is needed to accommodate a narrow pointed toe box profile.

The material from which the shoe is made is also significant. The most suitable upper material is leather. Leather has two properties which made it a superb choice for footwear uppers. It has both plasticity, meaning that it can be moulded into a shape which it can retain, and also elasticity, which means that it can stretch and return to that original shape. This is obviously useful in footwear manufacture, but also once worn, any leather footwear can be moulded using heat and moisture or other chemical solutions which allow the intrinsic fibres to change their alignment. Because of this plasticity, leather uppers when subjected to body heat and moisture gradually change to adopt the shape of the foot. Similarly, leather shoes can be stretched when placed over a stretching device, providing that heat and moisture or special stretching solutions are applied to the leather. This is useful if there is a small prominence on the foot which does not totally accord with the shape of the shoe as the shoe can be adjusted within useful limits. Leather will also give a degree of protection to the wearer from damp weather, especially if the leather is treated with wax polish or shoe cream. However, when leather shoes become wet, they should be dried away from direct heat otherwise their shape will change. This is the disadvantage of plasticity, in that the shoe in the presence of this moisture and heat will take on any shape imposed on it.

Shoe uppers may be made from a variety of other materials including woven and knitted fabrics and synthetic plastics. Woven fabrics in particular will need to contain seams or small pleats or gathers to ensure that they form a satisfactory shape for the upper, and seams and other irregularities in the upper can irritate and damage the feet. Some fabrics contain elastic and this can make adequate shoe uppers, however the elastic fabric may need to be reinforced in places by non-elastic stiffeners to ensure that the height required in the upper is maintained. Fabrics in general allow the feet to become wet in inclement weather conditions and tend to lack durability. Plastics maintain their shape and keep the feet dry, but they do not alter shape in any way to accommodate anomalies in foot shape and they are also occlusive. This means that any moisture generated from foot perspiration may not pass through the material and the foot can become slightly macerated providing an environment in which bacteria and dermatophytes may flourish.

Many shoe uppers are lined and this lining material should also be considered. Linings may be made of many different types of material: from thin leather to fur animal skin; from nylon to Gore-tex®; from plush weave fabrics to cotton; to those which absorb moisture such as Cambrelle®. The type of lining best suited to the patient is dependent again on the purpose for which the shoe is to be worn and the external environment in which the patient is active while wearing the footwear. In walking boots, for example, a Gore-tex® lining is useful as it allows moisture from the foot to evaporate while preventing external moisture penetrating to the foot. Fur linings will keep the foot warm in winter but do require that the shoe or boot is fitted properly as the lining occupies space within the footwear. Trainers, particularly those at the higher end of the market, often have a Cambrelle® lining which will help to absorb foot moisture. Gents' classic leather shoes often have a leather lining and this is useful if the wearer does not have high foot perspiration levels and does not live in a very warm climate. The issue with leather lining is that the lining is thin, and where there is excessive foot moisture, the leather can become hard and can split following repeated exposure to such moisture. Nylon lining often wears through at pressure points where the toes or nails may rub against it. This broken lining then causes an irritation against the foot.

Shoe outer sole materials have developed as technology has advanced over the last 40 years or so. Traditionally outer soles were made of leather. This is a durable material, and one which helps to keep the foot cool, but leather soles are not waterproof. They will absorb underfoot water and become wet. Leather also has little cushioning capability, and where people have high plantar pressure points, it should not be the soling material of choice. Leather outer soles also give little grip against external surfaces and can cause the wearer to slip. Other materials, both natural such as rubber, and synthetic such as ethylene vinyl acetate (EVA, which is a by-product of the petrochemical industry) are used for soling. Ethylene vinyl acetate has a shock-absorbing capability and so provides a counter to ground reaction force, but it can absorb water and become wet. Improved performance is offered by vulcanized composition rubber, by thermoplastic rubber and by microcellular polyurethane. These materials have good shock-absorbing capability and wear well. Table 1.3 provides some additional details.

Consideration also needs to be given to the terrain over which the patient will be walking as the outer sole of the shoe or boot needs to provide adequate grip for safety reasons. Footwear with a distinct sole pattern is best to give grip over uneven or slippery terrain whereas smooth soling makes for effortless transfer over even surfaces. One rider to this is in cases of people with shuffling gait, in particular the elderly who tend to wear slippers indoors. It is important that the risk of falling is minimized and a careful balance needs to be drawn between the ability of the sole to grip the surface and allowing the person's foot to move along that surface without too high a degree of friction, as this could also cause a fall. Studies of the incidence of falls in the elderly highlight that, even though therapeutic footwear may accommodate foot deformity, the outer soles are often slippery and may be devoid of any tread pattern. Moore et al (2002) suggest that although the smooth outer surface may be good for those who shuffle when they walk and trip easily in a thick-soled shoe, this type of outer sole can present the danger and liability of slipping in wet conditions. In this instance, for an older person, a fall may be worse than their original foot problem.

While footwear may damage feet causing lesions ranging from superficial corn and callous through to more permanent deformities of toes, it can also be used as an aid to foot function, can improve gait and relieve a host of painful symptoms. It can make the wearer more mobile, enable a range of specialist activities to be undertaken and can protect the wearer against harsh environmental conditions. While clinicians can prescribe footwear which may improve a patient's foot function, the footwear can only achieve the therapeutic aim if it is worn. Ultimately the patient makes the choice as to whether they wish to 'buy-in' to the therapeutic rationale and actually wear the shoes prescribed. Negotiating patient concordance is the most essential element of the therapeutic strategy. If patients find any aspect of the footwear unacceptable, they will not wear it. There will be resultant consequences – not only for the patient's own well-being, but also for the time, energy and effort that the clinician has devoted to the care, as well as for the budget which has funded the footwear. Patient concordance is vital (see Ch. 2 for more on concordance).

Table 1.3 Soling types and wear merits

Soling type	Recognition	Wear merits	Use
Resin rubber	Hard solid rubber feel.	Adequate wear performance at low thickness. Little cushioning capability.	Men's and women's formal footwear and general.
Vulcanized composition rubber	Solid rubber, more resilient than resin rubber.	Good to high durability. Good grip and all round performance.	Walking and sports footwear. Industrial applications. School wear.
Microcellular EVA	Lightweight, often brightly coloured. Sweet smell.	Adequate wear as thick soling, with good cushioning.	Casual shoes, sports through soles.
Microcellular rubber	Medium weight, dull colours. Distinctive smell (sometimes masked by vanilla).	Adequate wear as thick soling, with good cushioning.	Casual shoes, lower grades in slipper through soles.
Polyvinyl chloride (PVC)	Plastic feel, often has shiny finish. Distinctive smell.	Good all round performance.	General applications. School wear.
Thermoplastic rubber	High friction surface, resilient, often a 'pearly' or crepe appearance. Oily smell.	Good wear properties, including slip resistance, especially in cold conditions.	General, except for indoor sports (squash) or oil exposure risks. Tends to grip well, but maybe too well for certain patients.
Microcellular polyurethane	Medium density resilient, surface patterns may be 'pin-holed'.	Good wear properties, especially durability and grip, and cushions well. Lightweight.	General purpose, including sports, industrial and school wear.
Leather	Hard with distinctive smell.	Adequate for fashion shoes. Good customer appeal.	Formal shoes.
Plantation crepe	Translucent, difficult to distinguish from thermoplastic rubber.	Good grip and durability in the highest grades.	General purpose, school wear, unsuitable in cases of oil exposure risks.

References

Bestic L 2004 Try this for size. The Times April 21.

De Lateur BJ, Giaconi RM, Qestad K et al 1991 Footwear and posture: compensatory strategies for heel height. Am J Phys Med Rehabil 70:246–254.

Goonetilleke RS 1998 Designing to minimize discomfort. Ergon Des 6(3):12–19.

Grew F, de Neergaard M, Mitford S 2004 Shoes and pattens. London, Boydell Press.

Moore P, Taunton JE, Kalla TP 2002 If the shoe fits. Journal on Active Aging September/October, 50:17–19.

Janisse DJ, Wertsch JJ, Del Toro DR 1995 Foot orthoses and prescription shoes. In: Redford JB, Basmajian JV, Trautman P (eds) Orthotics: clinical practice and rehabilitation technology. Edinburgh, Churchill Livingstone.

McDowell C 1994 Shoes, fashion and fantasy. New York, Thames & Hudson.

Merriman LM, Tollafield DR 1997 Clinical skills in treating the foot. Edinburgh, Churchill Livingstone.

O'Keeffe L 1996 Shoes: a celebration of pumps, sandals, slippers and more. New York, Workman.

Peacock J 2005 Shoes: the complete sourcebook. New York, Thames & Hudson.

Rossi W, Tennant R 1993 Professional shoe fitting. New York, National Shoe Retailers Association.

World Footwear Publication 2006 Norms for shoe comfort (Editorial). World Footwear Publication May/June, 20(3):46–47.

Patient concordance

While clinicians may be able to offer sound advice about style and fit of footwear to patients, patients may either choose to take the advice and act on it, or may refuse to accept it. The decision is theirs and theirs alone. There has recently been much emphasis on the involvement of patients in their own health care. The term *empowerment* is now frequently used in the context of encouraging patient involvement. Empowerment has been described as 'returning power, knowledge, skills and other resources to the individual' (Rodwell 1996). This infers that patients must be fully informed, and make a decision about accepting or rejecting footwear advice on the basis of the knowledge they have about the effects on their foot health of ill-fitting or ill-designed footwear.

Much comment has been made about patient compliance and satisfaction with prescribed therapeutic footwear, although not very much work appears to have been done about how well patients follow advice about purchasing and wearing suitable retail footwear. Dissatisfaction with the cosmetic appearance of therapeutic footwear is a constant theme in the literature, with levels of dissatisfaction varying from 50% (Park & Craxford 1981), 40% (van de Weg 2002), 19.8% (Stewart 1996) and 18% (Neil 2002). Even though the degree of dissatisfaction varies, there are constant complaints around cosmesis and comfort. Patient comments particularly relate to:

- Limited number of styles
- Limited colour options
- Weight of the shoe
- Comfort and fit
- Ease of putting the shoe on
- Elevated foot temperature when wearing the shoe.

If we examine this further, the styles of therapeutic footwear are very similar to those of the retail styles advised by foot health practitioners as being the most suitable. Many colour options are available in therapeutic footwear – just look at the brochures. Therapeutic footwear is generally light in weight unless it includes a calliper or similar aid. The ease of donning the shoe may also be an issue for patients wearing suitable retail footwear, as that too should have a functional fastening. So how can compliance or concordance be improved?

Studies have also highlighted other common themes important in improving compliance. The cost of therapeutic and surgical footwear has been shown as being unrecognized by the patient. Patients often greatly underestimate the cost of therapeutic footwear provided for them and it has been suggested that charging a sum may help improve compliance (Emery & Borthwick 2002; Herold & Palmar 1992). If patients are to purchase suitable retail footwear for themselves, they will have to bear the financial burden, but there may well be issues around affordability, and practitioners should be sensitive to it. Many suitable shoes are available on the market at relatively low cost.

Another area highlighted as having potential for improving concordance is that of patient education. It is suggested that appropriate education will influence compliance and outcome (Baker & Letherdale 1999; Macfarlane & Jenson 2003; Neil 2002; van de Weg 2002). Education to change life-long patterns requires sensitivity in stressing its relevance to patients' lives (Neil 2002), though cause and effect relationships seem to have limited influence on a patient's decision regarding footwear (Macfarlane & Jenson 2003). The practitioner's understanding of the need for patient education has developed in recent years, and the value of evidence-based practice can be seen from both the practitioner's and the patients' perspective.

Health Belief Model

In examining the ways of achieving patient concordance, Beker (1974; abstracted from Banyard 1996), in his Health Belief Model, suggested that the likelihood of patients taking recommended action is influenced by their perception of the threat of the 'disease' with an associated cost–benefit analysis – the benefits of remaining in the current situation (continuing to wear the shoes they like and failing to improve their foot health) versus the costs of changing. Bear in mind that these costs are not only the financial costs involved in the purchase of suitable footwear, but the social and emotional costs of wearing shoes which may not match the patients' own body images and which may not match the dress

normally associated with their peers and with their social activities.

The health professional's view of susceptibility and severity and cost–benefit analysis may be very different from that of the patient. The clinician may be fully aware that a pressure lesion in a diabetic foot may lead to amputation, but in the mind of the patient, that amputation will never happen; after all, what the patient sees may be only a small open wound with no associated pain. The health professional may not be fully aware of the patient's emotional and social needs and expectations. Changing behaviour in a patient is a gradual process and is best taken in small steps, with reinforcement of positive actions and with achievement of outcomes given credit by the professional during clinical contact with the individual patient. Any suggested measures which patients have been unable to implement should be examined, discussed and modified in the light of their experiences. This gradual approach will help to establish when patients are ready and able to change their behaviour, before regaling them with full details of what you suggest they do to improve their condition, bearing in mind that compliance is a very abnormal behaviour pattern in normal adults (Day 2000).

Education Model

In the 1970s, the mode of achieving patient compliance was based on the Education Model, which basically involved clinicians imparting knowledge to patients in a didactic way, either verbally or by providing leaflets or written notes. This method results in information being passed to the patient, and hopefully achieves an increase in their knowledge base, but often this fails to change an individual's behaviour.

Stages of Change Model

The later-developed Stages of Change Model discusses the ability of an individual to recognize the need for change and the processes they go through to make that change (Fig. 2.1). This altered perception of risk, or susceptibility, has been recognized in the Health Belief Model. The model identifies that

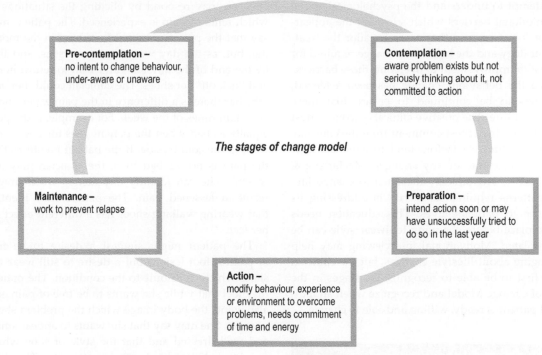

The stages of change model

Pre-contemplation – no intent to change behaviour, under-aware or unaware

Contemplation – aware problem exists but not seriously thinking about it, not committed to action

Maintenance – work to prevent relapse

Preparation – intend action soon or may have unsuccessfully tried to do so in the last year

Action – modify behaviour, experience or environment to overcome problems, needs commitment of time and energy

Figure 2.1 The Stages of Change Model.

it is important for the clinician to understand that patients have their own perception of their health. The clinician will have to consider:

- Perceived susceptibility: do patients believe their conditions have risks?
- Perceived severity: do patients understand/accept the severity of their conditions?
- Perceived benefits: are patients able to recognize the benefits of the treatment/course of action proposed to address their conditions?
- Perceived barriers: what might be the problems perceived by patients in adopting the planned treatment/course of action?
- Cues to action: what will prompt patients to remain true to the health belief and treatment/course of action?
- Self-efficacy: how will patients make this happen?

In applying this model to footwear, the first issues concern patients' perceptions of their foot conditions and whether they can identify the fact that their foot health is important to their general well-being, to their mobility levels, to their quality of life and to their social interactions. Do they understand that their conditions will not improve unless they take action, and, indeed, could deteriorate significantly. The example of the patient with diabetes and the seemingly unimportant foot lesion which might well be the trigger in the causal chain which leads to loss of the limb is relevant in this context. Can the patient see the link between choice of footwear and the lesion formation? Without understanding this connection, any attempt to change behaviour will founder. It may be that some patients will find that wearing suitable footwear which they consider to be ugly, unattractive and which makes them stand out from the norm is not acceptable at a given point in time, but with positive reinforcement from the clinician when the patient wears suitable footwear, and agreement with the patient about the benefits they have experienced, a gradual change should be achieved. Clinicians need to empathize with patients and attempt to understand the psychological, social and emotional barriers which surround the appearance of footwear, and they need to tailor the treatment strategy and the behaviour change required for foot health improvement to overcome those barriers.

Once the behaviour change has been achieved, work has to be continued to ensure that these changes endure. The positive clinical outcomes must be reinforced by honest comment from the clinician. Changes in lifestyle factors tend to have the lowest compliance rate of any changes (Macfarlane & Jensen 2003). The strategy designed to change lifelong patterns requires sensitivity in addressing its relevance to patients' lives. This education needs to take place before changing footwear style can be contemplated. Motivational interviewing may help in bringing about lifestyle changes, but the clinician needs first to be able to recognize the stages in the Stage of Change Model and recognize when an individual patient is ready, willing and able to change.

Motivational interviewing

Motivational interviewing may be one of the most effective ways of achieving behavioural change. This technique was developed in the 1980s in the treatment of problem alcohol drinkers. Rollnick & Miller (1995) describe it as: '… a directive, client-centred counselling style for eliciting behavioural change by helping clients to explore and resolve ambivalence'. The system is non-confrontational and non-persuasive and relies on patients identifying the need for change in their attitudes and behaviours.

At the heart of motivational interviewing is the examination and resolution of patients' ambivalence. Patients must be motivated to change, and the whole process relies on first identifying the patients' intrinsic values and their goals in order to stimulate the change.

For example, a woman may have a painful foot lesion which the clinician identifies as being caused by ill-fitting footwear. The patient may know that by attending the clinic regularly for debridement of the lesion, she can become pain free for short periods of time. However, she might identify that the condition is deteriorating and that more frequent debridement is necessary to relieve the pain. She may ask the clinician what the cause of the problem is, and the

clinician may respond by eliciting the situations in which relief of pain is experienced. The patient may say that the pain is minimal first thing in the morning, but, as the day wears on, it worsens, and that by the end of the day, she can't wait to return home and 'kick off' her shoes. The clinician could then ask whether there is a difference in the pain experienced at certain times of the week. For example, is the pain equally as bad when the patient goes for a leisurely walk in the countryside. If the patient identifies that the pain is not so bad then, the clinician may ask whether she can identify any factors which might result in lessened pain. The patient may identify that wearing walking shoes has a different effect on her feet.

The patient might suggest a desire to be free of painful foot lesions but a desire to still wear the shoes which contribute to the condition. The patient may feel that while she wants to be free of pain, she also wants the body image which the problem shoes give her. She may say that she wants to appear smart and well dressed and that the style of shoe which provides relief makes her feel unattractive. The clinician then needs to facilitate expression of both sides of this dilemma and guide the patient towards an acceptable solution which may trigger change. The counselling style should be patient centred, respectful, gentle, quiet, supportive, non-aggressive and non-confrontational.

It is tempting for the clinician to persuade patients that the problem is urgent and to try to make them see the benefits of changing their footwear. However, doing this will probably increase resistance to change and reduce the likelihood that patients will modify their footwear. The essence of motivational interviewing is that that ambivalence or lack of resolve is the principal obstacle to overcome in changing patients' attitudes to footwear. To the clinician, this can seem a very slow and tedious process, but patients must not be pushed, and unless patients are actually ready to change then the effort will be fruitless.

Readiness to change is a fluctuating product of interpersonal reaction between the patient and clinician. The clinician needs to be highly attentive and responsive to the patient's reactions. Any resistance to change shown by patients should be regarded not as a failing in them, but as feedback about the outcome of the way in which the clinician responded to them. This resistance in patients is an indicator that they are not ready to change and that the clinician needs to modify motivational strategies.

The relationship between the patient and clinician should become a partnership rather than that of recipient and expert roles, respectively. The clinician must always remember that patients have freedom of choice and may do as they wish, but will of course also need to accept the consequences of any actions they take.

The process is one of gradual change. The clinician must consistently reinforce even minor changes in behaviour which have had positive outcomes. If patients report that they have seen an improvement, the clinician should always give recognition to the behaviour which led to the improvement and should applaud it. Improvement will be slow and gradual but the clinician may wish to recall and remind patients of the progress they have made over time. Small changes may not be remembered by patients, but the clinician may be able to use some objective measures, such as visual analogue pain scales completed by patients at each visit, to remind them of the progress they have made.

In order to develop effective motivational interviewing techniques, the clinician will need to adopt a patient-centred approach, and will need to:

- Listen to patients and become empathic
- Accept patients' terms of reference
- Affirm the positive actions patients take
- Elicit and reinforce patients' own positive self-motivational statements, their problems, concerns and desire for change
- Monitor patients' readiness to change
- Allow them to change at their own pace, without imposing targets on them
- Affirm patients' freedom of choice.

Concordance is influenced by a large number of factors, economic, cultural, cosmetic and motivational. It is also interesting to note that a greater degree of compliance in footwear prescription is seen in men (Macfarlane & Jensen 2003), and that women express far more dissatisfaction with the footwear they receive (Stewart 1996). This can probably be explained by considering the range of footwear available for men and women commercially and the difference between this footwear and that prescribed.

Men in general are not as fashion conscious, and commercially available men's footwear bears a closer resemblance to prescribed footwear than does that for women.

What has also become evident is that, to achieve greater concordance, the patient needs to be involved in the very early stages of the prescribing process (Baker & Letherdale 1999) and that the prescriber needs to be fully aware of all the factors which will lead to a successful clinical outcome. Patients need to understand why particular features are significant; for example, why they might need a rocker sole, or why a boot style would be preferable to a shoe in meeting their foot health needs. They need to appreciate the features in shoe design which will allow a shoe of sufficient length and girth to stay on their foot during each stage of the gait cycle and why a functional fastening is necessary. They need to know the effects on their foot of raising the height of a heel. They need to be aware of the potentially damaging effects of including seams in the shoe upper, the effects that different shoe lining materials can have on their feet and to understand the necessity for specialist insole or orthotic materials. All such issues are those in which the patient should be consulted. There are other issues over which the patient can have the ultimate choice, such as the texture and colour of the shoe material and style of fastening. Although these seem few, they are perhaps the most important to the patient and the least significant to the clinician. It is, after all, the external appearance of their footwear that most patients are concerned with.

The multidisciplinary team

The involvement of multidisciplinary teams has been shown to improve results and increase patient satisfaction with footwear. The essential feature of multidisciplinary working is that the patient is seen as the central focus around which all other members of the team work. It provides a coordinated approach to patient care. Each member of the team should have access to and should contribute to the overall therapeutic rationale and strategy. This will enable each member to bring their own professional expertise to the benefit of the overall well-being of the patient. Taking an example from rheumatology, a patient with rheumatoid arthritis will have access to his general medical practitioner, to a specialist rheumatologist, a nurse specialist, occupational therapist, orthotist, podiatrist, physiotherapist, dietician, pharmacist and social worker. His general medical practitioner will have overall responsibility for his care, but will have referred him to other specialist services which he is unable to provide.

Looking at the roles of just a few of these specialisms, it can be seen that there may be areas in which therapies may overlap, and where there may on occasion be duplication or conflict. The occupational therapist will be concerned with the facilitation of the activities of daily living, such as washing, dressing, cooking, eating and working, and may suggest that the patient undertakes a regime to reduce pain and stress on the affected joints, including adapting movement patterns, using assistive devices and undertaking exercise, and may also prescribe splinting and insoles or orthoses. The physiotherapist may prescribe exercise therapy in an attempt to overcome the adverse effects of the condition on muscle strength, endurance and aerobic capacity, and may also prescribe splinting and insoles or orthoses. The podiatrist will be concerned with the way in which the patient's foot condition affects his overall mobility level, and will reduce painful superficial skin lesions and may provide footwear and insoles and/or orthoses. The orthotist may prescribe footwear and orthoses, and/or splinting.

If these professionals communicate with one another, an overall strategy can be developed which will include the expertise available from each. It is most important that the patient is given consistent information and advice; that one member of the team does not contradict the advice given by another. This is sometimes the case when a patient is prescribed footwear and orthoses. One professional may favour a particular type of orthotic device and may prescribe it for a patient. That same patient may be subsequently seen by a member of another profession who is unfamiliar with such orthotic prescriptions. It is essential that the orthotic device is not changed or modified by the second professional without referral to the prescriber, otherwise the patient will completely lose confidence in the prescription and in the clinicians involved. Similarly, a patient who has been provided with therapeutic footwear may attend the clinic and complain of the development of a new and painful lesion. A clinician who is unfamiliar with the footwear prescription may make an ill-considered comment and suggest that such lesions are usually caused by footwear. On further examination of the footwear, it is probably found that the therapeutic footwear prescribed has not caused the new lesion, but such a throw-away comment can cause patients to discard the footwear provided and revert to the damaging footwear which they used previously.

A fully functioning multidisciplinary team can bring a wide range of skills and can have a dramatic impact on patient care and well-being. Each team member can work to complement and enhance the skills of the other and improve the patient's quality of life. The occupational therapist can ensure that the patient has the assistance needed to manage everyday life; the physiotherapist can ensure that the patient's muscle strength and joint mobility levels remain at an optimal level; the podiatry and orthotic team can ensure that the patient's foot health is such that mobility can be maintained and that the patient has the footwear necessary to undertake the exercise required by the physiotherapist, that the patient is comfortable enough to be able to remain independent and can thus support the aims of the occupational therapist.

Teams providing foot care and footwear are becoming much more multidisciplinary in nature. Footwear was traditionally provided by a surgical appliance officer who had little contact with members of healthcare professions. Footwear prescription was derived without reference to associated care disciplines, and it was not unknown for the footwear provided to find a permanent home in the cupboard rather than on the feet of the patient. Fortunately the situation is changing, and several studies have examined the effectiveness of the multidisciplinary approach.

Satisfaction rates of two groups of patients were studied. One group was seen by a traditional surgical appliance clinic and the other group in a multidisciplinary clinic (Williams & Meacher 2001). Patients in the multidisciplinary group had a much higher satisfaction with footwear and greater pain reduction. This group all received education prior to the prescription process, and those assessed as having a 'positive attitude' had a high level of satisfaction. This group was also associated with continuous footwear usage. The effectiveness of a multidisciplinary approach was shown to be effective elsewhere (Emery & Borthwick

2002), suggesting that communication and consistency are vital to support change in behaviour.

Patients must receive a consistent message from all practitioners involved in their care. Contradicting opinions only act to confuse patients, especially those at the contemplation stage (Ley 1988). It may be that individual practitioners have their own values, but it is important to have shared goals based on evidence-based practice that have the best interests of the patient at heart. Lack of communication between professionals tends to cause a fragmented approach to care which often results in an unsatisfactory result (Emery & Borthwick 2002).

Regular review appointments have also been highlighted as improving compliance and satisfaction (Emery & Borthwick 2002; Williams & Meacher 2001). Those patients who have a review appointment booked or have written information advising them how to contact the clinic for advice also appear to achieve better outcomes.

If a patient is not sufficiently motivated to wear the recommended footwear, the footwear prescription needs to be reviewed. This is particularly so in the case of therapeutic (surgical) footwear where costs are high. It is pointless to provide this option if the patient will never wear it or will use it so infrequently that any therapeutic value is lost.

Conclusion

In considering the prescription of therapeutic footwear, the underlying foot pathology and foot shape will determine the type of footwear required – be it advising on retail footwear which patients may purchase for themselves, stock surgical footwear, modular surgical footwear or the fully bespoke footwear option. If patients' needs can be addressed by the retail option, they will have control and flexibility over footwear purchase. This option of course represents a cost saving for the NHS or for medical insurance companies. For patients who require more specialized footwear, the options are many. The variety of companies supplying footwear on different lasts and to different styles means that the choice available to patients has greatly increased in recent years, and this therapeutic footwear is now available in a wide variety of colours and styles. Style options have developed tremendously and

prescription footwear has become very much more cosmetically acceptable than it was a few years ago. By obtaining supplies from a variety of footwear manufacturers, all of whom use different last dimensions for each size available, the footwear needs of a greater number of people can be met from the most basic and least expensive form of therapeutic (surgical) footwear – stock footwear. This represents a huge cost saving on obtaining supply from only one manufacturer, as that manufacturer's stock footwear may fail to fit a number of patients who will then need to be prescribed the more expensive modular or bespoke range. Many of these factors resulted in the production of a booklet on therapeutic footwear by the Society of Chiropodists and Podiatrists (2004).

Other changes in the orthopaedic footwear industry have resulted in the production of footwear from computer-aided design/computer-aided manufacturing (CAD/CAM) systems. These systems speed up design and ensure quality of the product. Systems exist that are capable of manufacturing shoe lasts and designing shoe uppers to satisfy the most demanding cosmetic challenges. Production is rapid and accurate, but the finished product is only as good as the clinician's prescription.

The clinical effectiveness of orthopaedic footwear is heavily dependent on acceptability and actual use by the patient (Knowles & Boulton 1996). Thus if the ideal prescription process has been followed, the result should be a clinically effective shoe that also achieves patient satisfaction, so that the patient wears it. The greatest evidence of this comes from the use of therapeutic footwear in treating neuro-ischaemic feet in diabetes. There is some consensus of opinion among those involved in diabetic foot care that patients with a past history of ulceration and amputation, or both, are at significantly greater risk of repeat ulceration and amputation (Kumar et al 1994; Pecoraro et al 1990; Reiber et al 1992). It has been found that diabetic patients wearing protective footwear for more than 60% of the daytime reduced the ulcer recurrence rate by more than 50% (Chanteleau & Hagge 1993; Macfarlane & Jensen 2003).

Footwear provision is influenced by many factors that include the needs and wishes of the patient, the aims of the prescriber and financial considerations. If footwear is effective, the benefits to the patient are improved mobility, comfort and protection and generally improved well-being. The additional clinical benefits go as far as to address the devastating and resource-consuming foot problems such as ulceration; infection, gangrene and amputation can be prevented (Chanteleau et al 1990).

References

Baker N, Letherdale B 1999 Audit of special shoes: are they being worn? Diabetic Foot 2:100–104.

Beker B (abstracted from Banyard P) 1996 Applying psychology to health. London, Hodder & Stoughton.

Chanteleau E, Kushner T, Spraul M 1990 How effective is cushioned therapeutic footwear in protecting diabetic feet? A clinical study. Diabet Med 7:355–359.

Chanteleau E, Hagge P 1993 An audit of cushioned diabetic footwear: relation to patient compliance. Diabet Med 11(1):114–116.

Day JL 2000 Diabetic patient education: determinants of success. Diabet Metabol Res Rev 16(suppl 1):s70–s74.

Emery M, Borthwick A 2002 The orthopaedic footwear service: a survey of effectiveness. Diabetic Foot 5(1):45–50.

Herold DC, Palmer RG 1992 Questionnnaire study of the use of surgical shoes prescribed in a rheumatology outpatient clinic. J Rheumatol 19:1542–1544.

Knowles EA, Boulton AJM 1996 Do people with diabetes wear their prescribed footwear? Diabet Med 13:1064–1068.

Kumar S, Ashe HA, Parnell LN et al 1994 The prevalence of foot ulceration and its correlates in type 2 diabetic patients: a population-based study. Diabet Med 11:480–484.

Ley P 1988 Communicating with patients. London, Chapman & Hall.

Macfarlane DJ, Jensen JL 2003 Factors in diabetic footwear compliance. J Am Podiatr Med Assoc 93(6):485–491.

Neil JA 2002 Footwear practices of people with and without foot ulcers. Diabetic Foot 5(3):140–150.

Park C, Craxford AD 1981 Surgical footwear in rheumatoid arthritis: a patient acceptability study. Prosthet Orthot Int 5:33–36.

Pecoraro RE, Reiber GE, Burgess EM 1990 Pathways to diabetic limb amputation: basis for prevention. Diabetes Care 13:513.

Reiber GE, Pecoraro RE, Thomas DK 1992 Risk factors for amputation in patients with diabetes mellitus. Ann Intern Med 117:97–105.

Rodwell G 1996 An analysis of the concept of empowerment. J Adv Nurs 23(2):305–313.

Rollnick S, Miller WR 1995 What is motivational interviewing? Behavioural and Cognitive Psychotherapy 23:325–334.

Society of Chiropodists and Podiatrists 2004 Therapeutic footwear: 'quality in a team approach'. London, Society of Chiropodists and Podiatrists.

Stewart J 1996 Patient satisfaction with bespoke footwear in people with rheumatoid arthritis. J Br Podiatr Med 51:21–23.

Van de Weg FB 2002 Compliance with orthopaedic footwear in patients with diabetes. Diabetic Foot an de Weg 2002 Compliance with orthopaedic footwear in patients with diabetes. Diabetic Foot 5(1):32–36.

Williams A, Meacher K 2001 Shoes in the cupboard: the fate of prescribed footwear? Prost Orthot Int 25:53–59.

The last

The last is the model form or shape around which most footwear is made. The vast majority of manufacturing methods require a last on which to make footwear, although some very basic sandal styles, where the uppers are in the form of ties only, can be made without a last. The last determines the overall shape and fitting characteristics of a shoe or boot (Fig. 3.1).

The last will be made either of a plastic material or, in rare, special cases, may be made of wood, either of maple, redwood or of hornbeam. These are woods which are virtually knotless. As knots in wood are of a different density to the remainder of the wood, it is not possible to make smooth, durable lasts from woods which contain natural knots. Wooden lasts today are used mainly in the high-end,

high-cost, bespoke market. Lasts for the volume market are now made from recyclable polythene. This is more cost-effective as all the waste materials discarded during last manufacture can be reprocessed, as can the lasts, once they are finished with. A last is normally made with a hinge so that it can be easily removed from the footwear without causing any damage to the shoe and can be reused as many times as the factory chooses. This is usually until the related shoe design is obsolete.

The word 'lasting' actually means to pull a shoe upper tightly over a last and to secure it underneath the last. In the majority of manufacturing methods, the last remains inside the shoe during the manufacturing processes and this gives the shoe a defined shape. The inside dimensions of the finished footwear will conform to those of the last. An exception to this method is the 'sewn in sock' method of shoe construction where the completed upper is stitched to an insock and then forced onto a metal foot base to allow a moulded sole to be attached in an automated carousel machine. As soon as the sole is completed and set, the shoe is removed from the machine for final finishing so the shape of the shoe is not formed until almost the final process and is not held on the last for a long period of time. In volume manufacturing, the lasted upper with be passed through a tunnel where heat and moisture are applied to ensure

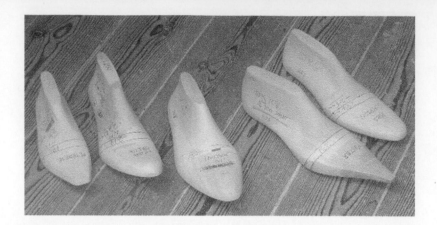

Figure 3.1 Selection of hand-crafted lasts for the retail market. (Reproduced with permission of Spring Line Lasts.)

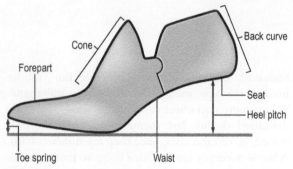

Figure 3.2 Outline diagram of parts of the last (profile view).

that the upper material then adopts the shape of the last. In traditional processes for hand-made bespoke footwear, the upper may be 'lasted' for up to ten days before being removed for finishing.

The last is vital to the manufacturing process for shoes, boots and most sandals, and in prescribing footwear, it is useful to understand the descriptive terminology applied to the parts of the last (Fig. 3.2):

- **Back curve**: the area that is shaped to fit closely to the heel of the foot.
- **Cone**: a solid shape, tapering to a narrower point at the top, above the top line of the upper.
- **Feather (line or edge)**: the boundary line around the upper where it joins the welt or the sole; the corresponding line around an insole or last.
- **Forepart**: the front part of the last from the waist forwards.

- **Heel pitch**: an angle between the axis and heel and baseline. If the heel is not vertical, damage may result.
- **Joint**: the main line of flexing of the foot, and hence of the shoe, occurs at this point which is therefore important in shoe fitting. It should correspond to the metatarso-phalangeal joints at the first and fifth metatarsal heads.
- **Seat**: the part of the shoe immediately below the heel of the foot. The seat angle is the difference between the seat position and the horizontal plane where the heel is attached. A levelling piece may be inserted here to provide a level surface for the heel to be attached, which blends in with the welt or the sole.
- **Toe spring**: the upward curvature or angle of the sole forepart, relative to ground level, when the shoe is on a level surface. It is related to the stiffness of the sole and height of the heel. It enables the wearer to proceed by a forward rolling action at the joint.
- **Waist**: the area anterior to the seat of the last.

The last is not a copy of the foot. It is shaped in such a way that it may produce a good-fitting shoe. In the retail sector, styling is influenced by fashion trends, and the resulting shoe shape may not necessarily be an ideal fitting shape. In the orthopaedic sector, the last is made from individual measurements and more accurately reflects the shape and size of the foot concerned.

The last versus the foot

There are essential differences between the last and the human foot that are worth considering, as a common misconception is that a bespoke shoe must surely be the perfect answer to foot pathologies. The last is a compromise and the most effective way of forming a shape on which functional footwear can be made (Table 3.1).

Lasts are complex structures made from many measurements that are statistically determined. The origins of these measurements are shrouded in the mists of time and it is difficult to establish exactly how, where and when they were gathered and who gathered them. Lasts are usually deeper in the mid-foot region, clipped in along the top line and flared and extended in the toe region. All this provides a shape which can apply appropriate tension when the shoe distorts as the fully-loaded foot takes its toll on the footwear during any level of activity.

Lasts are still made in the traditional way. The initial development of a new model is a highly-skilled craft. The success of the last depends upon the last maker's experience, his perception of the footwear design requirements and on his knowledge of fittings and measurements to ensure that the last will produce a good-fitting pair of shoes. Initial models and bespoke lasts are still crafted in wood. However, the large majority of bulk lasts are now made in plastic for improved durability. Lasts can be made to many specifications, with different hinges, plugs, plates and slots in toes according to the shoemaker's requirements (Fig. 3.3).

To make a bulk order, the initial model is taken and put in a copying lathe. The first stage is to rough turn the lasts, and then a hinge is fitted. After this, the lasts are fine turned on a second lathe. The lasts have been held in place in the lathe by toe and heel dogs. These now need to be removed and the toe and heels must be shaped according to the required templates. Plates can now be cut and attached and finally the lasts will be hand finished. Last manufacture is still a very skilled manual process (Figs 3.4–3.6).

The biggest development in the process over recent years has been the introduction of digitizing machines which allow a last to be effectively scanned and reproduced exactly on a computer screen. Software has been developed that enables the manufacturer to manipulate a last digitally – modifying heel height,

lengthening toes, adding sock allowances or boot back parts and more (courtesy of Spring Line Lasts).

One of the most important roles in the therapeutic bespoke manufacturing process is that of the last maker, who needs to produce an aesthetically acceptable shape on which a shoe can be made to accommodate a foot that is often far from being normal in shape.

To summarize, the last is not identical to the foot in shape or proportions, but a compromise of the two. It is used to form a shoe that must permit the foot to function in both static and dynamic modes.

Design and pattern cutting

The starting point of a new shoe is the initial design. The designer may also be the original pattern cutter, although some very large manufacturers may employ designers whose job is simply to design. Computer-aided design (CAD) is now regularly used by many designers to create new styles. These designers are able to build up a collection of upper shapes, lasts and sole designs as a library to draw from when creating new ideas. The computer allows them to produce a three-dimensional model of the design on the screen and enables them to view it from all angles before any patterns are cut or lasts produced. For mass production, this saves time and money in the early stages of development as the finished product can be seen digitally. Computer-aided design systems have many advantages, but to some they have one or two serious drawbacks.

World Footwear Publication (2006) published two articles on 'You will never achieve a perfect pattern' which highlight some of the technological downfalls of CAD. Foremost among these is the inaccuracy of the base pattern (forme) produced by three-dimensional CAD software from the user's last. The forme is responsible for the accuracy and quality of all footwear to be made on that last, and if this is inaccurate, the footwear made will fail to fit. For example, in a base pattern of 300 mm in length, in extreme cases there may be an error of 60–70 mm in the pitch at the back. This is described as 'deadened' (dragged down below their natural pitch) which results in difficult lasting and poor-quality footwear. To check this out, there is only one guaranteed method and that is to make either a drape or a simple court upper and

Table 3.1 Comparison of the last and the human foot

Comparison	Last	Human foot
Surfaces	Surfaces are smooth to enhance appearance of the shoe and to enable the upper to be moulded more easily to the shape.	Surfaces are variable, with bony prominences, and varying layers of skin, fat, muscle and even fluid to make a large variation in surface appearance.
Outline	The outline is regular and continuous with a sharp feather edge around the seat and forepart to assist lasting and give a clear, defined edge to the finished shoe.	Has no feather edge or sharp defined lines.
Substance	Hard and firm.	Softer surface and flexible.
Heel width	Narrower at the heel to ensure shoe fits snugly over the heel and does not slip.	Fleshy curved shape that changes on weight bearing.
Heel curves (comb)	Last curve is increased to help the grip at the back, but reduced at the sides to help the shoe fit around the quarters and topline. Dependent on the last maker for shape and fit.	Anatomical structure of bone and tendons that is very vulnerable if the heel fit is poor. Can be changed by deformity or conditions such as oedema.
Heel pitch	The pitch of the last is regulated by the height of the heel, which in turn is usually dictated by fashion.	Not normally present in the foot except in cases of deformity, e.g. congenital equinus.
Toes	Is longer than the foot in order to allow for foot extension during walking, and the shape may not allow room for the toes without extra length, e.g. pointed toe shape.	The foot is variable in its proportions and the length and shape of toes are particularly so. The extension of the foot during walking is also variable. Some need longer shoe length than others.
Toe profile	Depth gradually decreases to a feather edge on most lasts.	Toe profiles are very individual with no feather edge.
Toe depth	The last should be deeper than the foot to allow adequate room. Again dictated by fashion and all extremes are found.	No standard depth. Each foot is individual and in orthopaedics this is a critical area of fitting.
Toe spring	The shoe has to bend with the foot during walking. The spring in the last is shown by the height of the forepart when a heel is placed under the last. As a rule, high-heeled shoes require less toe spring than low-heeled shoes because a high-heeled shoe needs to flex less than a low-heeled shoe.	Toe spring is not present in the foot, however the foot does need to flex during walking. A compromise is made in the last between the heel height and the toe spring to allow foot flexion but a shoe can not flex as much as a foot.
Joint girth	Sometimes greater than the foot to allow foot flexion in the shoe. Dependent on upper material and style.	Static and dynamic measurements vary creating a fitting compromise.
Girth, size intervals and dimensions	Regular on lasts.	Irregular on feet.

(Continued)

Table 3.1 Continued

Comparison	Last	Human foot
Styling	Theoretically limitless, but in reality, needs to cope with the limits of foot shapes and function.	The foot is normally only modified in cases of surgery, for medical reasons and not cosmetic ones, although exceptions are known to fit feet into fashion shoes.
Function	Used for shoe making.	The foot is used for weight-bearing and propulsion.
Hinge	Last may have a single hinge in order to remove it from inside the shoe more easily.	The foot has no hinge but has many joints that move during the walking phase.

Figure 3.3 Hand-made prototype last.

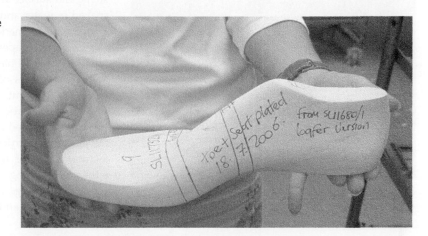

Figure 3.4 Copying lathe producing first 'pair' matching lasts. (Reproduced with permission of Spring Line Lasts.)

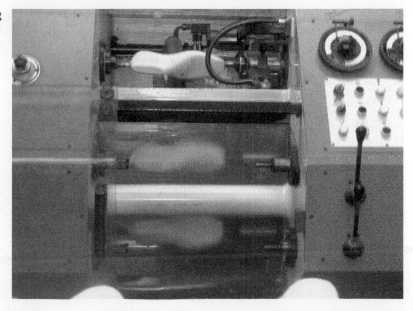

check it for fit onto the last. A drape can be fitted over the last by hand, whereas a court upper needs to be at least partly lasted. If the upper has a tight top line, no obvious gaping or straining in key areas, then it will be successful. However, as any CAD designer will admit, development of software for flattening is a highly fraught subject. The more successful systems have depended heavily on a deep understanding of how to flatten manually, and this knowledge is built into the CAD process. Without this knowledge, it becomes extremely difficult to define what is required, hence poorly-designed formes can be the result.

However, with expertise, it is still possible to obtain a very good pattern. This can be demonstrated by seaming the inside and outside formes at the front and back centre lines to produce a 'drape' that can be lasted by finger pressure only. This drape will not be perfect but will show the inaccuracies around the toe, seat and instep.

Formes were originally made by wrapping a piece of upper leather over the last and trimming around the edges to leave an approximation of the size, shape and surface area of the last. When uppers were soaked in water and hand lasted, this was sufficient. Formes can be made in several ways, including the use of slotted paper, plastic and car body masking tape, but they all have to be flattened to match them to the flat sheets of material from which the shoe uppers will be cut. This is where the real problems can occur. The process of flattening a forme will also tell an experienced craftsman a great deal about how the last and a particular upper will behave in manufacture. Areas of maximum distortion will appear either as creasing and pleating or undue stretching and straining. These can be corrected when the upper is lasted, and as long as the upper materials

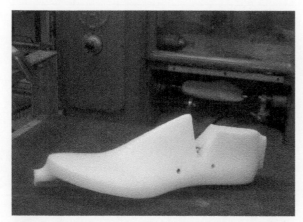

Figure 3.5 Last removed from lathe ready for finishing. (Reproduced with permission of Spring Line Lasts.)

Figure 3.6 Bespoke lasts with BS chart. (Reproduced with permission of Jane Saunders and Manning Bespoke Shoe Manufacturers.)

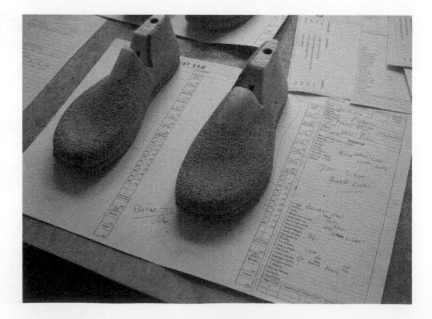

are soft and malleable, a good result can be achieved. It is essential that the 'reversibility' factor is clearly understood so that correction and compensation can be built into the patterns. The essence of reversibility in this instance is the ability of the upper to stretch at the points where the forme was creased or pleated, and to condense where the flattened forme was loose.

Shoe making can be described as the art of producing a three-dimensional, dynamic article from two-dimensional material; pattern making requires the conversion of the round curves of the last into the flat upper components and then back into the curved shape of the shoe. Therefore, at each stage, the designer needs to know and understand what the effects of the process will be and how to cope with them, and needs to develop techniques to compensate for the many errors which may occur in the transition from one state to another. This makes shoe making not quite so straightforward as many would like to believe.

Pump formes

The key to accurate patterns is to maintain the 'spring' of the last. The spring relates to the heel height and the specific requirement to meet the specific angulation and clip of the shoe top line within the upper of all the pattern pieces for any design made for that particular last. A method employed to achieve this is called the pump forme. This is the line that must be kept undistorted and correct on all types of footwear, including men's footwear, as it dictates the spring and pitch of the pattern (Fig. 3.7).

The pump forme has several advantages over the traditional full forme, and for every last there is an optimal base pattern and, if possible, all designs and their patterns to be made on that last should be developed from that pattern. The pattern maker creates a flat pattern that represents the area, size and shape of the last surface. If the process begins with a flat shape, then there will be less distortion in the flattening process which in turn provides greater accuracy in the base pattern made from the forme. The areas of greatest distortion are the toe, seat, inside waist and instep, and cone centre lines. It is no coincidence that these are the areas where lasting is most difficult, because any minor errors in the measuring of the last surface which may then be translated into the pattern have to be corrected at

Drape/court 'upper' for checking a forme's fit to the last

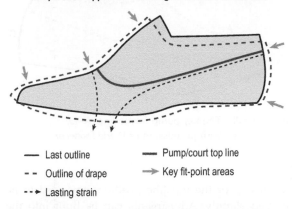

— Last outline   — Pump/court top line

-- Outline of drape   → Key fit-point areas

--→ Lasting strain

Typical deadening of a CAD forme compared to a tape forme

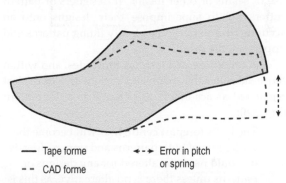

— Tape forme   ←-→ Error in pitch
-- CAD forme   or spring

Figure 3.7 Top drape/court upper checking a forme to fit the last. (Reproduced with permission of *World Footwear Publication* 2006.)

this point. When springing or deadening has to be introduced to make the pattern viable, the designer should be aware, if moving away from the accepted base shape, that there are will be implications for the success of the final footwear product.

The pump forme can be used to produce an accurate base pattern for any type of footwear, from heavy steel-capped safety boots to ladies' dress sandals or court shoes. Any additional design content can be grafted onto the base pattern once it has been proven. It is also important to realize that the forme must be made to fit the last without regard to style lines or future choice of construction method. It must be the best possible shape achievable, and when the style lines are added later to develop the design standard, modifications may be required. For example, the vamp point may need to be higher on

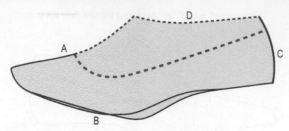

Figure 3.8 The key pump forme lines A–D. (Reproduced with permission of *World Footwear Publication* 2006.)

the instep or the top line position may need to be moved slightly. Adjustments can be built into the design standard and sectional patterns through the use of seams or other means. If designers or pattern cutters fail to superimpose their designs onto an accurate base pattern, then badly fitting patterns and uppers are the result.

The full forme of a last has four sides, and within those sides lies the shape and surface area of the last registered as accurately as possible as a flat pattern (Fig. 3.8):

A. The last's forepart centre line: will become the centre line of both patterns and uppers. Ideally it should never be altered for any designs or patterns unless there is no alternative, as this is the line that controls the pitch and spring of the patterns.

B. The feather line of the last. The general shape is important but it may be modified on subsequent patterns to cope with variations in upper thickness and stretch.

C. The back curve of the last. This can be varied slightly depending on the construction, stiffening materials and techniques for construction. The back point is also positioned on this line and its correct location is crucial to the ultimate comfort of the shoe.

D. The top edge of the last. It is unlikely that a design feature would use this line position, therefore it is not important at this stage, but if the designer wants to, it can be introduced later on in the process.

Crucially, one of the basic rules of footwear design is that if the upper design rises above the vamp point, the basic sectional patterns that are to be made should also rise on the same curve and angle. By using

stitched seams to build the shape of line A into the patterns, the resulting upper will produce a good fit. Where the curved line becomes straightened out at some point between the design concept and first patterns, the result will be a series of problems with the fit, fashion and ultimately the profitability of the finished product. This basic rule is not always fully understood and may be ignored by too many shoe makers leading to many poorly-designed uppers that have fitting problems.

No matter whether the pattern-making system is manual or computer-aided design/computer-aided manufacturing (CAD/CAM), base patterns are often distorted, possibly for the convenience of the user, but certainly to the detriment of the factory and ultimately the wearer. However, by understanding the principle behind the pump forme theory, that the vamp point also relates to the quarter or top line of the pump pattern, the designer may place design features correctly onto the base pattern without spoiling the final fit.

The basic features of a court shoe are to allow easy entry and exit for a normal foot without further adjustment. Footwear designed to rise higher up the instep, such as laced Oxford or Derby designs, should include an adjustment and entry/exit commencing on the pump shoe line (Fig. 3.9).

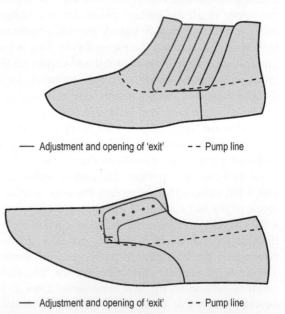

——— Adjustment and opening of 'exit'   – – Pump line

——— Adjustment and opening of 'exit'   – – Pump line

Figure 3.9 Diagram showing relationship between pump forme line and design features. (Reproduced with permission of *World Footwear Publication* 2006.)

For example, in the design of an elastic-sided boot, there is a close relationship between the pump top line and the positioning of the elastic panel, and this must be maintained even if the vamp section has to be deadened or sprung.

The traditional system of footwear production has three components: design and innovation, product development and product engineering. Where communication between the teams responsible for each component is minimal, there is a risk of the original concept losing its character or focus as each team concentrates on its own expertise. It is far better when the designer translates the original concept to the first set of patterns and trial 'pullover'. This ensures the concept of the design is fully understood and realized in terms of line, balance and general design effect. By combining various technical options while designing onto the last, computer screen or flat pattern, the modern designers of today develop improved skills in all areas. This should result in successful designs that work, fit and are economic to produce.

Grading

Once the sample design and pattern have been accepted for bulk production, the patterns need to be graded into the sizes and fittings in which the footwear will be made. Grading involves the enlargement or reduction of the sample base pattern proportionally to make a complete range of sizes to fit the graded last size range. The grading can be done by the CAD system if the CAD process has been used at the design stage. Computer-aided design is faster and more versatile than more traditional methods. The system produces all the size ranges, transfers the outlines onto a special press and will cut out the patterns digitally. This is very accurate and also allows the patterns to be stored digitally, reducing the space which would be needed to store traditionally-cut patterns. Where small quantities of footwear are being produced, the patterns are made from thick board with a brass-bound edge for hand cutting (Fig. 3.10).

Where large quantities are to be produced, steel knives are made to be used with a press. This is much more costly initially, but the knives stand up to constant use and make the whole manufacturing process more economic due to the large quantity being made. More modern factories now use laser cutting or water-jet cutting to speed up the cutting process. With these techniques, many thicknesses of material may be cut at once, thus saving time and reducing labour costs.

Figure 3.10 Pattern grading: a set of traditional patterns. (Reproduced with permission of Spring Line Lasts.)

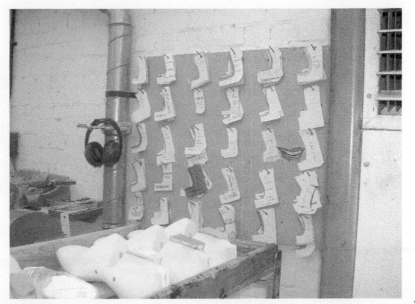

Cutting (clicking)

The term *clicking* arose from the action of the press clicking the knives through the leather with a distinct sound. The majority of uppers are cut by press, although hand cutting is still practised, especially for bespoke items. The 'clickers' are highly skilled workers who need to be very familiar with the properties of the tanned leather hides or other materials they work with. They need to understand how the material stretches in different directions, as this is vital to the lasting process and the wear properties of the finished item. They also need to be economic in how the leather is used, choosing the best part of the leather (the back part of the animal) for the vamp, and cutting it so that its natural stretch characteristics are in the appropriate position within the vamp of the finished shoe. The remainder of the upper material is often cut using a 'lay pattern' which allows for as many sections as possible to be cut from the material, with the different thicknesses being used appropriately for other sections of the uppers (Fig. 3.11).

Closing

The component parts of the shoe uppers need to be combined by sewing or adhering, or both, before going on to be lasted. The sections are each marked up in the positions where they are to be joined, any decoration is added, and any edges that will be folded or have trims will be thinned (skived) to ensure that seams are kept as flat as possible. This is done either by hand with a very sharp knife or on a skiving wheel, which takes a thin layer from the underside of the leather to reduce bulk before stitching the pieces together. The sections are stitched together, and linings attached by hand on a post-type sewing machine. This is a machine with a small base under the needle that allows the leather to be moved in any direction. The vamp and quarters are sewn together and the tongue (if separate), appliqués, caps and collars are added according to the style (Fig. 3.12).

Lasting and making

The prepared uppers are then sent to the lasting area where they are matched up with the correct size last. The toe puffs are glued into the toe area and the upper is pulled over the toe of the last, most often by a lasting machine, which is set to apply the correct pressure, consistently producing a repeatable action. Hand lasting is still practised mainly for bespoke items. It is a skill which requires much practice to perfect and is very much more time consuming than machine lasting (Fig. 3.13).

Figure 3.11 Clicking with hand press and metal knives. (Reproduced with permission of Klaveness Portugal.)

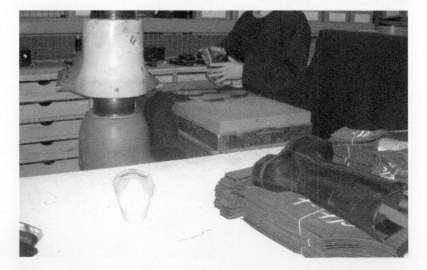

The counters are inserted into the quarters and lasted by a separate back-part machine which either heats or cools the counter material, depending on which type has been selected. This gives the all important grip and heel shape to the quarter. Quality footwear is then 'heat set' in a special chamber to retain the last shape. It moves on a slow-moving belt through the heat setter and at the other end is ready for the final finishing processes (Fig. 3.14).

The footwear is now at the rough fit stage, where a bespoke item will be returned to the prescriber for fitting onto the feet of the person they are intended for. The fitter will note down and also mark the position of any required alterations on the shoe with an effaceable pen. If necessary, the footwear will then be modified on return to the factory. Once the fitting is

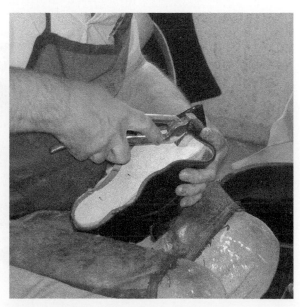

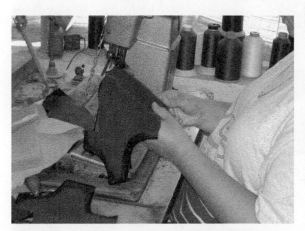

Figure 3.12 Closing on a post sewing machine. (Reproduced with permission of Jane Saunders and Manning Bespoke Shoe Manufacturers.)

Figure 3.13 Hand lasting is a specialized skill. (Reproduced with permission of Jane Saunders and Manning Bespoke Shoe Manufacturers.)

Figure 3.14 Heat-setting machine. (Reproduced with permission of Klaveness Portugal.)

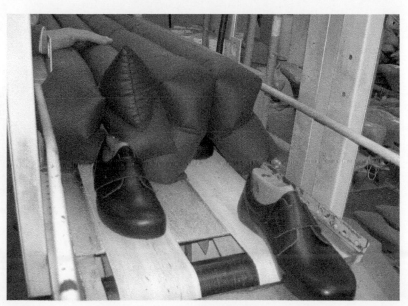

perfect, the shoe will go through the finishing process. Any necessary adjustments must be made at this fitting stage. Once the final soling process has been completed, the footwear cannot be adjusted. At this point, the shoe may go back and forwards more than once in order to check the changes are correct for final finishing.

The finishing process will include thinning down the lasting margin. This is the excess leather of the upper material which has been pulled under the feather edge onto the bottom of the last and fixed to the midsole at the lasting stage of the shoe. This excess leather will be scoured or roughened and adhesive will be applied to it. The bulk of the excess

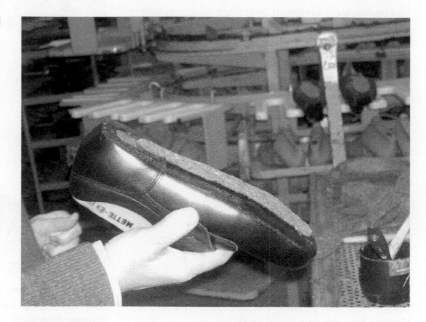

Figure 3.15 Upper leather skived and bottom filler in place ready for sole unit. (Reproduced with permission of Klaveness Portugal.)

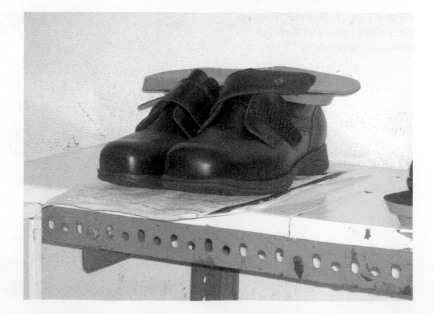

Figure 3.16 Finished footwear ready for final check and despatch. (Reproduced with permission of Klaveness Portugal.)

leather must be reduced in order to fix the sole unit onto a flattened surface. As there is still a slight ridge between the midsole and the skived leather, a bottom filler of cork, cork composite or felt wool padding is usually added at this stage to level the surface and also to give the sole some spring or bounce (Fig. 3.15).

Lasting and upper pattern design is a complex process which requires skill. Many of those skills involved have been traditionally learned, and while modern technology has been introduced to the process, there are circumstances where it fails to meet the craft levels developed by expert last makers and pattern designers (Fig. 3.16).

Acknowledgements

With thanks to the following manufacturers:

Spring Line Precision Last Manufacturers, Spring Line Ltd, Pond Wood Close, Moulton Park, Northampton NN3 6RT, UK; tel: +44 (0)160 464 4961; fax: +44 (0)160 449 5090.

Jane Saunders and Manning Bespoke Shoe Manufacturers, 1070–1072 London Road, Thornton Heath, Surrey CR7 7ND, UK; tel: +44 (0)208 684 2364/2584; fax: +44 (0)208 665 5968.

Klaveness UK, 14 Woodland Avenue, Narborough, Leicester LE19 3FF, UK; tel: +44 (0)116 286 6290; e-mail: klaveness@aol.com.

Reference

World Footwear Publication 2006 You will never achieve a perfect pattern (part 1). World Footwear Publication May/June 20(3):32, 33. (Part 2: September/October 20(5):18–20.)

Footwear components and construction methods

Chapter contents

Shoe anatomy
Footwear materials
The footwear manufacturing process
Conclusion

Footwear manufacture is complex and labour intensive. Despite recent massive strides in technology, the footwear industry still requires much manpower to undertake many of the processes involved in footwear manufacture. This high manpower requirement makes footwear an expensive item, particularly so in orthopaedic footwear when volumes are low and when individual lasts and components are required for patients with unusual foot shapes.

Shoe anatomy

Shoes are constructed from a number of separate pieces of material that are individually cut out and stitched or adhered together. The pieces required to make a shoe include uppers, linings, stiffeners, midsole, outsole and heel components. The number of pieces required for the shoe depends on the style, as some designs, like a trainer, have many more individual pieces than a simple Mary Jane, or court shoe style (Fig. 4.1).

The terminology applied to each area of the shoe is also applied to the corresponding pattern pieces. There are numerous ways in which a shoe can be designed and constructed, but the relevant upper components are still given the same name even if their shape differs because of shoe design.

The vamp

This is the part of the upper covering the front part of the shoe from the toe as far as the quarters. The term *vamp* may also be applied to the material between the toe cap and the quarters, where the shoe design includes a separate toe cap.

The vamp can often consist of a single piece of upper material, but can also be made up of two or more pieces stitched together, for example in the brogue shoe. Men's laced shoes tend to be made in two basic styles, the Oxford (Bal) and the Gibson or Derby (Blucher) (Figs 4.2–4.4).

The Oxford or Bal has a vamp which overlies the base of the quarters. The facings are set to meet exactly and the tongue is cut as an individual pattern piece and is attached separately. In this style, the opening for the foot is restricted due to the way the facings are stitched down.

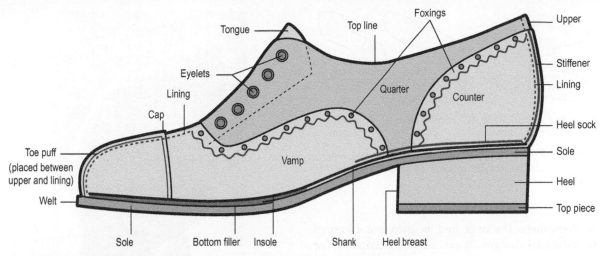

Figure 4.1 A gent's Goodyear welted shoe showing components and positions.

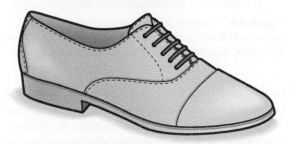

Figure 4.2 Line drawing of traditional Oxford or Bal style.

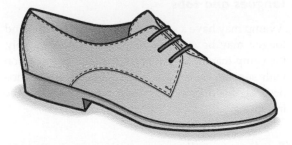

Figure 4.3 Line drawing of a simple Gibson or Derby (Blucher) style.

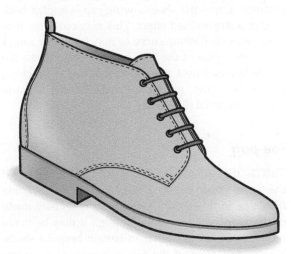

Figure 4.4 Line drawing of basic Derby Boot style.

The Gibson lace and the Derby or Blucher have a quarter which overlies the vamp. The facings are stitched onto the vamp and the number of eyelets included in the fastening determines their alignment on the vamp. The facings can be opened out and the tongue taken back to allow easy entry of the foot into the shoe, thus making this style very versatile.

The tongue may form part of the vamp, being cut in one piece with the vamp, or may be cut separately and then attached to the vamp. The tongue may also be padded. Cushioning material can be included between the tongue upper and its lining for extra comfort.

Toe caps and wing caps

The toe cap is an additional piece of material extending forwards from the vamp to the toe of the shoe. It is attached and placed over the toe stiffener.

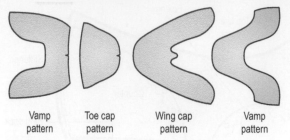

Vamp pattern Toe cap pattern Wing cap pattern Vamp pattern

Figure 4.5 Vamp pattern pieces for toe cap and wing cap. (Reproduced with permission of Rossi & Tennant 1993.)

It strengthens the area and is therefore favoured in industrial designs. It can also be decorative, for example in a brogue shoe.

A conventional toe cap is straight edged and set squarely across the shoe; a wing cap is angled back to give a streamlined effect. This may cover the toes in an intricate flowing curve or may lie simply round the feather edge of the last. In some designs, the toe cap is imitated by a row or double row of stitching across the vamp, giving the illusion of a separate piece of material (Fig. 4.5).

Toe puff

This is the stiffener placed under the toe part of the vamp or toe cap to ensure that the shoe retains its shape in this area. The toe puff is usually made of thermoplastic material, although it may be made of strong blocking leather in certain bespoke shoes. Where protection of the toes is required, for example in industrial safety footwear, the toe puff may be made of metal. Toe puffs in retail footwear usually extend through the vamp to cover the tops (dorsum) of the toes. However, in certain types of therapeutic footwear, rim toe puffs can be requested. These hold up the front of the shoe but do not extend back over the dorsum of the toes. They are particularly useful where patients have toe deformities which might be irritated by a hard stiffener covering them.

Mudguards

These are designed to protect the side wall of the shoe upper and are stitched to it to provide a double layer. Mudguards may be made of leather and may

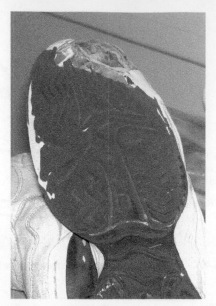

Figure 4.6 Example of ten days' wear on a cheap trainer sole from cerebral palsy-affected gait. (Reproduced with permission of Mile End Hospital Footwear Centre.)

be mistaken for a simple wing cap. They might also be made from a much tougher material such as neolite, if the wear is likely to be excessive, for example in a patient with cerebral palsy who has severe toe drag when walking (Fig. 4.6).

Tongues and tabs

A vamp may have a separate tongue or the vamp and tongue may be cut in a single piece. Alternatively, the vamp may be in two parts, that is, a centre apron with separate side wall pieces, and, in some shoe designs, this may include a separate tab to cover the instep.

Top line or collar

The top of the shoe that surrounds the opening for the foot is called the top line or collar. This may be finished with a simple turned lining, a casing for a lace to pull through or with the addition of a padded collar for comfort and protection. The top fit is important in ensuring that the shoe stays on the foot. Gaping of the top line or twisting or rubbing clearly indicate a functional defect that needs to be corrected if the shoe is to allow the foot to function properly.

Feather edge

The lower extremity where the shoe upper meets the outsole is called the feather edge. When shoe upper patterns are cut, they include an additional margin at the feather edge which provides enough material to permit the upper to be turned under the last and attached to the insole. This is known as the lasting allowance.

Quarters

Most shoes have two quarters and these are the two sections which form the back, outside part of the upper and lay over the instep to close the shoe as facings (Fig. 4.7). The two quarters are known as the outside quarter and the inside quarter. Quarters can also be simple or complicated. In some designs, the facings (where the eyelets of a lace-up shoe are positioned) may be separate pieces. While the basic shoe is normally made up of two quarters joined at the back, it is possible to eliminate this seam and cut the back in one piece. This piece is usually joined at the waist to the vamp or wings but an insertion may be included.

Less common is the division of the quarter into foxings. These foxings enclose the heel and provide an insertion at the waist. This insertion will certainly comprise part of the feather line. For example, foxings and insertions are normal in a brogue Oxford shoe, which has perforations along the various edges as a design feature (see Fig. 4.1).

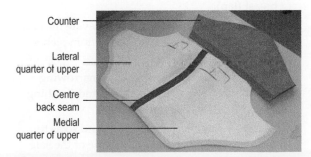

Counter

Lateral quarter of upper

Centre back seam

Medial quarter of upper

Figure 4.7 Quarters and counter stiffener pieces ready to be stitched to vamp. (Reproduced with permission of TayCare Medical Ltd.)

Counters

The counter is a reinforcement placed between the outside and the lining at the back of the quarters to prevent the upper from collapsing and to hold the heel of the foot securely (see Fig. 4.7). Not all shoes have a counter as part of their construction. The absence of counters results in a shoe with a back which is very soft and pliable and which offers no support to control the rear foot. As a consequence, the heel of the foot will often deform the back of counterless shoes.

Appliqués

The parts of the shoe described above are all separate pieces which will be joined together to make a whole component, for example a whole vamp or quarter. Each component performs an individual function essential to the composition of the shoe.

Shoe styles can be varied by using duplicate pattern pieces attached on top of the completed vamp or quarters. These extra pieces, called appliqués, do not perform functions essential to the composition of the shoe but do alter its appearance. They also add strength to the shoe by providing a double layer on the upper, and can be used to cover seams that might be subject to strain in lasting and in wear.

In the retail sector, many seemingly individual parts of the shoe may be found to be appliqués, for example toe caps, foxings and counters. Although more material is used in forming appliqués, this may not increase the cost. It is possible to use the appliqué to disguise or to strengthen inferior leather. The use of appliqués is not normal practice in orthopaedic construction, although appliqués are used especially for strength and protection where hard wear is likely to damage the upper very quickly. By applying either a mudguard or double toe caps, the wear properties can be effectively enhanced.

Saddles and bars

The vamp may have a saddle or bar across it from joint to joint that could have two purposes:

1. To reinforce the shoe, especially at the entry where it takes continual strain from flexing.

2. To cover a seam or gusset. This may be a vamp/quarter seam or could be the seam joining an apron to a tab or tongue.

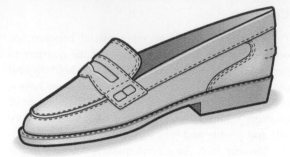

Figure 4.8 Line drawing of a half saddle decoration to vamp. (Reproduced with permission of Rossi & Tennant 1993.)

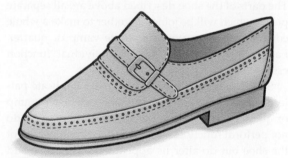

Figure 4.9 Line drawing of a buckle and bar arrangement to a high-vamp shoe. (Reproduced with permission of Rossi & Tennant 1993.)

A bar is usually used to secure the shoe to the foot and is adjustable. It may also be decorative and be used to cover a seam (Figs 4.8 and 4.9).

Heels

Heels are one of the most variable parts of a shoe design. The height and shape of the heel gives the shoe a distinctive style, and heels have been exploited and made the focus of design features throughout history. There are several heel shapes in current common use and they are classified according to how they are positioned in relation to the sole (Rama 1961) (Fig. 4.10):

- Cuban heel: a high heel, either covered with wood or leather, sloping and with an approximately rectangular profile when viewed from either side.
- French heel: a flat, close-seat heel with a slight forward pitch which is very curved in the breast.

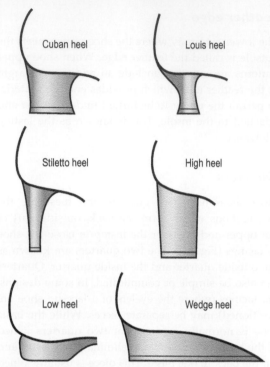

Figure 4.10 Comparison of different heel shapes. (Reproduced with permission of Rossi & Tennant 1993.)

- High heel: a heel which gives considerable elevation to the seat and has an angle between the planes of the seat and the top piece.
- Hour-glass or waisted heel: a heel with a narrow central portion, widening out again towards the base.
- Louis heel: a high, very curved heel in which the breast is covered by an extension of the sole (the breast flap).
- Low heel: a heel which does not elevate the seat very much and has the top and bottom planes more or less parallel.
- Spike or stiletto heel: a Louis heel narrowing considerably towards the bottom and finishing with a very small top piece.
- Wedge heel: a heel extended forward so as to continue without a break in the line of the sole.

Heels can be made of a variety of materials including leather, wood, plastics, cork and rubber. The heels of women's shoes are designed in numerous shapes and heights with added details such as jewel trims, colour contrasting and texture for endless variety. Men's heels on the whole remain a standard shape and height, although changing fashions do bring in more variation, particularly in the heels of boots and casual shoes.

Heel height and heel design are an integral part of last design, and the height and shape of the heel must be determined before the last is engineered and the last prototype developed. Heel height also has a direct relationship with toe spring, and changing the height of a heel will alter the position of the treadline of the shoe and so also change the elevation of the toe of the shoe from the ground. Where shoes are to be made with higher heels, the actual position and pitch of the heel under the shoe must be decided in the first phase of the design stage to ensure that the shoe is properly balanced and has stability. Where a shoe is made with incorrect balance or incorrect pitch, the heel of the shoe may buckle under and break. The way the shoe reacts during wear will change the way in which it grips the heel of the foot and the consequent effect on toe spring will cause the shoe to flex in an incorrect position.

The position and shape of the heel can give the shoe a different style, so a simple pump style upper with a flat heel looks quite different to one with a French heel. The heel can be placed forward, central or set back giving a very different appearance to the profile of the shoe. This heel position should not be confused with the heel pitch. Heel pitch is the slant or angle of the heel under the shoe, which can be used very effectively to create an optical illusion. The greater the slant of the heel, the shorter the shoe will appear to be. Hence high-heeled shoes have such appeal, especially for larger ladies' shoe sizes, as they can flatter and disguise the width or length of the foot (Rossi & Tennant 1993). In wear, the shoe heel position and style also affect the body's centre of gravity. When the heel height is raised, compensatory action is required to prevent the body tilting forward. This requires the knees and the hips to flex, giving a lumbar lordosis, more prominent gluteal area and resulting in an altered gait pattern.

Measuring the height of the heel is a simple yet often misunderstood concept. The reason for measuring the heel height is varied but, in therapeutic terms, is mostly required for adding a raise to treat limb length discrepancy, in the use of callipers of a predetermined length or in the case of a prosthetic limb where it is vital that the heel height is accurate on each pair of shoes worn, as the prosthesis will be made to wear footwear of a specific heel height.

The established way to measure a heel as done by a last maker or heel maker is to measure the breast side of the heel at a point which would be directly beneath the malleolus in wear. The height should *not* be measured through the centre of the heel nor from the very back of the shoe. Frequently the heel height is measured at the back of the heel. This gives an inaccurate measurement as the height at the back of the heel will be higher than the heel breast measurement. The heel breast height measurement is the designated heel height for the shoe design (Fig. 4.11).

Heel tread and associated wear marks are very useful in determining a diagnosis. Normal heel wear is seen at the posterio-lateral aspect of the heel top piece. This reflects the angle at which the calcaneus strikes the ground during gait. A flat or low-heeled shoe with a broad heel shows clearer wear marks than higher heeled shoes with narrower heel bases. In such shoes, for example the high stiletto heeled type, there is a very small surface contact area and wear patterns will not be easily examined because of the size of the area in ground contact. Wear marks placed central to the back of the top piece suggest

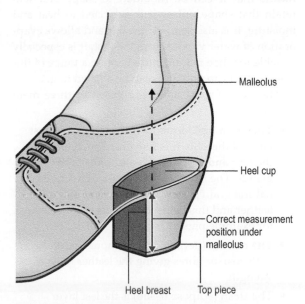

Figure 4.11 Anatomy of the heel and where to measure heel height correctly.

functional foot anomalies and a biomechanical examination might be indicated.

Footwear materials

Upper materials

Footwear uppers can be manufactured from a variety of different materials; some natural, such as leathers, and some synthetic. Most leathers are suitable for shoe making, including the skin of any animal, bird, fish or reptile, although only that from cattle and a few other farm animals are used commercially (Shoe and Allied Trades Research Association (SATRA) 1973). Synthetic alternatives have been invented and are widely incorporated into ladies' fashion footwear, mainly because the cost to produce them is lower than that of natural leather products. Synthetics commonly used include polyurethane coated fabrics, polyvinyl chloride (PVC) coated fabrics and poromerics. Finally, woven fabrics, knitted fabrics and rubber are also used for uppers, linings or trims.

Leathers

Leather is the preserved hide of animals, and is the most effective material for footwear manufacture due to its properties of plasticity and elasticity. This means that it can be moulded to shape and will retain that shape unless it is subjected to heat and moisture. It is also semi-permeable and allows evaporation of water vapour from the foot. It is especially suitable for shoe manufacture because a range of finishes, colours and textures can be applied to it.

The skin of most animals consists of three main layers:

- **The grain** (epidermis) which is the outermost layer of the skin. It is fine fibred and contains the hair and hair follicles and some of the sweat glands. The hair follicles leave a characteristic natural grain pattern on the surface of the leather and this helps identify its original source, for example pigskin, sealskin, calfskin, etc.
- **The corium** (dermis) is the fibrous middle layer with coarser fibres giving the leather most of its strength.
- **The flesh** (adipose tissue) is the last layer found between the corium and the muscle of the animal, and is of little value in the finished

product and is partly or completely removed (SATRA 1973).

The animal skin which is to become leather suitable for footwear needs to be preserved to prevent it from decaying, and this is done by a process called tanning. This process preserves the natural appearance, strength and flexibility of the leather. The preparation for turning skins/pelts into leather involves several processes before tanning can begin. Both the top and undersurfaces need to be cleaned. The hair is then removed by means of a blunt knife or machine. Wool is loosened from sheepskin by hanging the skin in a warm, moist atmosphere where the epidermis will begin to putrefy, facilitating the removal of the wool. Any remaining hairs or wool and epithelial debris are removed from the grain side either by immersing the skin in a solution of lime or brushing a solution of slaked lime and sodium sulphide onto the surface. Fatty substances and tissue left on the flesh side are removed either by hand, with a large two-handled knife, or by machine, which passes the skins under sharp-bladed cylinders. Finally the skins go through a series of cleaning processes before the tanning begins.

Methods of tanning

The two most common methods of tanning are vegetable tanning and mineral or chrome tanning. For special leather finishes, other tanning methods are used. These include:

- Oil: cod liver oil for chamois leather.
- Aldehyde: formaldehyde or similar organic compounds are used to produce soft suede leather.
- Syntans: complex organic chemicals similar in action to vegetable tans, which may be used in conjunction with vegetable or chrome tanning as either a pretreatment or post-treatment.
- Retan or combination tanning: this involves the use of one form of tanning followed by another. Where vegetable tanning is followed by chrome tanning, the process is known as semi-chrome. Where chrome tanning is followed by vegetable tanning, the process is known as chrome retan.

Vegetable tanning involves the use of vegetable extracts mainly from trees and shrubs, such as:

- Trees: chestnut, oak, quebracho
- Shrubs: sumac and gambier

- Fruit/nuts: myrobalans (nuts) and valonia (acorn cups). These are generally used for sole leathers rather than upper leathers.

Mineral or chrome tanning makes use of the salts of chrome, aluminium or zirconium as the main tanning chemicals. The latter two are used for white leather finishes. Finally the leather is dyed or given a surface finish or treatment to improve the appearance, cover any blemishes, produce a special effect, protect the leather and/or improve water resistance. A high percentage of uppers are chrome tanned.

Dyeing following this process is carried out using a large rotating drum in which the skin is immersed until the required penetration of dye is achieved. Additional colour enhancements can be achieved by staining and brushing using a soft-haired brush on open or coarse grained leather or by using a sponge on closer grained leathers. Spray dyeing is another quick and easy method of applying dye and is used to great effect, producing a variety of modern patterns and colours.

Finishes to the leather can be varied to create unique styles. Familiar ones include:

- Patent or wet look: originally the very high gloss was based on linseed oil, but today is applied as a plastic coating of polyvinyl chloride or polyurethane.
- Glazing: leathers that require a high gloss are sometimes glazed. Casein is used as a film-forming agent which is then polished by steel cylinders or hot plating.
- Aniline: a clear aniline dye and wax finish allows the natural colour and grain pattern to show.
- Rub-off: helps to give the leather an antique type finish and is achieved by treating the leather with a light coloured base coat and then adding darker cellulose lacquers on top. The lacquers are selectively rubbed off using a brush and cutting wax. This process can be done once the shoes are made up or before the leather patterns are cut.
- Pearlized, metallic gold and silver finishes and embossing and printing are a few of the treatments that can be applied to the tanned animal skin before it is ready for selling on to the footwear manufacturing trade.

Types of upper leather

Once tanned, many thick skins are split into several thinner sheets of leather. The uppermost split is usually the most durable, while lower-level splits may be used for items such as lining where less strength is required. The types of leather most commonly used in footwear manufacture are:

- **Calf**: skins from young animals which produce high-quality leather which is tanned and sold as whole skins. It has good wearing properties and retains its shape well.
- **Softee**: leather that has been softened during the tanning process and then drummed to break down the fibres to soften it further is known as 'softee' leather. This is very soft to wear but can soon become creased and appear shabby in wear. It is quite often chosen for bespoke shoes.
- **Suede**: this is split from the back of the leather skin and has a raised nap surface. It will not be as strong as full-grain leather because of the splitting process, but makes a pleasant soft shoe that is rather prone to staining easily.
- **Nubuck**: a full-grain leather with top surface lightly buffed during the manufacture resulting in a fine-napped surface. It is an imitation of buckskin (deer hide) which is not so readily available and is very expensive. Nubuck is harder wearing than suede and has similar properties.
- **Waxy**: this is made from side leather taken from larger animals and tanned using a higher proportion of oils to give a waxy appearance and feel. The specification can be customized to produce a variety of differing waxy leathers according to the type of application.
- **Side**: the skins from adult animals that are firmer and tougher than calf which can have endless amounts of surface treatments and colours applied, making it a very popular and versatile material. This leather is not always suitable for orthopaedic footwear unless extra hard-wearing shoes are required.

Therapeutic footwear manufacturers select leathers that are particularly suited to orthopaedic footwear, which combine both wear quality and appearance, and are available in various weights for both men's and ladies' shoes plus heavy-duty work wear. Most manufacturers have swatches available on request to show patients for colour and texture selection.

The permeability of leather means that it cannot be completely waterproof, although most leathers are sufficiently water repellent for normal wear. Water resistance can be improved by special treatments, such as spraying a silicone finish onto the leather, and can be further enhanced by using special construction methods such as Goodyear welt.

Synthetic materials

Synthetic materials are less permeable to water vapour than leather, and tend to return to their original shape after use so cannot adapt or reshape to the foot as leather might. However they are cheaper materials to use as they are man-made and readily available. They are of standard quality throughout, making shoe pattern cutting easier. The availability of leather can be variable. Recent events such as the bovine spongiform encephalopathy (BSE) crisis in the UK caused many cattle carcasses to be completely destroyed, thus reducing the hides available to the leather industry and increasing the cost of leather.

The commonest synthetic materials and their features include:

- **Polyurethane coated fabrics**: these have a synthetic layer applied to a fabric base and can have a similar appearance to leather, are soft, light-weight, comfortable to wear but prone to abrasion damage.

- **Polyvinyl chloride coated fabrics**: made from a solid or cellular layer of PVC onto a fabric base. This is inexpensive, has good abrasion resistance and is impermeable to water vapour.

- **Poromerics**: a class of man-made materials that has been developed specially for the footwear industry. The poromerics have a leather-like appearance and are similar to the firmer leathers like calf and side rather than the softer ones. Poromerics vary considerably in their structure, most having a fairly thick, porous polyurethane surface which is equivalent to the grain layer of leather. Most have a textile base, woven or non-woven, which is impregnated with polymer. Poromerics generally are not as permeable to moisture as leather and can therefore be less comfortable for some wearers. They also do not mould to the foot as leather does, and

this should be considered when fitting shoes, because the shoes must be of adequate size and fit initially as the fit will not improve with wear (SATRA 1973).

Neither synthetic nor fabric materials are normally used in orthopaedic footwear. The exceptions may be some linings or certain types of footwear designed for indoor use, or in cases where the patient has an allergy to leather or chrome. In such cases, synthetics can be invaluable.

Linings

It is usual for a shoe upper to be partly or completely lined. The main functions of lining the shoe are to improve its appearance, to increase comfort where softness or protection is needed and to increase the durability of the footwear. The main materials used for linings are:

- **Leather and shearling** (wool sheepskin). Leather is still frequently used in bespoke footwear for the lining, but in retail footwear, it has mostly been replaced by synthetic materials (except for the most expensive fashion items). Where leather is used, it is generally vegetable tanned calf, kid goat or sheep. In some ladies' expensive, all-leather shoes, the linings may be a chrome tanned or semi-chrome goat, Persian or sheep, or a suede, and may be dyed to a colour which matches the upper.

- **Shearling**. This is used in winter boots and some good quality slippers, but there is also a range of imitation shearlings available which can be used as a substitute in either bespoke or commercial manufacturing.

- **Cotton and rayon fabrics**. These were very common for vamp linings at one time, but have been replaced with foam-backed linings or other synthetic contemporary materials.

- **Contemporary materials**. Many new types of man-made materials are now available, mainly developed for the sports footwear industry. Modern technology has produced high-end wicking textiles that reduce friction, heat and moisture in ways that leather cannot. These include materials such as Gore-tex®, and Sympatex®. Washable, durable and hard-wearing textiles like moleskin are now being offered in bespoke and stock footwear items alongside traditional leather. Research is ongoing into the development of new materials and techniques. Each footwear manufacturer uses different lining materials and each will provide details of their range.

Counter linings

Where heel counter stiffeners are used, they need to be lined. Generally, suede leather or similar material with some nap helps to grip the back of the foot and retain it firmly within the shoe. Reversed leather counter linings are frequently prescribed in semi-bespoke and bespoke footwear because the sueded side of the leather offers a better grip than the smoother grain side.

Quarter and full linings

More expensive retail shoes and most stock and bespoke shoes have a quarter lining that extends to the facings. A full lining also covers the vamp and can be whole cut, reducing the seams within the shoe to an absolute minimum and offering the best protection for vulnerable feet (Fig 4.12).

Backers

In addition to the stiffeners and linings, some styles need reinforcing in certain areas. This is achieved by sticking a fabric 'backer' to the reverse side of the upper under the lining. The throat of an apron-fronted shoe or the facings of a lace-up shoe are examples of positions where a backer might be useful for increasing the durability of the shoe.

Features of uppers in orthopaedic footwear

In orthopaedic manufacture, upper components may be modified to ensure that the shoe or boot meets the prescription requirement, maintains its integrity and wears well. For example, it is often preferable that the vamp is one single piece of leather without seams to ensure that possible irritation to the foot is kept to a minimum. Seams in footwear can be the cause of lesion formation where they occur over a joint or bony prominence. The toe puff may be either in winged form, where it reinforces the front part of the vamp of the shoe and also provides stiffening over the dorsum of the toes, or in the form of a rim, where it stiffens only the front part of the vamp of the shoe and does not provide a hard covering

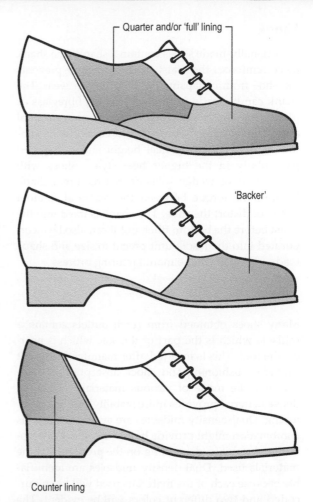

Figure 4.12 Different shoe lining positions. (Reproduced with permission of Society of Shoe Fitters.)

over the tops of the toes. This rim puff is particularly useful for orthopaedic footwear where a patient has toe deformities. The soft leather contained in the vamp may then form a non-irritant covering over the dorsum of the toes. The quarters should contain no seams next to the foot, and the heel counters contained within the quarters may be reinforced or may be extended forward through to the waist of the shoe, either medially, laterally or both, or may be heightened to include stiffening of the area surrounding the ankle and the malleoli. This is particularly useful in boots and where a patient has ankle instability. The shoe lining should also be chosen to be made of a soft material with minimal seams. Each manufacturer will have a range of linings from which to choose, bearing in mind that each patient's needs will be different.

49

Shank

Traditionally-made shoes contain a shank. The shank piece reinforces the waist of the shoe and prevents the shoe from collapsing or distorting in wear. The shank can be made from wood, metal, fibreglass or plastic and consists of a strip of the chosen material approximately 10 cm long and 1.5 cm wide. Its contour is determined by heel height and is required particularly in the higher heel styles. Shoes with lower heels or wedge soles do not require a shank because the torque between the rear and forefoot does not distort the shoe. The shank is fixed into the waist before the bottom filler, but it can also be incorporated into the insole unit precut to size and shape ready to be used in the manufacturing process.

Midsole

Many shoes obtained from retail outlets contain a midsole which is the part of the sole which is nearest the foot. This is inserted after manufacture and it provides cushioning and shock absorption. A midsole may be made of various materials. Heavy or dense material provides more stability, but less cushioning. Dual-density midsoles are available, and this combination might provide both some shock absorption and stability, depending on the properties of the materials used. Dual-density midsoles are identifiable because each of the materials used will be colour-coded and two different colors will be evident. The midsole is usually covered by an inlay with the manufacturer's logo and perhaps sizing detail imprinted on it. Midsoles are not often found in orthopaedic footwear, but it may be useful to consider their properties when advising patients to obtain retail footwear to treat foot pathologies.

The footwear manufacturing process

There are usually five stages in the footwear manufacturing process (Chiropody Review 2007) and these processes are known as clicking, closing, lasting, sole preparation and attachment, and finishing. The first stage in the manufacture of all but the simplest sandal is to make the last. This is the model around which shoes are made. The shoe will take on the exact shape and dimensions of the last on which it

is made. In the case of the volume market for retail footwear and of stock orthopaedic footwear, the last will be standard for each size, width and girth fitting. The manufacturer will have a supply of lasts, each designed for specific shoe styles and shapes, and will reuse them for the manufacture of subsequent pairs of shoes of that particular style, size and fitting.

In the case of modular footwear manufacture, where only a very few changes from the standard shoe size are required, an existing standard last will be taken and modifications added to it to accommodate the footwear prescription received by the footwear manufacturer. A simple example here would be a case of hallux valgus where the addition of a bunion pocket might be required to accommodate the medial eminence on the first metatarsal head of the foot. In order for the shoe to contain this additional pocket, the last will need to be modified so that it provides the exact required shape around which the shoe will be moulded. The modification to the last is usually made by covering it with thin thermoplastic sheet material, such as acrylonitrile butadiene styrene (ABS), which is heated then moulded to fit exactly over the dimensions of the upper part of the last. An addition of material over the area where the bunion pocket will sit is then adhered on top of the ABS shell. All such additions are usually made of cork, and in the case of hallux valgus, would take the form of a dome shape which would exactly represent the depth required in the footwear to accommodate the prominence on the medial aspect of the first metatarsal head. The added cork material is bevelled and machined to exactly match the required shape. The last, complete with its ABS cover containing the added modification, is then used as the base on which the shoe is manufactured. Once the footwear is completed, the ABS mould with the cork modification is removed from the last, labelled and retained separately. The last then goes back into stock for use on other footwear of standard size. When the patient requires a repeat pair of shoes made to the same prescription, the ABS shell is added once more to the same standard last and adhered in place so that another pair of shoes with the same modification can be made.

Many other modifications can be made to lasts in this way, for example extra toe depth for hammered toes or additional girth in the midfoot to accommodate bony prominences, but lasts can never be made smaller. Therefore, when prescribing modifications, it is always necessary to choose a smaller last and to add to it, rather than taking a large last and subtracting from it. More detail on this is contained in Chapter 9.

The last

For bespoke footwear, a last will be made which reflects an appropriate shape for footwear for each of an individual patient's feet. The need to have an individual last made is one of the high costs involved in the manufacture of bespoke footwear. This last will be made either from a special foot scan, from a draft of the foot or from a draft plus an impression of the foot (see Ch. 8). The last may be made entirely manually by skilled craftsmen or by a computer-aided design/computer-aided manufacturing (CAD/CAM) system. The most commonly used CAD/CAM system is that supplied by Shoemaster (www.shoemaster.co.uk). This allows skilled operators to scan the feet and match each foot with the closest existing last contained within the CAD/CAM software library and to modify the last appropriately. More commonly, CAD/CAM technicians will not use the direct foot scanning facility, but will extract data from drafts or from impressions of feet and then use the same system to select and modify existing lasts, and then design a new last based on the modifications. Once the computer-assisted design modification (the CAD element) is complete, a computer-assisted milling machine (the CAM element) will produce the last. The last will be made either of a plastic material or, in rare, special cases, may be made of wood, either of redwood or of hornbeam; woods which are virtually knotless. As knots in wood are of a different density to the remainder of the wood, it is not possible to make smooth, durable lasts from woods which contain natural knots.

Pattern design

The next stage in the process is to design the patterns for the upper of the shoe or boot. The number of pattern pieces required for the upper will depend on the design. The basic shoe upper will contain at least three pattern pieces. A traditional lace-up shoe will usually need pattern pieces for the medial and lateral quarters and for the vamp. However, if the design is more intricate, a larger number of pieces may be required for the vamp or for each quarter. It should

be borne in mind that the simpler the style, the fewer the pieces of upper pattern required and therefore the fewer the seams required within the footwear. Footwear uppers with few seams are usually preferred for people with foot pathologies because seams can irritate foot joints and bony prominences such as those on the dorsum of deformed toes.

In the case of bespoke footwear, individual paper patterns will be made for each upper piece, and those patterns will be placed onto the leather and the upper components cut by hand using a sharp scalpel or knife. CAD/CAM is also available for upper pattern design and to cut upper pieces. CAD/CAM systems can be either linked to last design and can perform the entire pattern design process or can be used to cut out patterns designed in other ways (see Ch. 3).

Clicking and pattern cutting

The actual cutting of upper pattern pieces is known as 'clicking'. In the volume footwear industry, metal cutters will be made for each pattern piece in each size and width fitting. These cutters look almost like pastry cutters but have sharp cutting edges. The process is known as 'clicking' because the cutter is pressed into the upper material using a compressed air, hand-operated press known as a 'clicker'. Where the shoe uppers are made of leather, the cutters are placed with precision on an appropriate part of an animal hide suitable for use in the specific upper section to be cut. This is an extremely skilled task, as to use a hide economically with little waste takes much expertise. The craftsman cutter will use his skill to cut certain parts of the shoe from parts of the skin with specific features. Leather is a natural material and will contain many scars where the animal has injured itself during its lifetime or where it has suffered from skin lesions. These marks in the hide need to be avoided. Similarly, parts of the hide, for example in the belly area, will be thinner than those on other parts, for example the back of the animal. The cutter needs to know which part of the skin is best suited to particular parts of the shoe. Leather is an expensive material and skilled cutters can cut the hide with minimal wastage (Fig. 4.13).

The art of pattern cutting is highly skilled, especially where leather is the chosen upper material. Even when CAD/CAM is used, the cutter may guide

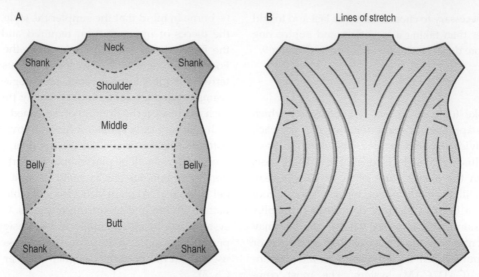

A

Neck

Shank Shank

Shoulder

Middle

Belly Belly

Butt

Shank Shank

B Lines of stretch

Figure 4.13 Areas of a leather skin and the natural stretch directions. (Reproduced with permission of Society of Shoe Fitters.)

Figure 4.14 Hand cutting a set of upper and lining patterns. (Reproduced with permission of County Footwear.)

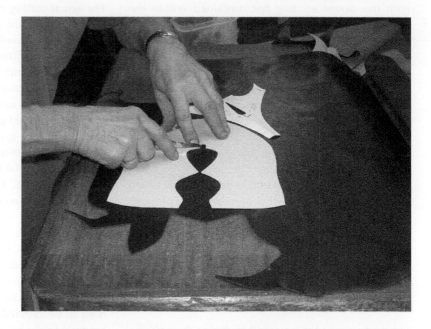

the cutting machine to the best part of the skin for the particular piece of the pattern (Fig. 4.14).

Closing

Each pattern piece is cut with a seam allowance. The size of the seam allowance will vary according to whether the seam is joining upper parts together or is to join the upper to the sole of the shoe. The allowance to join the upper to the sole is much greater and will be about 2.5 cm all around the edge of the upper. Using such a large allowance is helpful in facilitating any later adjustments to the size of the shoe following fitting onto the patient's foot, before the shoe

Figure 4.15 Uppers closed awaiting lasting.

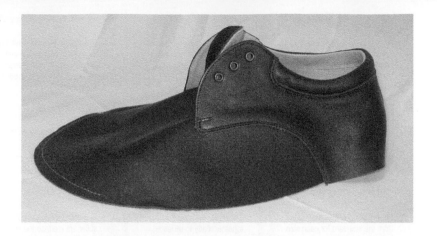

is finished. The edges of the upper pattern pieces to be joined to each other are then thinned down to make a neat seam join and are sewn together. The components to be seamed together are also sometimes reinforced with adhesive before stitching. The shoe upper lining will similarly be cut, using pattern cutters, scalpels or knives, and the lining pieces will be sewn together. The lining will be attached to the shoe upper, and any eyelets, straps or other fastenings will also be added. This stage in the process is known as 'closing' (Fig. 4.15).

The upper preparation to this stage is similar no matter which type of shoe construction process is used. There are many types of construction in use and the method of choice is determined by the shoe style, the amount of flexibility required in the finished shoe and the type of material to be used for the footwear outer sole.

Lasting

The shoe patterns will have been prepared to match the last shape and dimensions (Fig. 4.16) (see Ch. 3 for more details on lasts). The next stage in the manufacturing process involves the attachment of the shoe upper to the last. The shoe will take on the shape of the last using various processes involving the application of heat and moisture. The upper materials must have two properties: those of plasticity (mouldability) and elasticity (the ability to return to the shape achieved in manufacture under normal wear conditions).

No matter the type of construction selected, the first stage in the process is to attach an insole to the undersurface of the chosen last. The insole quality affects the wear and performance of the shoe markedly. During gait, the forepart of the insole needs to be flexible to flex with the foot, but the waist and seat areas need more firmness hence the necessity of the addition of the shank to add this extra strength (see later). The forepart of the insole must have the right degree of softness and flexion but also resist abrasion and cracking, particularly at the flex line. It also needs to be resistant to the damaging effects of sweat.

The types of material used to make insole boards have changed with new technology and with the availability of new materials. Many are composition materials, often made by bonding the fine dust or waste of leathers or synthetics which become recycled in flat sheets that can be precut into various insole shapes.

Bespoke footwear tends to use traditional materials throughout and the insoles frequently used are made from vegetable-tanned belly or shoulder leather. Although these are long lasting, they are also heavy and fairly stiff. Newer materials such as Bontex® are light-weight, durable and cheaper so have the advantage over traditional materials. Leatherboard, a reconstituted material made from scraps of leather fibre bonded with rubber, is used frequently. Leatherboard is similar to leather in both appearance and performance and is used in all types of footwear for through soles or two-part insoles.

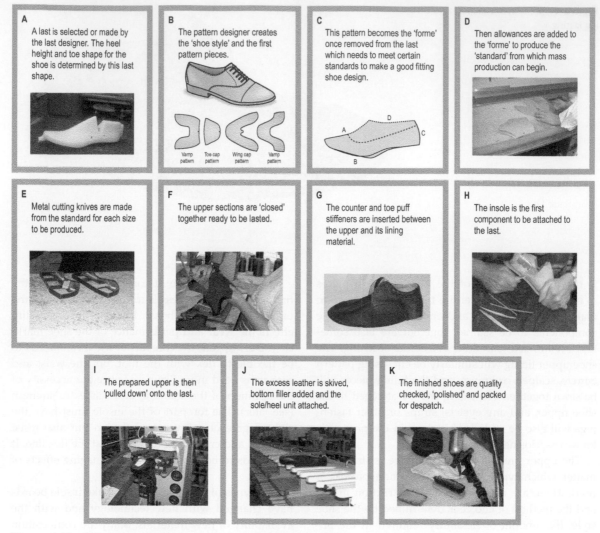

A A last is selected or made by the last designer. The heel height and toe shape for the shoe is determined by this last shape.

B The pattern designer creates the 'shoe style' and the first pattern pieces.

Vamp pattern Toe cap pattern Wing cap pattern Vamp pattern

C This pattern becomes the 'forme' once removed from the last which needs to meet certain standards to make a good fitting shoe design.

D Then allowances are added to the 'forme' to produce the 'standard' from which mass production can begin.

E Metal cutting knives are made from the standard for each size to be produced.

F The upper sections are 'closed' together ready to be lasted.

G The counter and toe puff stiffeners are inserted between the upper and its lining material.

H The insole is the first component to be attached to the last.

I The prepared upper is then 'pulled down' onto the last.

J The excess leather is skived, bottom filler added and the sole/heel unit attached.

K The finished shoes are quality checked, 'polished' and packed for despatch.

Figure 4.16 "Shoe construction laid out as a simplified procedure."

Insole boards have also been made from wood pulp and rubber and a combination of both leather and wood pulp fibres. This mixed board uses lower grade scrap and is used in the cheap casual footwear to reduce production costs.

Insoles are sometimes made from carbon fibre which is highly durable, very light but not flexible, but is very useful in prescription items where protection from movement is necessary. Carbon fibre needs careful shaping to reflect the bottom of the last to create the correct toe spring.

Two main operations follow the attachment of the insole: the first is lasting when the upper sections are shaped to the last and insole; the second is known as bottoming, or sole preparation and attachment where the sole is attached to the upper. Shoe constructions are usually identified by the method of 'bottoming' used (SATRA 1973). The process of bottoming will determine price, quality and performance of the shoe.

There are several methods of shoe construction that affect the overall stiffness of the shoe. To identify which has been used in the manufacture of a particular shoe, remove the insert. You will notice that the shoe is constructed using either a slip last or a board last. In a slip-lasted shoe, the fabric of the shoe is sewn together. There will be stitching running down the middle of the inside of the shoe. In a board-lasted shoe, the bottom of the shoe is covered with leatherboard. Some shoes are combination lasted. In this kind of shoe, the part of the shoe toward the heel is covered with leatherboard and the part toward the toe is stitched. Slip-lasted shoes tend to be more flexible while board-lasted shoes tend to be stiffer. It is possible to use a combination of slip-lasting and board-lasting where, for example, firmness is required in the rear part of the shoe (board lasted) and flexibility in the forepart (slip lasted).

Sole preparation and attachment

This will vary according to the construction method used. The most common construction methods are detailed in the sections that follow.

The cemented or stuck-on construction

The cemented or stuck-on construction is the most popular construction, both in the volume footwear industry and in orthopaedic footwear manufacturing. In this construction process, the upper is prepared and an inner sole for the shoe or boot will also be prepared. This inner sole will match the dimensions of the undersurface of the last and may be made of a variety of materials, the most popular of which is leatherboard (made of reconstituted leather off-cuts and particles). The next stage in the manufacturing process is lasting. The last will have the inner sole accurately positioned and placed against its underside. The stiffening elements for the toe box and for the heel counter will be positioned in place between the upper and its lining. These stiffening elements include the toe puff, which is the stiffener which gives extra strength and firmness to the area of the shoes over the toes, and the heel counters which give strength, shape and form to the back part of the shoe upper which surrounds the heel. The stiffeners are now thermoplastic but were traditionally made of belly leather. Adhesive will be added to the edge of the upper to be placed under the inner sole. These components are pulled tightly around the last and attached to the inner sole by the adhesive. The upper material will become mouldable and will retain the new shape of the last with the application

of heat and moisture. The entire unit will be passed through a machine which subjects it to heat and steam so that it will take on and retain the shape of the last. This particular process speeds up the production considerably, as a hand-made shoe could take up to ten days to dry and attain the shape of the last before being ready for the next stage in the manufacturing process.

Once the footwear has been lasted, the bottom surface of the upper is scoured to reduce the bulk and allow a smooth surface for the outer sole to be attached. The shank (if used) and filler (wool felt or multicork) will be inserted and the outer sole is then attached using a cementing adhesive. For this reason, the construction is known as cemented construction, or stuck-on construction.

This construction is most commonly used for light-weight, flexible footwear and, in particular, for ladies' fashion shoes. Other applications include men's and ladies' walking shoes, casuals and children's shoes.

The stages in the process for cemented construction

1. Upper, lining and inner sole prepared.
2. Cement applied to the lasting edge of the upper and inner sole.
3. Stiffener inserted between the upper and lining, and in the heel area (heel counter).
4. Last inserted and inner sole accurately positioned to feather edge.
5. Shank and filler inserted.
6. Undersurface scoured.
7. Sole attached with cement.
8. Heel attached.
9. Shoe removed from last.
10. Inner sole lining inserted.

This basic procedure is used for most methods of shoe construction (Fig. 4.17).

Bonwelt is a variation on cemented construction with the distinguishing feature being a strip of welting attached by stitching or adhered to the top edge of the insole. The shoe is then flat lasted. This is not a true welt construction (when the welt is attached to the rib of the insole) but gives a similar appearance.

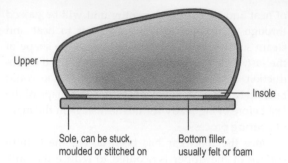

Figure 4.17 Cross-section through vamp of flat-lasted cemented construction.

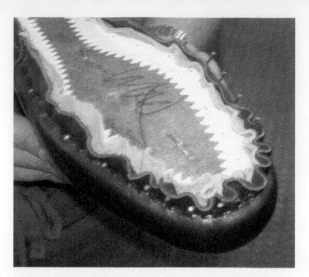

Figure 4.18 Welted construction showing the shoe upper and lining stitched to a walled insole. The welt will also be attached to this walled insole. (Reproduced with permission of Jane Saunders & Manning.)

Welted construction

This is the traditional method of manufacture for well-made, waterproof walking shoes, particularly for men's shoes. The uppers are made in the method described above but a special insole is used which features an upstanding wall. During lasting, the upper and the lining are secured to this wall. A strip of leather known as the *welt* is then sewn in to combine the welt, upper and lining to the wall of the insole. After the welt has been stitched, the sole is stuck to the shoe bottom and lock stitched into place through the welt. This is an indirect attachment, as the sole is not directly attached to the upper.

For high-quality dress and town shoes, the top section (or welt) is chain stitched to the upper and insole rib at the point where it curves under the last. This is supplemented by a lock stitch outer seam bonding the welt and outer sole. The outer sole is then sewn to the welt around the edge. The 'Goodyear' welted construction is a traditional method of manufacture, taking its name from the inventor who mechanized the original hand-sewn method.

The essence of this construction is that the upper is shaped over the last and secured by sewing a strip of leather or 'welt' to the upper and inner sole. The cavity formed by the welt is then filled with a cork compound which is highly flexible and resilient. The process is then completed by attaching a sole to the welt.

Goodyear welt creates heavier, less flexible footwear. The stitched construction allows the shoe to be repaired many times by replacing the sole.

The very nature of this method of shoemaking is lengthy and labour intensive but the resultant shoe is strong and durable (Fig. 4.18).

The stitchdown, flanged or Veldtschoen construction

This construction also features a welt but it is a cheaper method of construction than the traditional welted method. Veldtschoen construction is used to produce light-weight, flexible soled shoes for children and also for some casual adult footwear. Traditional desert boots are also manufactured using this construction.

In Veldtshoen construction, the upper is prepared in the usual way but a special insole known as the runner, which is wider than the base of the last, is used. The upper is flanged (turned outwards) over the edge of this runner rather than being turned under the last. The upper is adhered and stitched to the runner and this stitching becomes a feature of the design. An outer sole is then adhered in place over the runner.

This is the only method where the upper material is flanged during the lasting process and is attached by adhesive to a laminated 'runner' which takes the place of the inner sole. After lasting, the upper and runner are lock stitched together, close to the feather edge. The sole and heel are then stuck to the bottom of the runner.

There may be variations on this construction, such as the 'polyveldt', where a polyurethane sole–heel wedge-shaped unit, which has a sole and heel area which is deeper than the welt, contains the stitching (Fig. 4.19).

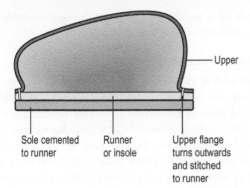

Figure 4.19 — labels: Sole cemented to runner | Runner or insole | Upper flange turns outwards and stitched to runner | Upper

Figure 4.19 Cross-section through vamp of stitch-down construction.

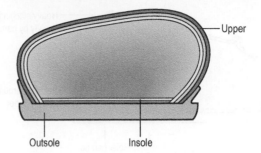

Figure 4.20 — labels: Upper | Outsole | Insole

Figure 4.20 Cross section through vamp of Strobel construction.

Force lasting or Strobel construction

Force lasting has evolved from sport shoes and trainers but is increasingly used in other footwear. The Strobel-stitched method (or sewn-in sock) describes one of many force-lasting techniques. The upper is prepared in the usual way but is then sewn directly to a sock by means of an overlooking machine (Strobel stitcher). The upper stitched to the sock is then pulled or forced onto a last. Premoulded flexible soles with raised walls made of the same material are attached to completely cover the seam. This technique is sometimes known as the Californian process or slip lasting.

The construction gives a flexible light-weight shoe which can accommodate feet of varying widths and proportions because of the way in which the flexible outer sole walls cup the upper. The flexibility of the sole unit also makes the heel-to-ball and toe-to-ball relationship less significant for shoe fitting as the treadline position is also flexible. The soling material used in this construction will have viscosity and elasticity and will provide a high degree of cushioning, thus ameliorating the effect of ground reaction force against the foot. These factors of ease of fit and cushioning capability may be one reason why trainers have become so popular as the footwear of choice among a large number of the population (Fig. 4.20).

Moccasin construction

Thought to be the oldest shoe construction, this consists of a single upper layer section, which covers both the upper and sole of the foot. The upper

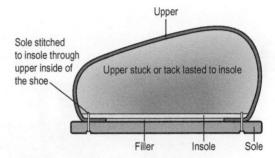

Figure 4.21 — labels: Upper | Sole stitched to insole through upper inside of the shoe | Upper stuck or tack lasted to insole | Filler | Insole | Sole

Figure 4.21 Cross-section through vamp of machine-sewn construction.

piece is placed under the last and extends up and around the last to form the quarters and vamp, and is then joined to an apron top part. This apron is then stitched to the gathered edges of the vamp piece which covers the sole. If required, a sole can be stuck or stitched direct to the upper, though the original moccasin did not have a separate sole. This method is used for flexible fashion footwear, particularly slippers and light-weight casuals. The 'imitation' moccasin version which has become more available has the visual appearance of a moccasin but does not have the wrap-around construction of the genuine moccasin. This version uses less leather by eliminating the wrap, consequently it is much cheaper to produce but has limited wear quality (Fig. 4.21).

Blake sewn is a variation of the moccasin construction. It is a method in which the sole is attached to the upper and insole directly by a single chain-stitched seam. Blake-stitched shoes have an upper, an insole and a sole like a welted shoe, but without the welt. The insole and upper are attached to the last. Then the sole is adhered in place and a single

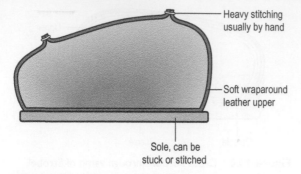

Figure 4.22 Cross-section through vamp of moccasin construction.

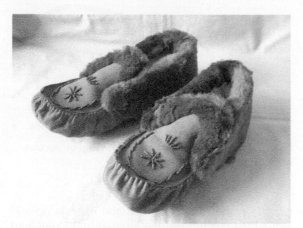

Figure 4.23 Samples of child's moccasins, early twentieth century. (Reproduced with permission of Northampton Museum.)

row of machine stitching is used to stitch through and attach the sole, the insole and the upper. The one advantage of this method is that it can make for a very light, thin-soled shoe. However, Blake-stitched shoes are not as water resistant, as durable or as easily repaired as a welted shoe. If the manufacturer has not covered the insole with a full-length insole cover, you can recognize a Blake-stitched shoe by looking inside it. You will see a single row of stitching around the forepart of the shoe (Figs 4.22 and 4.23).

Blake stitching and moccasin constructions are used primarily by Italian shoemakers. A traditional moccasin is made without an insole. The upper leather wraps all the way around the foot and is sewn by hand to a flat vamp that sits on top of the toes and instep. The sole is then sewn directly to the

upper on a machine. The most famous example of this method is the classic Gucci slip-on.

Moulded construction

In moulded construction, the upper is placed on its last and is then placed into a mould. The sole is formed around the lasted upper by injecting liquid synthetic soling material (PVC, urethane) into the mould. Alternatively, the sole may be vulcanized by using an uncured rubber 'slab' and converting the rubber into a stable compound by heat and pressure.

Whichever process is used, when the material in the mould cools, the sole–upper bonding is complete. These methods combine the upper permanently into the sole and such shoes cannot therefore be repaired easily. Moulded methods can be used to make most types of footwear.

The vulcanizing process is undertaken in the following stages

1. Upper and lining prepared.
2. Inner sole attached to the last.
3. Upper tacked or stuck onto last.
4. Upper processed with heat and steam to adopt the shape of the last.
5. If a shank and filler are to be used, they are attached.
6. Shoe slipped from 'making last' onto special metal last.
7. Rubber blank is placed onto the sole mould in a vulcanizing machine.
8. Applied heat and pressure from the vulcanizing machine melts the rubber blank, which then flows to fill the mould evenly and vulcanizes itself to the bottom of the shoe.

The injection-moulding process follows steps 1–5 as above, but then liquid PVC or polyurethane with a catalyst is poured into a mould which is directly held against the bottom of the shoe to form the sole and heel unit.

Certain footwear may have the appearance of injection moulding but may not have gone through this exact process. Many companies now purchase premade thermoplastic rubber soles and adhere them to prepared and lasted upper units, thus essentially using the cemented construction method but using soling material which has the properties of those available through the moulding process (Fig. 4.24).

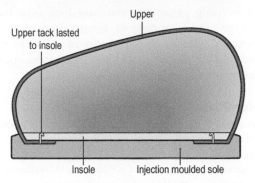

Figure 4.24   Cross-section through vamp of injection-moulded soling.

Turn shoe construction

In this construction, the upper is stitched to the sole in a reversed position and then turned inside out to conceal the stitching. This is the construction used especially in the manufacture of ballet shoes, but also in some cycling and running shoes, and demonstrates the skill and finesse that is possible in producing footwear for specialist use.

In ballet shoe construction, the upper comprises a single piece, seamless vamp and two quarters joined together with a backstrap. The uppers are made using an upper layer of either soft leather or satin, and another two layers of lining which are usually woven cotton material. The pieces of the upper are stitched together and the quarters are joined by a piece of material known as the backstrap. This covers and strengthens the back seam.

A sole is cut from a sheet of leather and contains a groove about 0.25 inch in from the edge. This groove will accommodate the stitching and the bulk of the edge of the upper material. The sole is pinned onto the last and the upper is placed over it. The upper is pleated and stitched to the sole ensuring that it sits within the groove previously cut into the sole.

During construction, the shoe is inside out on the last. It is now removed from the last, turned the right way, fitted with an insole and put back onto the same last. This process is called 'turning', giving rise to the term 'turn shoe'.

Ballet shoes may be made with or without toe blocks, dependent on whether the dancer is performing on pointe. The toe block is usually made of burlap, a dense, fibrous material made of either jute or vegetable fibres. This is impregnated with glue and has to be baked in a special oven at 60°C (140°F) for 14 hours to develop and maintain its hardness (www.pointeshoe.co.uk) (Fig. 4.25).

Pegged, riveted or screwed shoe (e.g. protective safety footwear, Army boot)

The upper is prepared and lasted in the usual way. Strong toe puff stiffeners are inserted into the toe area. These stiffeners may sometimes be metal to provide protection for the toes in situations where crush injuries may be possible. The construction of such rigid soled footwear traditionally involves the use of an inner sole which is attached to a middle sole and then attached to an outer sole. All three soles are then bonded or riveted together (Fig. 4.26).

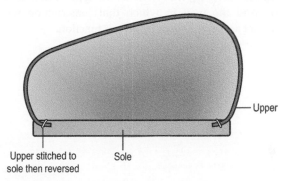

Figure 4.25   Cross-section through vamp of a turn shoe.

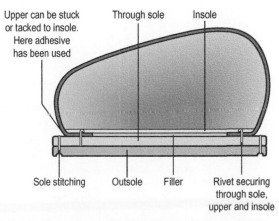

Figure 4.26   Cross-section through vamp of riveted sole.

Footwear such as this may have one of two types of soling material:

- Rubber, which is hard wearing, has good slip resistance and a heat resistance of up to 300°C.
- Polyurethane, which is lighter in weight and has good slip resistance properties and has heat resistance of up to 120°C (Society of Chiropodists and Podiatrists 2007).

Conclusion

Footwear manufacture is a complex, labour-intensive and time-consuming process. When prescribing footwear, it is important to understand the properties of each of the components of the shoe, of the various materials available, as well as the type of construction and the way in which that construction will interact and enhance or limit foot function.

If advising patients to purchase their own footwear, an understanding of construction methods commonly used for certain types of footwear will again provide a basis on which to develop an appropriate therapeutic strategy.

References

Chiropody Review 2007 How shoes are made (technical article). Chiropody Review 64(4):23.

Rama L 1961 Footwear industry technical vocabulary. Paris, Organisation for Economic Cooperation and Development.

Rossi W, Tennant R 1993 Professional shoe fitting. New York, National Shoe Retailers Association, pp 45–46, 72.

Shoe and Allied Trades Research Association (SATRA) 1973 Footwear, construction and materials. Northamptonshire, SATRA.

Shoe and Allied Trades Research Association 1997 How shoes are made. Northamptonshire, SATRA.

Society of Chiropodists and Podiatrists 2007 Workplace footwear. A practical guide for podiatrists looking after working feet. London, Society of Chiropodists and Podiatrists.

Retail footwear

Chapter contents

Retail footwear is a complex area in its own right and it may be surprising to find it included in a specialist text such as this. However a thorough and up-to-date knowledge of technological developments and therapeutic options which become available from such a wide-ranging footwear supply is extremely useful in practice. The market is continually changing, and keeping up with what's new, innovative, useful or even discontinued when advising clients on purchasing their footwear, cannot be emphasized too strongly. A strong knowledge base is essential to the clinician's practice, professionalism and credibility. This chapter examines the concepts of using retail footwear as a therapeutic strategy, the information about footwear which may be obtained from a retail

supplier, the assessment of 'good fit' by examining fitting principles in depth, and discusses taking measurements for footwear and shoe size systems.

The ability to assess accurately the fit of any shoe, be it retail or prescription, is essential as it underpins and provides the basis of a footwear evaluation programme. Without this understanding, practice will be undermined and advice will be meaningless.

Therapeutic applications for retail footwear

A shoe is much more than just a foot covering. It has many roles, of which protection, comfort, fashion, performance in sport and improved foot health are the main elements.

It appears that the majority of people with foot problems will *not* connect this to their footwear, may deny any relationship between their foot health and their footwear (Foster 2006; Rossi & Tennant 1984) and may fail to relate the discomfort they feel when wearing footwear with the actual shoe.

For the majority of patients, retail footwear may be used effectively to improve foot function and foot health. However, practitioners may be reticent about giving advice and guidance to patients about their footwear because of insufficient knowledge and understanding about the basics of shoe fitting and styling.

There is a huge range of footwear outlets throughout most developed countries. A number of them specialize in footwear for particular activities or in size ranges such as extra narrow, extra large, etc. However, when patients require specifics such as these, they may not be aware of what is available. It is therefore important that the practitioner has the information readily available so that the patient may be guided to the source of suitable footwear. The majority of patients are not only willing to purchase the correct type of footwear or fitting recommended, but are also grateful for the advice and guidance. However, this does require that the practitioner is knowledgeable about footwear styling and sizing and is able to approach and advise patients in a manner which is helpful to, rather than being critical of, their previous choice of footwear.

The *Oxford English Dictionary* defines the word 'therapeutic' as: 'Of or pertaining to the treatment of disease'. Footwear can be used to successfully treat the symptoms of diseases which affect the feet and, when appropriately prescribed, footwear should be considered as a therapy. However, most people cannot perceive their own footwear in this way and, perhaps even more significantly, many professionals also fail to appreciate the value of footwear in improving and maintaining foot health.

In conditions such as diabetes or arthritis, where the feet are vulnerable or showing classic signs of damage, footwear will have an important role to play in improving the environment which surrounds the foot. Many practitioners may wish to treat such conditions with orthoses, insoles or inlays, but generally in normal depth retail footwear there will be insufficient accommodation for such devices. Adding extra bulk, in the form of inlays, orthoses or dressings into a shoe that was not designed to accommodate it, will cause pressure elsewhere on the foot, distort the upper and greatly diminish the effectiveness of the orthotic or inlay prescription. Every prescription for orthotics should be derived only after considering the footwear within which they are to be worn. Footwear and orthoses must be considered to be a single therapeutic entity (see Ch. 7).

Assessing the foot for signs of trauma, shape, deformity, depth and limitation in function is part of a foot specialist's professional skills, and it is only a small shift to apply the same criteria to the consideration of footwear. Most practitioners will examine a patient's footwear for signs of abnormal wear, creasing or general fit and suitability. However this is only one part of the equation. Understanding and evaluating the fit and function of the footwear, and identifying the means of addressing any anomalies in a practical and affordable manner and in a way that appeals to the patient, are challenging but achievable, given that all the necessary information is at hand.

There are now many more extra wide and deep fittings available in the retail sector (some now as wide as a prescription option, which until recently was not available to purchase readily). Many manufacturers produce shoes and sandals with extra inlays that may be removed so that prescribed orthotics may fit adequately. There are also styles that allow for better foot protection, better entry for wide bunion joints or with additional depth to accommodate clawed toes. Other common pathological features may also readily be accommodated within retail footwear, and shoes that are specifically designed for accommodating oedema, such as those with stretch vamps and larger heel seat width, may be easily found. Also helpful for patients who have difficulty in bending or using their hands, shoes with Velcro® fastening instead of laces are readily available. Other features include shoes with built-in rocker soles and shoes with ready-made orthotics.

There are numerous sports designs for the active person to choose from. The investment into sports footwear by large brands is quite staggering, and as more research is undertaken, new materials, designs and technology make for a large range of footwear choices. Much of the development is aimed at the professional sports player, but the general public also benefits from the investment as brands make their latest developments available across the market segments. By comparison, the retail footwear industry has been slow to research and undertake technological developments. Coupled with this, the demand for sports footwear has increased dramatically and it is interesting to see how the popularity of the styling has become a fashion trend.

It is important that those who offer footwear advice should be familiar with the entire spectrum of retail footwear. There may well be very many more options on the retail shelf, via mail order or the Internet than may be initially recognized, but the practitioner should be aware of them and should be able to use them as they form a very useful adjunctive treatment.

Retail footwear outlets and suppliers

Local directories, Internet searches and local shop research are helpful in identifying sources of retail footwear with specific features. Most large department stores will have a footwear section and specialist retailers such as sports shops will carry a wide range of running/walking shoes and boots. It is helpful for the practitioner to visit personally and discover what choices each store offers to the public. However, it is useful to frame some fundamental questions in order to make a clear comparison between suppliers and to build up a useful list of local footwear sources. The following points are important to consider:

- Brands: does the supplier carry more than just one brand? It may be that independent retailers carry a very small range from a variety of manufacturers, whereas a 'named brand' shop will have a comprehensive selection of their styles, colours and sizes.
- Size range stocked: does the outlet stock the average size range or do they cater for extra small and/or larger ladies'/men's ranges (i.e. ladies' sizes 2, 3, 8–10; and men's sizes 5–7, 12–15)?
- Does the outlet stock half sizes or are only whole sizes available?
- What range of fittings is available: wide or extra wide D, E, EE, EEE, etc.; narrow AA, A or B? (Shoe suppliers in the USA carry a much wider range of width fittings than their counterparts in the UK: see Table 5.2, p. 82.)
- What types of shoes are stocked: does the range focus solely on current fashion or does the outlet also stock leisure shoes, sports, smart wear, work/safety or a combination of all types?
- Gender and age specific: does the retailer supply only ladies' shoes, only children's shoes or do they cater for all ages and genders?
- Measuring and fitting service: is this available for children only, or is the service also available for adults?

- Are the fitters professionally trained? For example, in the UK, there is a professional qualification leading to Membership of the Society of Shoe Fitters (MSSF). In the USA, the National Shoe Retailers Association (NSRA) is recognized in shoe retailing, and the Pedorthic Footwear Association (PFA) offers more specialized fitting. Outlets will display the logo of the association to which they are affiliated. The associations themselves also have Web sites and lists of members which can be easily accessed (see p. 84).
- Special order service: will the retailer place an order for a colour or size for a customer, without additional charge and without an obligation to purchase?
- Odd size service: will the retailer help by supplying a pair of shoes with right and left of different size without the necessity of buying one pair in each size. If the retailer requires that two pairs are purchased, is there a willingness to offer them at a discounted price?
- Home visiting: is a home visiting service available for house-bound people locally. If so, does this service incur an extra charge and an obligation to buy?
- Returns policy: does the retailer display the returns policy in the store, and advise as to what is appropriate for returns? It may be necessary for the patient to use a store which will exchange unworn footwear in cases where the clinician needs to examine it for fit and suitability. This may be necessary for footwear which needs to be raised to accommodate a limb length discrepancy or needs to accommodate orthotics. If the patient purchases footwear which proves to be unsuitable for purposes such as these, will the retailer exchange the footwear or refund the purchase price?

It is useful to keep a list of stores which meet the specific needs identified by the healthcare professional for a range of patients. Ideally, the practitioner might visit stores at quiet times and meet the manager or proprietor to discuss the professional interest in their business. It is useful to forge a link with the retailer who may then correctly interpret the footwear prescription needs of the patient. Cooperation from the shop staff is essential to support patients who are prepared to go out and buy new shoes as part of their foot treatment. Time taken by the foot health professional in discussing with retail staff the features required in footwear is time well spent. This relationship works conversely too, as shoe fitters quite frequently come across severe foot problems and can, if asked, recommend a local foot health practitioner.

Having completed a local search of footwear suppliers within a reasonable travelling distance for patients, it is useful to prepare a list of suppliers' addresses and telephone numbers and to identify the type of footwear that each specializes in. The large majority of patients will require footwear advice as part of their treatment strategy. A footwear evaluation should become part of the comprehensive foot health assessment undertaken at the initial consultation and at regular intervals thereafter. A list of suppliers of footwear appropriate for their needs is a useful resource to provide for patients.

Mail order and Internet purchases

There is an increasing number of mail order and Internet sites selling footwear. The obvious advantage is the convenience of shopping from home or office, well outside normal store opening hours. It is also useful for patients to try the shoes over a longer time period than they would be able to do in store. The disadvantages are that purchasers have to make an estimation of their size and fitting, they cannot see the true colour or overall shape from illustrations, and they also need to be prepared to return the shoes if they are ultimately unsuitable. When researching mail order suppliers, it is worth checking the following points:

- Are the shoes only available by mail order or are there outlets where the footwear can be tried? Some manufacturers have factory outlet stores or may have special sale days when shoes may be tried. They may have a catalogue available in addition to the information on their Web site.
- Is the cost of postage and packing included or extra?
- What is the company's returns policy: is there a time limit; is there a fee payable to return the footwear for exchange? Some companies charge a handling fee.
- The delivery time scale is important and needs to be identified.
- It is also worth identifying the cost of phone calls to the mail order supplier. Some may be high while others may charge local rates or may even be free of charge.
- Some companies offer advice to the customer about size and fittings to enable the best choice of size with first time orders. Some offer a size template to help with accuracy.
- There may also be a choice of payment options, but it is worth evaluating whether these are secure.

It is useful for the practitioner to have collected a variety of mail order catalogues, and to prepare a comparison of choice, variety, price, fittings, etc. Additionally, many suppliers will send out single samples for examination of quality of materials, construction and overall style features. This is useful as a demonstration aid to patients.

Shoes available via the Internet are often from international suppliers, and many sources are overseas. The source of footwear will determine the size system used. The US size system is different to both the English size system and the Continental system (see p. 81). Unless the practitioner can easily convert the size from one system to another, this size variation may cause difficulties when buying shoes on the Internet and could result in expensive return costs. However, the advantages of accessing the specialist suppliers, such as those with very narrow fittings or extra larger sizes which can be difficult to find in retail outlets, may outweigh the initial difficulty, always providing that a clear idea of size or conversion can be established. Once the customer has found their ideal size and fitting, future purchases are then easily made.

As with obtaining the mail order catalogues for reference, it is useful to be familiar with Internet sources, discovering the choice and variety available and preparing a list of the best sites to pass on to patients. Such searches need to be updated regularly as new Internet suppliers become available virtually every week. Some Internet suppliers will also send out samples which are useful for clinical reference.

Principles of shoe fitting

A full understanding of the principles of shoe fitting is essential so that the clinician may offer clear and confident advice or guidance about choosing suitable footwear styles, heel height, shape and retaining mechanisms (fastenings).

Examining the patient's existing footwear by looking at creases and wear marks will tell much about foot function, and the choice of style will say quite a lot about the patient's ability to choose suitable footwear. This section examines all the principles of shoe fitting in depth, taking each fitting point and examining its contribution to the overall shoe fit. These fitting principles can be applied to check worn footwear as well as in fitting new retail or prescription items.

Overall length

The overall length of the shoe, boot or sandal is measured from the back of the heel to the longest toe (which may be either the first, second or third toe). This is subdivided into two specific length features: the heel-to-ball measurement and the ball-to-toe length. Beginning with the overall length, the fitter must check that the shoe is long enough to accommodate all the toes and not assume that the first toe (hallux) is the longest. There also needs to be additional space to allow for the elongation which takes place when the foot is loaded with body weight during the stance phase of the gait cycle.

There is no fixed rule for the amount of space required at the end of the toe box, but generally 1 cm (0.5 inch) (Alpert et al 1998) is considered sufficient. The amount of space available within a shoe can vary with styling and can be affected by the shape and taper of the shoe. This may add extra length to the style and is effectively 'unused' space. Styles that have a very pointed toe come into this category. The length of the lesser toes should also be checked, as these also need extension room and are often compromised in the very pointed toe shaped footwear which may be fashionable. Where prescription/therapeutic footwear has been fitted, there should certainly be adequate toe width (length and width of the lesser toes) whatever the foot profile presented, because the prescription often has to accommodate a misshapen foot comfortably in the shoe.

In general, the lower the heel height, the more toe extension space is required as the foot tends to move through the full range of tri-planar motion. Normal pronation may be inhibited when the heel is raised. This includes dorsiflexion, abduction and eversion. If the dorsiflexion is reduced because of an elevated heel height, when it takes place from a more plantarflexed position, then the other components of tri-planar pronation are also reduced and foot elongation is inhibited. Shoe styles that have low heels, such as laced walking shoes or moccasins, will need to contain slightly more extension room for the foot as they allow the foot to move through its full range of movement (Rossi & Tennant 1984). Conversely, the higher the heel height, the less space is required as the foot barely extends, as pronatory motion is inhibited. In these styles, the vamp is cut in such a way that no creases form due to the lack of extension movement of the foot. Therefore, styles such as high-heeled court shoes are very popular as the neat vamp reduces the visual length of the foot, making it appear smaller. In addition, the shape and the appearance of this style of shoe is retained for longer.

Another feature which will affect foot elongation is ligamentous laxity and hypermobility. A foot which is hypermobile contained within a flat shoe may require a half size added to the length for full extension, to reduce damage to the foot – including deformation of the toes, the development of callous and nail trauma.

Children's shoes require specific growth room and that allowance should be made when measuring the correct size. Most children's shoe sizes include extra length for growth within the size measured on the gauge designed for that specific brand of footwear (see Ch. 6).

Heel-to-ball length and flex angle

The heel-to-ball length is the first subdivision of the overall length measurement and is significant in successful shoe fitting. The joint at the base of the hallux (first metatarsal joint or ball joint) must fit to the widest part of the shoe where the shoe is designed to flex across the metatarsal heads from 1–5; sometimes called the 'ball pocket' (Alpert et al 1998). Correct positioning will ensure that the foot and shoe bend together. The fitter needs to be proficient at determining the exact position of the ball joint inside the shoe by feeling where the metatarso-phalangeal joint flexes and also by feeling for the position of the fifth metatarsal head across the flex line of the shoe (Figs 5.1 and 5.2).

The shoe (and last) have been designed to flex on a precise angle across the ball joints (first–fifth metatarsals). The flexion angle within the shoe should match the angle between the first and fifth metatarsal heads of the foot. This is essential to allow the shoe to function correctly from its tread line. It is also essential for the comfort of the wearer. If the ball joint position is too far forward, the shoe flexes further forward than it should and the toes are crowded into the toe box. When too far back, the result is again that the tread is misplaced, often at a point where the shoe cannot flex at all. This causes excessive vamp creasing and discomfort in the foot. On full weight-bearing, the ball of the foot should be positioned in the widest part of the outer sole; at the point immediately distal to the narrowing of the insole into the waist and shank area of the shoe (Fig. 5.3).

Both the first and fifth metatarsals need to be positioned exactly so that the foot and shoe work in harmony together. Where this is either too far forward or too far back, the shoe may appear to fit overall but it will never be comfortable, often causing a tiredness when wearing the shoe that is often unexplained because the shoe seems to be long enough in overall length. Where the angle of flexion is unusual, for example in the case of a short fifth ray, or is compromised, for example where a joint is fixed such as in hallux rigidus, noticeable diagonal creases form across the vamp of the shoe (Fig. 5.4).

The skill of assessment of heel-to-ball length cannot be emphasized too strongly. It is absolutely essential in determining the good fit of a shoe. If a shoe does not correctly fit both overall length and heel-to-ball length, then the fitter should seek to find a shoe made on a last design which better matches the anatomical features and flexion points of the foot.

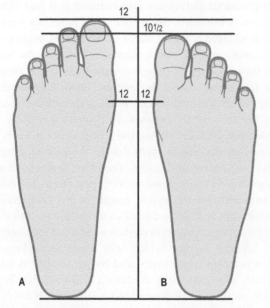

Figure 5.1 Different overall length feet but same heel-to-ball measurement. (Reproduced with permission of Rossi & Tennant 1984.)

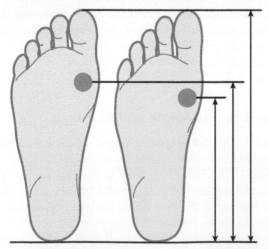

Figure 5.2 Same overall length feet but different heel-to-ball measurement. (Reproduced with permission of Rossi & Tennant 1984.)

Ball joint-to-toe length

The ball joint-to-toe length is variable in every foot, therefore the fitter must not assume that if the heel-to-ball length is correct that the toe length is automatically correct. The lengths of toes also vary. They can be short and stubby, average or very long and thin. Where overall length of the toes is either very short or long, it is helpful to try different lasts to achieve the best fit (Figs 5.5–5.8).

In time, the skilled observation of foot shapes will enable the practitioner to determine which feet are easily fitted and those that need specialist lasts. Several common foot pathologies, such as hallux valgus and hallux rigidus, can sometimes partly be

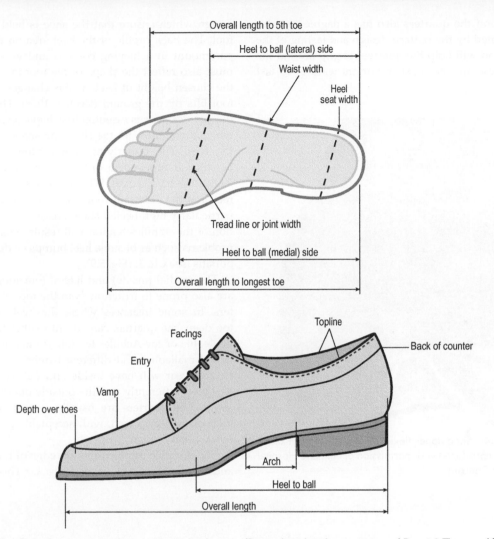

Figure 5.3 Shoe fitting points: plantar view and side view. (Reproduced with permission of Rossi & Tennant 1984.)

the result of a disproportional foot which does not fit the average last proportions. Badly fitting footwear worn over a number of years can lead to trauma to the first metatarso-phalangeal joint.

Having satisfied the first fitting points of over-all length and heel-to-ball length, the next check is that the toe length is satisfactory, allowing sufficient extension space to *all* the toes.

Heel and seat fit

The fit of the back quarters, top line and heel seat influences not only the fit of the heel, but the fit of

the entire shoe, partly because the foot will function differently within a high-heeled shoe to the way in which it will pronate within a low-heeled shoe. This is partly due to the last proportions of the heel area and partly due to the style of the shoe. Ultimately, the aim is to achieve a snug fit around the heel. However, in low-heeled styles, there should be an allowance for the slight movement required by foot pronation (Alpert et al 1998).

When a last is designed, it is thinned down in the region which corresponds to the infra-malleoli area of the foot. This reduction on the last helps to wedge the shoe counter onto the rear foot. The top line around the quarters also has a degree of tightness created by the pattern design and lasting of the upper, and will help the quarters to grip around the heel. These are the most important features in last

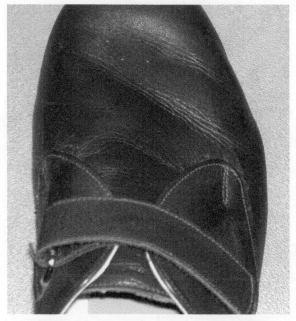

Figure 5.4 Shoe upper flexion crease caused by hallux rigidus. (Reproduced with permission of Mile End Hospital Footwear Centre.)

design which ensure that the shoe is held onto the foot. The back profile of the heel area on the last is paramount in achieving comfort and good grip. It must also reflect the shape of the foot in relation to the chosen height of heel, as this changes when the foot lifts off the ground (Ceeney 1958). The skill of the last designer is essential to achieve a shoe shape which accommodates the changing shape of a walking foot. The underlying foot anatomy needs to be fully understood in order to achieve this shape (called the back curve). Where this design is not correct, and the fitter fails to identify this when fitting a particularly high-heeled shoe, pressure on the insertion of the Achilles tendon will result, often causing problems such as blisters, heel bumps or deep tissue bursitis (see Ch. 3) (Fig. 5.9).

The medial (inside) and lateral (outside) malleoli are also prone to irritation from the top of the quarters. In some instances where the heel counter is too deep, the quarters can cut into either the lateral malleolus or the Achilles tendon. As the medial and lateral malleoli are at different heights, better quality footwear will have inside and outside quarters designed differently and the outside quarter will be lower. The quarters are usually curved under the malleoli and grip well, with acceptable pressure on the Achilles tendon.

The distance between the top edge of the counter and the heel seat is known as the *pocket*. This is where

Figure 5.5 Three right feet, each size 5 in length but different width fittings. Each suits a different style. (Reproduced with permission of Hotter Shoes.)

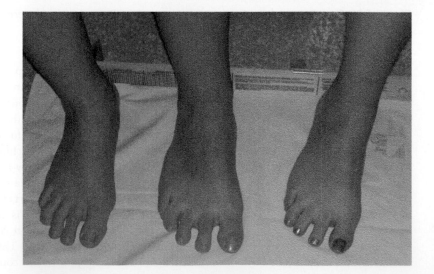

Figure 5.6 Narrow width foot suits a Mary Jane style. (Reproduced with permission of Hotter Shoes.)

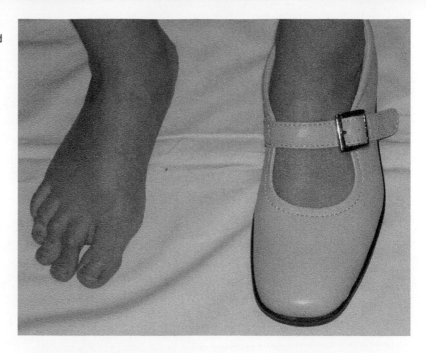

Figure 5.7 Medium width foot suits Velcro® fastening style. (Reproduced with permission of Hotter Shoes.)

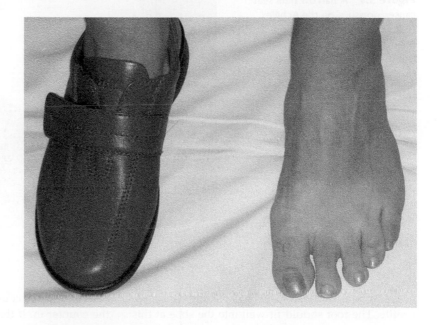

the heel of the foot locates. The measurements in this area are precise on the last and will vary in accordance with the external heel height, style and size of the shoe. However, if they are not always followed carefully by the manufacturer in the actual making up of the pattern, a faulty back part can result. This can cause heel slippage or excess pressure at the back of the foot (Rossi & Tennant 1984) (see Ch. 12).

The heel of the foot is a very complex shape, and the 'seat' or width of the plantar surface of the heel

Figure 5.8 Wide foot suits a lace style best. (Reproduced with permission of Hotter Shoes.)

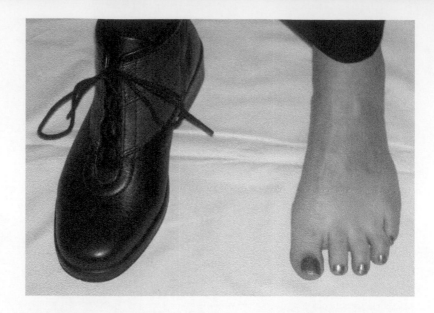

Figure 5.9 A narrow heel seat causes pressure on the Achilles tendon as the foot forces the counter outwards at the seat and in at the back of the top line. (Reproduced with permission of Mile End Hospital Footwear Centre.)

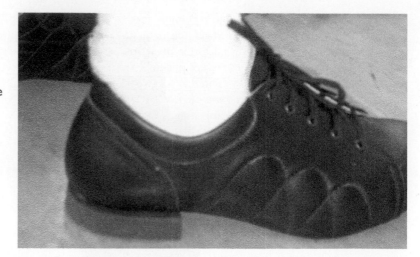

needs to be considered as well as the retro-calcaneal profile. The foot should fit well into the shoe at this point, across the width of the heel seat (see Fig. 5.3).

Where the seat is too narrow, the flesh may bulge up over the counter and it will feel very tight, but the shoe may also be too short or too narrow. Conversely, if the heel fit is too loose, the shoe may be too long or too wide, and where it is too wide in the seat, the shoe is likely to slip off the foot. By palpating the foot around the counter, it may be possible to pinch the counter in. If this is a noticeable amount, it suggests that the seat is too wide. Alternatively, by gripping the back of the shoe and gently pulling it down, the ease with which it slips off the foot indicates how loose the seat may be. If the shoe has a removable inlay, it is very helpful to place the heel of the foot on it and observe if there is a gap around the foot or if the foot overhangs the sides of the inlay (Fig. 5.10).

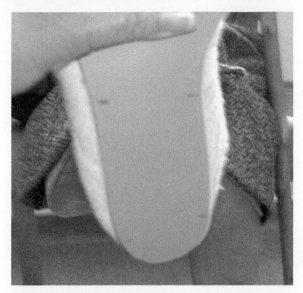

Figure 5.10 Inlay from narrow heel shoe demonstrates seat width required. (Reproduced with permission of Mile End Hospital Footwear Centre.)

The consequences of poor heel seat width can be significant. Where it is too narrow, for example, the flesh will force the quarters away from the stiffener, exposing the hard ridge of the heel seat. The skin will be irritated by this ridge and eventually form a protective layer of callous. This callous can often become very hard and painful and can damage hosiery. The longer this situation continues, the worse the lesions become.

Another commonly seen problem is the formation of heel bumps. These can be caused when the back top line of the shoe grips into the flesh too firmly, causing irritation which may initially cause blistering but over time will cause damage to deeper tissue, resulting in fibrosis, bursae and heel bumps. To avoid discomfort and rubbing, the patient's future choice of footwear is likely to focus on the comfort obtained from backless shoes, or from footwear with very soft unstructured counters.

In the high-heeled, slip-on styles, the heel seat is usually narrow in order to help grip the foot. Where the wearer has a thick-set ankle, or is overweight, the width of the heel of the foot will gradually break down the counter, affecting the fit of the shoe and spoiling its appearance. This will have an effect on gait and the patient will be unstable, particularly where the heel and top piece are very narrow. This

can be the cause of falls or trips, particularly in the elderly (Ceeney 1958).

In so many instances, the wearer will declare that a lower heel height cannot be worn, however it is perfectly possible to improve stability by changing the shape of the heel, if not the height. By changing a narrow or tapered heel shape to a block shape, it is possible to increase the surface area by more than twice the amount, improving ground surface contact and stability easily, without insisting on a flat shoe, which in many cases would not be tolerated after a lifetime of wearing heels (Fig. 5.11).

Where the heel seat is too wide, the shoe is not held securely onto the foot and will slip up and down with every step. This leads to possible irritation of the skin and blisters which eventually harden up; also the wearer can 'slop about', scuffing the heels along the ground rather than picking the foot and shoe up properly. In addition, there will be a tendency to claw the toes excessively in an effort to grip and keep the shoe on the foot. This toe clawing may become a permanent deformity and can lead to other possible long-term foot disorders (Ceeney 1958).

The construction of the back quarters will also affect how the shoe fits to the heel of the foot. Many retail shoe designs have removed the counter stiffener, creating a very soft flexible back to the shoe. This is often found in the cheaper imports, but is also quite common in footwear sold in the high street chain stores.

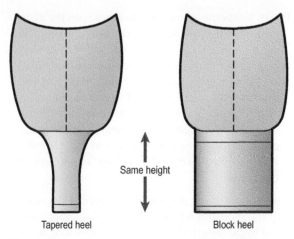

Tapered heel   Same height   Block heel

Figure 5.11 Heels are the same height but different shapes. This demonstrates an increase in ground surface area with a broader heel shape and, therefore, greater stability in walking.

71

The absence of the counter makes the quarters soft and helps the comfort factor, but in consequence there is a lack of control around the heel of the foot. The soft-backed shoe cannot be held onto the foot as securely as one which is well constructed with firm heel counters.

The same problem occurs in sandals with back straps, and when these are worn for long periods of time, the wearer may become intolerant of a shoe with a normal counter which may then feel too stiff or too hard. Firm heel counters are helpful in controlling heel motion and help to reduce calcaneal eversion and medial tilt. Wearing footwear without these counters can allow certain foot types to pronate excessively and can lead to inversion sprains at the ankle. Optimal foot function is assisted by wearing footwear with firm heel counters, and patients should be advised to ensure that their shoes have firm support in this area.

Instep, waist and arch fit

It is helpful to first define these terms, as some confusion may arise with terminology.

Instep: refers to the *foot* within the shoe and encompasses the whole girth of the foot around the 'arch' and onto the dorsum. The natural shape of the foot affects this area considerably in shoe fitting, particularly in cases such as pes cavus, pes planus or in conditions such as Charcot-Marie-Tooth disease and in fixed valgus deformity.

Waist: this is the area of the shoe between the distal portion of the heel seat and the area immediately behind the ball flex point. It is affected by the heel height, and in most well-made footwear is supported by a shank placed between the insole and the outer sole construction. It has both medial and lateral edges that need to be the correct width to support the weight-bearing surfaces of the foot, particularly on the lateral side. The waist is influenced by the width of the heel seat and is proportional to it.

Arch fit: this is the inner undercut area of the waist of the shoe and refers to the fit of the upper material to the longitudinal arch of the foot as it sits in the shoe (Fig. 5.12).

These three areas are interdependent, and an understanding of how to check the fit of the shoe in these

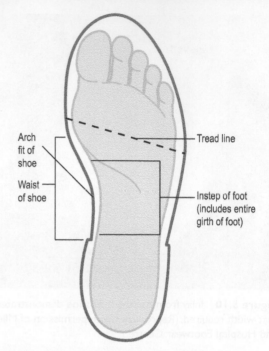

Figure 5.12 Relationship between instep of foot and waist of shoe. (Modified with permission of Rossi & Tennant 1984.)

areas, and when to alter the last selection is vital in fitting all styles, but especially so in certain types of footwear such as boots, high-vamp styles without a fastening and loafers.

The aim is that the foot should fill the volume of the footwear correctly so that there are neither wrinkles, nor torsion creases in the leather of the footwear at the arch or along the lateral side of the quarter. Too much room here will make the fastening ineffective in holding the foot in its correct position; too little can cause compression on the dorsum leading to circulation problems. In boot styles where there is no fastening, the instep fit is vital to comfort and for retaining the foot in the correct internal position within the boot.

The upper material should 'hug' the instep of the foot as snugly as possible when the shoe is correctly fastened. The length of the waist should be the same as the instep of the foot. Where this is not so, it is likely that the heel-to-ball fitting is incorrect. This is another way of checking that essential heel-to-ball fit (Alpert et al 1998).

The height of the instep should correspond to the arch fit and not distort it, and the waist should support the outside/lateral surface of the foot along

Figure 5.13 A high-arched foot and facings that are too far apart cause poor fitting of the shoe. (Reproduced with permission of Prince Philip Hospital, Llanelli.)

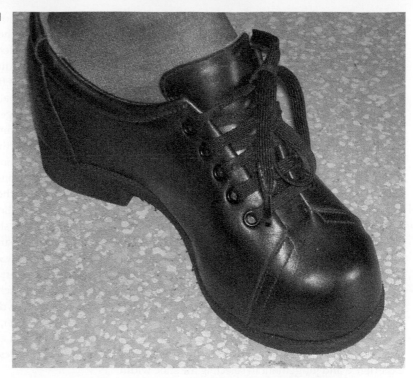

the fifth metatarsal. The lateral side of the foot should not overhang this edge, nor push the upper out over the outer sole. If it does, then the waist is too narrow and probably the heel seat also, therefore a change to a last of wider rear foot proportions is necessary.

Low instep

Feet with a very low instep or which are hypermobile can cause quite a lot of stress on the shoe arch fit. The use of orthoses to control and support such feet may serve a dual purpose of helping to improve shoe fit and foot function. Trying a selection of shoes made on different lasts will be the best way of obtaining optimal shoe fit, and an adaptation to footwear such as a long inside counter or medial extended heel may also be very useful.

High instep

Shoe fit may also be compromised in feet which are highly arched. In such cases, the foot may not contact the waist of the shoe, the length of the longitudinal arch may be incorrect or the volume may be

insufficient. This will be evident as the facings will fail to meet properly across the fastening of the shoe and will be pulled too far apart (Fig. 5.13).

Generally, the fastening of a shoe will allow a certain amount of latitude in accommodating the girth of the instep and a small space between the facings is always desirable in a Gibson/Blucher style. However the Oxford/Bal styling requires very accurate fitting of the instep as it is stitched at the base of the facings under the vamp and allows little tolerance.

The pes cavus foot is also affected by external heel height. Such a foot will fail to make adequate contact with the shoe insole of a higher heeled shoe style and may not be held adequately by the quarters, so a change in heel height may also be very helpful (see p. 71).

Joint width and vamp

The foot is dynamic and changes in shape during the gait cycle, causing the width and girth to alter continuously. There are three key situations that affect the width across the first to fifth metatarsal joints: non-weight-bearing, weight-bearing including activity, and thermal conditions, for example excessive heat or extreme cold. The average foot will normally expand by about 5% over the course of a day. This amounts to one shoe size in volume. The foot will expand as much as 7–8% after vigorous exercise or during very warm or humid conditions. This is the equivalent of 1.5 shoe sizes. Where a circulatory pathology exists, the foot could expand by 10% during the day, causing considerable pressure inside the shoe by the end of the day. This can often lead to the development of pressure lesions, or to injury of the skin and soft tissue if the footwear cuts into the swelling (Rossi & Tennant 1984).

The shoe, although fitted initially non-weight-bearing, must provide adequate width for the foot during activity, and for conditions where thermal variation may be a factor. During initial shoe selection, fit during activity is briefly observed by walking around in the store. However this is usually only a token of what the wearer will actually be doing during normal wear, and accurate fitting is a matter of experience and judgement in selecting the shoe width that will best accommodate all of these situations.

The fitter needs to check the tightness of the leather across the vamp, particularly over the joint area, so that it is neither too tight nor too roomy. The width of the foot inside the shoe needs to be checked so that it does not cause the vamp leather to splay out over the width of the outer sole, particularly at the first toe joint, a problem often seen with hallux valgus or tailor's bunion affecting the fifth metatarso-phalangeal joint. The most effective way of checking fit is to check the foot dimensions against the shoe inlay. If the shoe does not have a removable one, it is possible to quickly make a template of the inner dimensions of the shoe by placing the shoe on card or paper, drawing around its outline and cutting out the shape just within the outline to make a small allowance for seams. Place the foot onto the insole or insole template and then check the match between the foot width and the internal shoe width across the joint area, overall length and toe shape. Using removable inlays as a fitting aid is quick and effective, as several checks can be made this way. This inlay provides the internal dimension of the shoe and is particularly useful when the wearer has neuropathy and cannot be relied upon to feel the fit of the shoe properly (Fig. 5.14).

Adequate knowledge of the patient's medical history will be helpful, as conditions such as neuropathy and oedema may cause fitting issues. Where the foot swells diurnally, it may be subject to pressure or tightness from the footwear by the end of the day. Where a patient has sensory neuropathy, the shoe may damage the feet without the patient being aware of the trauma (see Ch. 12).

Finally, subjective factors cannot be ignored and the personal choice on width fitting comfort of the wearer should also be considered; therefore asking the wearer to comment on the comfort of the shoe is essential. It can be problematic when the wearer insists on a loose-fitting shoe or a shoe of excessive length or tightness and is not prepared to be guided by an expert. In these cases, professionalism is paramount to discourage such bad practices. Conscientious retailers will refuse to sell such an item to the customer as they have no wish to deal with potential complaints after the sale. However, this is rare, sadly, partly due to the shortage of such expertise in the retail sector and the need to make sales.

Top line

The shoe should fit snugly around the heel and onto the dorsum of the foot at the top line. Variation in styles alters the position and closeness of the top line and there are particular differences between the top line in slip-on styles and lace ups. Excessive gaping of the top line may indicate a faulty fit, and making the shoe on a different last, or in a different style or fitting, may be necessary.

Certain biomechanical anomalies, for example excessive pronation, will also cause gaping of the top line, particularly on the lateral side, whereas conditions such as posterior tibial tendon dysfunction may cause gaping on the medial side of the shoe top line. By correcting the foot position within the shoe with a simple orthotic, it is possible to eliminate the gaping. This is especially the case when fitting the extra depth therapeutic footwear where there will be adequate accommodation for the orthotic. This orthotic will also, of course, help the foot to function more effectively.

The pattern designer's understanding of foot function is paramount to the design of the whole shoe, but in particular to the facings. For example, a lace Gibson style can be designed in several ways

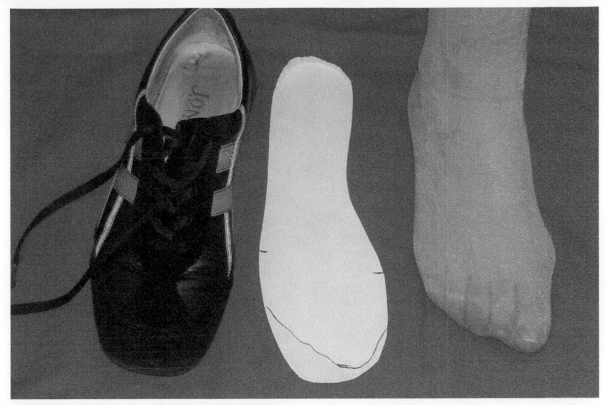

Figure 5.14 Comparison of a shoe, its inlay and the foot side by side. Checking the inlay under the foot is a helpful fitting tool. (Reproduced with permission of Mile End Hospital Footwear Centre.)

and the design may well affect the top line grip (Rossi & Tennant 1984).

Figure 5.15 shows how different shapes of the top line affects the direction of grip into the foot. The skill in fitting is to know which shape works with which foot shape, and to choose the correct style of facing for the low-arch foot or the high-arch foot. Both designs can work well when correctly fitted. This is where giving advice about choosing a lace shoe can be confusing, if the shoe fitter has little understanding in the context of varying foot shapes (see Ch. 1).

Low-heeled shoes do require a minimal amount of open and close bellows style action of the top line as part of the character of the shoe style. This is necessary to accommodate the heel-to-toe action that is more pronounced in a flat shoe than in a high-heeled style. This again highlights the difference in the shod static foot and the shod walking foot and how shoe fit changes with movement. If the correct style of facings has been chosen, the shoe will fit closely when the

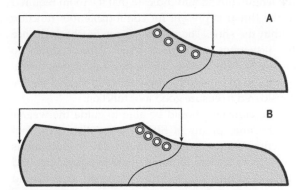

Figure 5.15 Outline drawings to demonstrate short and long vamp sections. (Reproduced with permission of Rossi & Tennant 1984.)

foot is at rest. With a slip-on style, without the benefit of an adjustable fastening, the fit of the top line must be accurately predesigned into the pattern, otherwise the result is a 'grinning' top line with excess gaping on flexion of the foot. The skill of the designer and trial fitting of new designs are essential here to avoid mass producing a 'faulty fit' style, which fails to fit however skilled the fitter may be.

The throat or 'entry'

The throat is the entry point for the foot into the vamp. The position of the entry is determined by the length of the vamp and type of facings. These can be long or short, depending on the style. In low-heeled lace styles, the throat fit deserves particular attention, as it will be altered considerably by the position of the base of the facings, the stay stitching and by particular design variations such as in Oxford and Gibson facings (also known as Bal and Blucher in the USA) (Rossi & Tennant 1984).

During weight-bearing and walking, the foot extends forwards along the waist and instep of the shoe, so throat room is required to accommodate this extension in addition to the extension room required at the toe end of the shoe. In a low-heeled Oxford or Gibson shoe with the shoe unlaced, the wearer should be able to slide the foot forward inside the shoe and have a space at the back of the shoe sufficient to insert a slim finger or pencil (for adults, 4–6 mm; for children, see Ch. 6). This gap does not necessarily indicate that the shoe is too big in the heel fit or too long in the length, but should indicate that the room required in the throat is present for comfortable foot function within the shoe. The overall fit can be checked once the fastenings are correctly tied. It is necessary to ensure that the space allows the smallest heel movement, but the subjective view of the fit should also be considered to ensure good foot function.

The clinician should be able to guide the wearer on the finer points of fitting, especially where foot function is already compromised. The overall aim is to improve or maintain adequate foot function, and the well-fitting and carefully designed shoe should enhance that function.

Patterns and styles

Patterns have a tremendous influence on shoe fit, as has become evident in the sections above. This applies especially to the ease of getting the foot into the shoe and keeping it on securely. There are many variations of long and short vamp designs and,

generally, the rounder the toe, the shorter the vamp, and conversely the more tapered the toe, the longer the vamp will be. Vamp length is determined by the shoes' overall design especially in the retail industry, but in bespoke footwear, vamp length is determined by the last maker following instructions from the clinician. The clinician will have supplied the outlines and measurements of the foot and will have chosen the shoe style.

As the foot flexes, natural vamp creasing occurs. The toe spring designed into the last will keep this creasing to a minimum (see p. 28). The higher the heel, the less creasing occurs as the flex action required of the foot is reduced by increasing heel height.

Choosing the correct style is vital in the clinical situation, especially if severe foot deformity is present, otherwise the shoe may not fit onto the foot. How to use styles to the best advantage is explored fully in Chapter 1.

Summary of fitting principles

1. Overall length.
2. Heel-to-ball length and flex angle.
3. Ball joint-to-toe length.
4. Heel and seat fit.
5. Instep, waist and arch fit.
6. Joint width and vamp.
7. Top line grip.
8. The throat or 'entry'.
9. Patterns and styles.

Measurement and size systems

This section explores the various methods of foot measurement and the types of measuring equipment available. It examines the numerous size systems that have been developed worldwide, and evaluates how they compare and the means of conversion from one system to another.

Taking a foot measurement can be as simple as using a last maker's tape measure, or as complex as the hand-drawn chart for a bespoke item or the use of the latest computer-aided design/computer-aided manufacturing (CAD/CAM) scanning system that records hundreds of measurements in a split second to reproduce a three-dimensional image on the computer screen.

There are many methods for measuring feet and each method will determine how many measurements are actually taken. The choice of method will depend on how the information will be used: for example, measuring for a bespoke shoe requires many more detailed measurements than being measured by a shop assistant for a pair of retail shoes (Peet & Weston 2001).

Therefore, having decided the purpose of the measurement, selecting the appropriate method is important for the outcome. For example, a survey of, say, children's shoe sizes will require a different approach to measuring and then testing a new last design before a production run is set up (see p. 79 on population surveys).

Measuring devices

When it comes to using any type of measuring device, it is essential to understand the measurement scale impressed on it. The scale may be marked as either shoe size or foot size, or it may not be clear at first glance what the scale is actually measuring. The device may be marked for weight-on or weight-off use. Many measuring devices are made for specific manufacturers or brands, particularly in the children's retail sector. These devices are designed to measure for that specific brand only and may not match another brand exactly on size scale or width fitting. Generally, retail shoe fitters are trained to use a specific device by the manufacturer: they will understand how to read the scale and obtain the correct information from it. Measuring a foot on the wrong scale may lead to an incorrect shoe fitting. Parents should beware of taking their children to have their feet measured in a specialist shop and then transferring that measurement size to footwear from, perhaps, a chain store. It is unlikely that the sizes from the two sources will be the same.

Last maker's size stick and tape

The simplest form of measuring device is a size stick. Correctly named the *last maker's* size stick, it is usually a box wood device similar to a ruler with one fixed end and a sliding arm. It normally indicates foot size only and it is necessary to convert the measurement to shoe size by adding an allowance. The amount to be added depends on whether it is used weight-on or weight-off and can be from 1.5 to 3 sizes. While the size is indicated on the top of the stick, measurements in millimetres are often indicated on the reverse side. Size sticks are rarely used in retail outlets but are often used by experienced fitters for bespoke items (Peet & Weston 2001).

To use the size stick correctly, the foot should be placed on the floor at 90° to the leg. Usually, the client is seated and the knee is also flexed at 90°. This position is semi-weight-bearing, meaning that there is some pressure through the foot. The fixed arm is placed at the back of the heel and the stick is laid on the floor along the medial side of the foot. The sliding arm is moved to contact the longest toe. The stick should be removed carefully to read the measurement inside the sliding arm, and the necessary additions are then made. In the position described, 2 sizes are usually added to the reading, however if the foot is hypermobile then 2.5 sizes will be needed to reach the correct shoe size. The stick can also be used to measure length in millimetres, either by markings on the back or by placing a tape measure between the arms. Apart from overall length, the stick can be used to measure joint width, heel width and toe height by placing it appropriately on the foot. In addition to these measures, it is normal to use a last maker's tape measure to determine the girth of the joints and of the instep. A standard tape measure can be substituted, but the last maker's one is shorter and has shoe sizes marked on one side and cm/mm on the other side.

The basic measurements of length, joint girth and instep are the first measures used by clinicians to determine the type of footwear required to meet the patient's needs. The guide provided by basic measurements will indicate whether, with detailed advice, the patient is likely to be able to obtain suitable footwear from retail sources, whether specialist wide or deep shoes will be needed, or whether the patient has feet well outside normal size ranges and will need a bespoke item. The size stick and tape measure are easily carried about and versatile in use but require training to use correctly.

Devices for retail use are numerous and varied. Some measure both feet at once, such as the flat board style device with a centre spine and a width conversion scale. This makes it possible to compare the left and right feet. Some board type devices measure a single foot only, but all have a reference point for the placement of the heel, generally a low wall or curved plastic heel stop, and some incorporate their own tape measure attached on a sliding bar (Peet & Weston 2001).

Most devices available are designed by individual shoe manufacturers to use with their own brand of shoes for both adults' and children's ranges. A qualified fitter soon learns the relationship between the different brands and fittings in the shop, and ensures that the correct device is used wherever possible.

All devices should be used according to the manufacturers' instructions, and if weight-on, the client should be instructed to stand upright and look straight ahead with the weight evenly on both feet (Russell & Hardy 1988).

Electronic devices

There are also several types of electronic measuring devices in retail stores. Their sophistication and colourful presentation look impressive. Children think they're more fun than a standard shoe gauge, but essentially they only record two measurements, length and width. They work by either moving sensors against the foot, or by using photo cells to record foot length and width. They eliminate the skill required by the fitter in using a gauge correctly and are usually brand orientated.

The Brannock Device®

The Brannock Device® records three measurements. In addition to length and width, it also measures heel-to-ball length. The reasoning is that heel-to-ball measurement is more important than total length (Peet & Weston 2001). Where the foot is disproportional, this gauge can help to find the best overall fitting to accommodate the heel-to-ball length. The device contains an extra sliding side piece which has to be lined up to the ball joint, and pointer lines which marry up with shoe sizes on a scale. This may not always match up with the length measurement taken from the front of the foot. Where there is a discrepancy, the heel-to-ball length is used, as this should help to find the best heel-to-ball length fit. It also has a width indicator bar to the outside of the foot which helps to establish the required width fitting. The gauge is reversible, with the right and left

heel position clearly marked at each end of the gauge. The Brannock gauge is not made for a specific range of shoes, but does give the experienced fitter a good guide for choosing a length and width fitting. These gauges are separately available for men's, ladies' and children's sizes, and in both US and English size systems. The Brannock Device® is much more popular in the USA as the size range is far greater than in the UK, and because it helps the fitter to find the best size more efficiently from a much wider choice. For up-to-date guidelines on using the Brannock Device®, visit their Web site at http://brannock.com (Tippet 2007) (Fig. 5.16; also see p. 80 on sizing systems).

Scanning devices

These are the latest advance in technology. They use either a photo system of several cameras or laser scanning to record thousands of measurements of the whole foot. These are sent directly to a computer to create an image of the foot in three dimensions. The data collected can be used in many ways, and lasts and orthotics can be individually designed and modified using a computer modelling program, sent to a remote milling machine and produced in an accurate, rapid and efficient way. This technology will have many applications and is gradually being added to many different production systems, including bespoke suppliers. The scanners are rather costly and, because they are highly sensitive, difficult to move around at present, but in the foreseeable future they will become more widespread and user friendly. Interpretation of the data they generate requires great expertise, but this technology will provide an extremely useful tool and has the potential to save much time in a clinical situation.

Measuring for bespoke footwear

Due to the complexity of the foot shape, a bespoke item of footwear may need to be made. This will require the prescriber to take many more measurements than the basic length, joint and instep girth. The way in which these measurements are recorded will vary according to the country, type of training received and requirements of the manufacturer involved in making the footwear. Generally, recording measurements for footwear involves

Figure 5.16 Variety of measurement gauges. From the left: last maker's size stick, used in bespoke measuring; Ken Hall brand gauge for therapeutic footwear; Piedro children's size gauge; Brannock Device® incorporating heel-to-ball length and width as well as length. (Reproduced with permission of Mile End Hospital Footwear Centre, with thanks to the various manufacturers.)

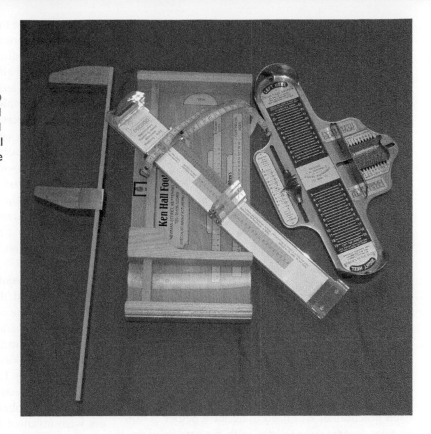

drawing round the foot, making an outline, taking various measurements and recording them on the outline. Additionally, a cast of the foot may be made and photographs taken. These foot plans, which are also called charts or drafts, vary enormously in both quality and detail, and from the many examples used in factories both in the UK and Europe, the 'British Standard Method 5943' appears to be the most comprehensive system for recording foot measurements. This is fully explored in Chapter 11.

Population surveys: ensuring validity and reliability of measurements

To ensure that measurements are taken accurately and reflect those they represent on the foot, some basic considerations need to be adhered to. Peet & Weston (2001) recommend the following rules.

Location of the foot

It is essential that the foot is accurately located onto the measuring device as instructed by the manufacturer, for example the heel should be accurately positioned into a cup or back stop.

Reference points

Where measures require a specific position on the foot, for example 1–5 joint girth, this point must be accurately located every time. By measuring the foot without footwear or hosiery, reference points can be more accurately located.

Weight-on or weight-off measures

Different devices will require the foot to be placed in different positions. Some ask that the foot should be fully weight-bearing and others semi-weight-bearing, such as when using the angled measuring stool. It is important to use the device correctly to obtain accurate measurement information. The foot changes considerably in dimension from non-weight-bearing to full weight-bearing. The degree of change varies from person to person, making it very difficult to predict precisely how much each foot will lengthen or broaden when under body load. This creates quite a dilemma, as the most accurate information should be gained from weight-on measurement, but the majority of shoe manufacturers work from non-weight-bearing measurements and add allowances for foot extension to obtain the correct size. So, depending on the purpose, it is important to choose the measurement method carefully.

Underfoot surface

It is recommended that the foot is placed on a firm surface for measurement taking. A soft, springy surface will cause the girth measurement to change, reducing it as the foot becomes more rounded due to the softer surface.

Effect of hose

Each practitioner will need to decide whether or not to take foot measurements with hosiery in place. Tight hose can cause compression and thick hose will increase all the measurements. If it is decided to measure with hosiery in place, ensure that each subject wears the type of hose they expect to wear in the footwear for which they are being measured. Ensure also that the hosiery is of the correct size.

Global shoe sizing systems

Over the centuries, worldwide, numerous ways of making shoes have evolved, and with them a variety of size systems have also been developed. The twentieth century has seen some dramatic advances in nutrition and health care; consequently, people are growing taller and larger. Similarly, feet have also become larger and wider (Russell & Hardy 1988). It is interesting to compare shoe sizes of the seventeenth and eighteenth centuries with the early twentieth century and note how much larger the feet of the twenty-first century population have become.

The history of the origins of shoe sizing is rather muddled. Historically, the majority of shoes were made for the wealthy by a local cordwainer. The less wealthy made their own footwear and would 'cobble' (hence the term 'cobbler' for a shoe repairer) together leather pieces into a simple shape. It was not thought necessary to create shoe sizes until about 150 years ago, when a sizing system began to emerge that became established and accepted by the Guild of Shoemakers. This was recorded in the *Illustrated Handbook of the Foot* by Robert Gardiner in 1856, where the 'one-third of an inch' scale was the system generally deemed acceptable in the UK. Thus, each shoe size increased one-third of an inch but there were no half sizes at this point (Rossi & Tennant 1984).

In the fourteenth century, King Edward II of England decreed that 3 barleycorns placed end to end would be the official measurement for an 'inch', therefore each barley corn represented one-third of an inch and 12 inches equalled '1 foot' (=36 barley corns), but he is not accredited with starting shoe sizes at this time. However, the system of using barley corns as a measure did exist for many centuries, being an easily obtainable grain until eventually rulers were invented that measured inches (Russell & Hardy 1988).

Finally, in 1880, the world's first proper shoe sizing system was invented by an American, Edwin B Simpson. His amazing system detailed proportional measurements for lasts, to include length, ball width, waist and heel. Shoe sizes were then derived from these last sizes. He set up individual systems for infants', children's, women's and men's lasts. His system used the one-third of an inch measurement for each size and he introduced half sizes for the first time. The proportional increases in each rising size, for the ball, waist and instep, became the first step towards better shoe fit (Rossi & Tennant 1984). For further reading about the history of shoe sizes, see Rossi & Tennant 1984.

Today, there are essentially four main sizing systems used around the world (Table 5.1). These are:

1. The English system
2. The American system
3. The Continental or Paris points system
4. The Japanese or centimetre system.

Table 5.1 Variations between starting points and measurements in shoe size systems (data modified from Parker et al 2001)

	English	American	Continental	Japanese
Length scale starts at:	4 inches = 0	$3\frac{1}{12}$ inches = 0	0	0
	Children: 2–13 $\frac{1}{2}$	Children: 2 $\frac{1}{2}$–13 $\frac{1}{2}$	Continues with no break to maximum size 47	Continues with no break to maximum size 29 $\frac{1}{2}$
	Adults: 1–12	Adults: 3 $\frac{1}{2}$–13		
Intervals of:	$\frac{1}{3}$ inch (8.47 mm)	$\frac{1}{3}$ inch (8.47 mm)	$\frac{2}{3}$ cm (6.67 mm)	10 mm
Half size intervals	$\frac{1}{6}$ inch (4.23 mm)	$\frac{1}{6}$ inch (4.23 mm)	Very rare but $\frac{1}{3}$ cm (3.33 mm)	5 mm
Width fittings: interval between sizes	$\frac{1}{4}$ inch (6.35 mm)	$\frac{1}{4}$ inch (6.35 mm)	5 mm	60% of length
Interval between fittings	$\frac{1}{4}$ inch (6.35 mm)	$\frac{1}{4}$ inch (6.35 mm)	5 mm	6 mm girth increase between fittings

Conversion

Table 5.2 sets out a conversion between the four main global size systems, however it is not quite so straightforward to convert all sizes because of variations within the systems that occur in some countries of manufacture. Particular care is needed using the Continental or Paris points system because of the method used for measuring lasts. Footwear from Spain or South America is sometimes marked one or two sizes smaller than expected in other European countries using the *same sizing system*. It is therefore useful to know the country of origin of the footwear (Parker et al 2001).

The American system is also confusing because, although using inches, they start one-twelfth of an inch smaller than the English system, causing the American size to be one-quarter of a size smaller. This is further complicated because the actual size scale marked on the footwear is much larger. Women's shoes tend to be 1.5 sizes larger, but men's shoes are only 1 size larger than the equivalent English fitting. By using the conversion chart shown in Table 5.2, a woman's English 5 becomes 6.5 American; a men's English 8 becomes 9 American (Parker et al 2001).

Although there are established size systems around the world, there are many more variations of the size scales than it is possible to list. This is because of the numerous small manufacturing businesses in every country making footwear. Some manufacture for their own local market only, but many export their goods. It is impossible to regulate all these relatively small businesses (Tippet 2007).

Traditionally, a last is designed and made up and tried, usually in one size, often a ladies' size 4. Once it is accepted as being a good fit, the last is scaled up and down for larger or smaller sizes, and the smallest is given the lowest size number, for example 3, and the remainder of the sizes follow on. It is not matched exactly to any size scale despite there being perfectly good scales available, hence there are slight variations in the actual size of the shoe which the last represents when the finished footwear is tried on in a store. There is consequently much confusion over sizes.

Another way to consider footwear sizing is to liken it to the difference in buying a dress or trousers (pants) from one large high street shop compared to another. Shoppers often find that they can fit into a size smaller in one store, although the garment size labels indicate the use of a similar clothes sizing system.

Table 5.2 Shoe size conversion chart

| UK sizes | Paris points | USA sizes | | | Japanese |
		Men	Women	Children	
2	18			2 ½	10
2 ½	18 ½			3	10 ½
3	19			3 ½	11
3 ½	19 ½			4	11 ½
4	20 ½			4 ½	12
4 ½	21			5	12 ½
5	21 ½			5 ½	12 ½
5 ½	22			6	13
6	23			6 ½	13 ½
6 ½	23 ½			7	14
7	24			7 ½	14 ½
7 ½	25			8	15
8	25 ½			8 ½	15
8 ½	26			9	15 ½
9	26 ½			9 ½	16
9 ½	27 ½			10	16 ½
10	28			10 ½	17
10 ½	28 ½			11	17 ½
11	29			11½	18
11 ½	30			12	18
12	30 ½			12 ½	18 ½
12 ½	31			13	19
13	32			13 ½	19 ½
13 ½	32 ½			1	20

(Continued)

Table 5.2 Continued

| UK sizes | Paris points | USA sizes | | | Japanese |
		Men	Women	Children	
1	33			1 ½	20 ½
1 ½	33 ½			2	20 ½
2	34 ½		3 ½	2 ½	21
2 ½	35		4	3	21 ½
3	35 ½		4 ½	3 ½	22
3 ½	36		5	4	22 ½
4	37		5 ½	4 ½	23
4 ½	37 ½		6	5	23 ½
5	38	6	6 ½	5 ½	23 ½
5 ½	38 ½	6 ½	7	6	24
6	39 ½	7	7 ½	6 ½	24 ½
6 ½	40	7 ½	8	7	25
7	40 ½	8	8 ½	7 ½	25 ½
7 ½	41 ½	8 ½	9		26
8	42	9	9 ½		26
8 ½	42 ½	9 ½	10		26 ½
9	43	10	10 ½		27
9 ½	44	10 ½	11		27 ½
10	44 ½	11	11 ½		28
10 ½	45	11 ½	12		28 ½
11	45 ½	12			29
11 ½	46 ½	12 ½			29
12	47	13			29 ½
13	48	14	14 ½		
14	48 ½	15	15 ½		

(Continued)

Table 5.2 Continued

UK sizes	Paris points	USA sizes			Japanese
		Men	Women	Children	
15	49 ½	16	16 ½		
16	51	17	17 ½		
17	52	18	18 ½		
18	53 ½	19	19 ½		

Conclusion

Experience is required to finally establish that the footwear is the most appropriate fitting and size for a foot. Whatever size scale is printed inside the footwear, or whatever size is measured on a gauge, there is no substitute for the valuable experience of an expert in shoe fitting who can ensure that the shoe and the foot complement each other in size, form and function.

References

Alpert T, Boettge B, Bowman M et al 1998 Testing for fit. In: National Shoe Retailers Association/Pedorthic Footwear Association. When the shoe fits: the basics of professional shoe fitting (student course book). USA, Fairchild.

Ceeney E 1958 In: Seat and heel. An introduction to shoe fitting. London, Pitman.

Foster A 2006 Podiatric assessment and management of the diabetic foot. Edinburgh, Churchill Livingstone.

Parker K, Tailby S, Weston A 2001 Settling footwear complaints. Northamptonshire, Shoe and Allied Trades Research Association.

Peet M, Weston A 2001 Modern shoemaking No. 60: fitting. Northamptonshire, Shoe and Allied Trades Research Association.

Rossi W, Tennant R 1984 In: Advanced principles of shoe fitting. Professional shoe fitting. New York, National Shoe Retailers Association.

Russell L, Hardy B 1988 In healthy feet. London, Macdonald Optima.

Tippit B 2007 The size gamble. World Footwear Publication. May/June 21(3):19–21.

Suggested reading

http://scholar.google.com. Search under sports footwear research.

Organizations

National Shoe Retailers Association, 7150 Columbia Gateway Drive, Suite G, Columbia, Maryland 21046–1151, USA; tel: +1 410 381 8282; e-mail: info@nsra.org; Web site: www.nsra.org.

Pedorthic Footwear Association, 2025 M Street, NW, Suite 800, Washington DC 20036, USA; tel: +1 202 367 2145; Web site: www.pedorthics.org.

Society of Shoe Fitters, The Anchorage, Admirals Walk, Hingham, Norfolk NR9 4JL, UK; tel: +44 (0)195 385 1171; e-mail: secretary@shoefitters-uk.org.

Shoes for special purposes

Chapter contents

Alongside everyday footwear styles, there are also numerous designs for footwear to be used in particular circumstances or when undertaking particular activities. This chapter considers footwear for children, for sports activities and for protection in industrial environments. Such footwear has been the subject of considerable development in recent years and each type is specialized in its design features, manufacturing methods and fittings. Footwear for children, when properly fitted, allows the foot to develop normally, and with advances in styling and manufacture, fewer children than ever before have foot problems. As therapeutic footwear prescribing advances, understanding and accessing the types of footwear which enables patients with foot pathologies to undertake work, social and leisure activities are becoming possible. Clinicians can now make best use of technological developments and new materials, and these, along with research findings and product testing, make the subject interesting, challenging and progressive and provide patients with a therapy which enhances their foot health and improves their lifestyles.

Children's shoes

Shoe styles for children tend to follow the fashion trends for adults, more so in regards to shape rather than the materials used. However, the needs of children's feet are specific and change with different stages of learning to walk. Ignoring these specific requirements can hinder the healthy development of the foot and lead to problems in adulthood.

(World Footwear Publication 2005)

Development

Newborn feet are very soft, like a 'bag of soft tissue and cartilage', and contain only three bones evident on X-ray (calcaneus, talus and cuboid). The limbs and feet are very active and the infant performs lots of wriggling and kicking that builds up strength ready for standing and walking a few months after birth. The foot is very pliable and can be easily distorted by stretch fabric hosiery/clothing and pram/cot shoes, if these become tight. The practice of dressing a baby, including shoes, has become fashionable to the extent that the little shoes are sold with the outfit to match; however it has more to do with the image of the infant by a mother and the fantasy idea that wearing shoes so young will, in some way, help the walking process to develop. Nature does a far better job unheeded by modern trends and baby shoes should be discouraged.

The rate of growth is very rapid at this stage of development and, for the child, the gradual adaptation from the horizontal to a vertical position is the end result of a long process of both physical and mental development. Walking helps every baby to develop confidence in its environment and in itself and encourages exploration of its surroundings. At about 9–12 months of age, the crawling and walking stage begins to develop, although this can be as late as 16 months in some children. In terms of foot development, sensory awareness is most acute between 9 and 12 months as the baby begins to walk (World Footwear Publication 2005). The sensitivity allows the child to collect the information it requires in terms of balance, stability and ambulation, and it is therefore vital that footwear does not hinder this development in any way. Babies start to build up strength in the limbs and muscle groups by exercising. This is mainly by pulling themselves up to a standing position and learning to balance, using anything they can to hold onto until they eventually begin to walk unaided.

The baby is very unstable, with no toe control for balance, and the legs are very bandy and wobbly. They stand with feet wide apart for stability (Fig. 6.1). The feet are in-flared, with the big toe abducted

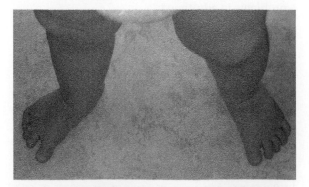

Figure 6.1 A toddler just starting to fully weight-bear. The first toes are abducted and the lesser toes claw the floor for grip and balance. The stance is very wide and the knees are locked for more stability.

from the midline of the foot, and they appear flat footed. As there is a limited amount of solid bone in the foot at this stage, there is no proper arch evident. Once the child can take a number of steps unaided and wants to walk outdoors, then shoes should be sought. During this period, infants should wear structured shoes that assist them in finding their balance and develop their confidence, and yet the shoe should also offer reasonable flexibility in the sole to allow the foot to develop in its natural way. The concept of including in the footwear support around the malleoli (ankle bones) or in the sole – by means of a shank – is now called into question as not necessarily beneficial to the very young foot. It has been suggested that such support might cause some damage if the foot is too restricted (Rossi & Tennant 1993).

Footwear criteria for toddlers: ages 1–3 (sizes 18–23 Continental; sizes 1–6 English, approximately)

The uppers in this age group are generally high cut and many European styles stop just at the malleoli to ensure the foot is well supported. For some children, particularly if they are tall and perhaps slightly heavy, a degree of ankle support can be important to help control the ankle joint and allow good foot posture, but this must be selected on an individual basis. The length of the shoe must not hinder the growth of the foot, but at the same time, too much space at the front of the shoe can also have a negative effect on the growth of a child's foot as the flexion point of the shoe will not be positioned correctly to the metatarsal joint (heel-to-ball fit). The front of the shoe requires volume around the perimeter of the joint and some growth space beyond the toes. This should be no more than 7–10 mm, equating with 2 shoe sizes (World Footwear Publication 2005).

Infants' feet have relatively large big toes at this stage in development, and it is necessary to ensure that there is sufficient room for this toe to function as it is abducted from the midline, requiring extra width on the medial border of the shoe. The back height of the shoe should be proportional to the average measurements of the shoe size. If it is too low, the foot will not be held correctly in the shoe. If it is too high, damage to the Achilles tendon could result. The instep of the shoe needs to follow the natural line of a baby's foot, fitting closely to the foot

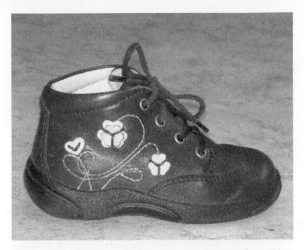

Figure 6.2 Toddlers' high-top lace-style shoe for ankle stability, with a padded top line and flexible sole for maximum flexion with the soft foot. The upper and lining are leather.

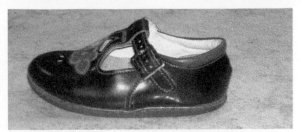

Figure 6.3 A classic toddlers' early walking shoe. It has no heel, the sole is completely flat and there is a generous toe spring. The strap and buckle fasten high on the dorsum to hold the foot securely back into the heel counter.

The length of the shoe is just as important as for toddlers, allowing growth room at the back, instep and toe in moderate proportions. The vamp and toe shape should allow space around the joint area and be of sufficient depth not to damage the soft cartilaginous toes or toe nails. The back height and instep shape are the same as for the toddlers' age group (Fig. 6.3).

but not raising or actively supporting the arch area of the foot because the arch is not yet formed at this early stage. The shoe instep shape helps to position the forefoot correctly inside the shoe (Fig. 6.2).

Toddlers from 1 to 2.5 years run or 'toddle' rather than walk. They need to develop balance and muscle coordination. They appear to have bandy legs at first, but this slowly changes as they strengthen, to look almost 'knock kneed' by 2.5 to 3 years.

Footwear criteria for infants: ages 3–5 (sizes 24–27 Continental; sizes 7–10 English, approximately)

By the age of 3, the long arch should be developing and the knees should be front facing. At age 3 to 4, the legs straighten so that the knees are not 'knocked together'. By age 5, the heel-to-toe gait should be evident and walking and running should be well-established and coordinated. The foot shape should be neither in-flared nor out-flared at the toes and a small arch should be visible. In comparison with the earlier age group, children at this age are more dynamic and confident. However, the foot is still weak and it is important to allow for this in the shoe design.

The uppers of shoes are often cut lower for this age group than for toddlers. However, good all-round structure should be incorporated into the style and the shoe should contain a functional fastening to retain the growing foot back into the heel counter.

Footwear criteria for boys and girls: ages 5–7 (sizes 27–33 Continental; sizes 9–1 English, approximately)

Between the ages of 5 and 7 years, the foot becomes more structured and defined in its shape. The arch is beginning to form and the foot has good flexibility. The difference between boys' and girls' feet starts to become evident now and it is necessary to have specific shoe lasts for each sex. The differences can be noted around the instep proportions and the size of the first metatarsal joint. At this stage, style starts to influence the choices made in the shoe shop, and with fashion trends becoming influential, choosing well is a balance between what is good for the growing foot and the latest trend. Sadly many parents are unaware of the potential damage that can be done to the young growing foot by poor footwear. Sales assistants are more interested in sales volume than foot health, which makes a dynamic combination for potential future foot problems if fashion and the child's wishes overrule. All the requirements previously mentioned are still relevant, but last shape matters especially as the foot becomes more out-flared (a straight first toe position, no longer abducted). This change in last shape can go too far, mimicking adults' shoe shapes and putting pressure on the still soft bone structure of the medial side of the foot, and it can start the process

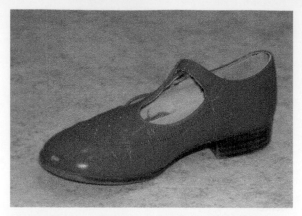

Figure 6.4 A traditional child's shoe made with a low, wide heel and very stable sole with good toe spring. The strap and buckle are positioned high on the dorsum to hold the foot back in the counter. The form is virtually straight lasted allowing plenty of room for all the toes with no in-flare to the first metatarsal joint.

of developing a hallux valgus deformity which may then appear fully in later years.

Girls' feet develop faster than boys' feet from now on, and by age 10, girls have achieved 90% of total foot growth and most achieve full adult shoe size by age 14. They tend to have a growth spurt around 10 to 11 years. At age 10, boys reach 82% of total foot growth, with a growth spurt at about 14 years and final growth at around 16 to 18 years. Even though the rate of growth has slowed down from infancy, the need to have children regularly measured to check their shoe size cannot be overemphasized as children tend to grow in 'spurts' rather than steadily like an infant. The regular check of every 6 to 8 weeks is a good rule of thumb; coinciding with school holidays and midterm breaks helps parents/carers to maintain this as a regular event. Hence the majority of children's shoe shops are very busy just before the start of a new term (Fig. 6.4).

Rate of growth

At birth, the foot contains 22 partially formed bones, primarily made up of cartilage. These gradually form solid bone following an ossification timetable that is not completed until between the ages of 18 and 24 years of age. The foot then possesses all fully formed 26 bones of the adult foot.

The rate of growth drops rapidly from infancy to 4 to 5 years. The foot takes 4 years to double its birth

length, and at age 2 years, the shoe size doubled will give a good indication of the adult shoe size to come.

Numerous muscles, tendons and ligaments are also developing and sometimes these can be the cause of gait problems if they are too tight, limiting movements such as proper heel contact or in-toeing. The most common developmental conditions relate to position of the feet and knees and are briefly covered below. For more in-depth study, please refer to a specialist podopaediatrics text.

Bow leg (genu varum)

Bow leg of some degree involving femur, fibula and tibia is a common finding at birth and is associated with normal development to approximately 2 years. Most bow legs are transitory in nature and, unless associated with a disease, correct themselves by the age of 2 years (Fig. 6.5).

Knock knee (genu valgum)

Knock knee is also part of the normal developmental growth pattern of a child's limbs. This usually becomes apparent at the age of 2 years, reaches maximum deformity at 4 years and tends to disappear at 6 to 7 years of age (Fig. 6.6).

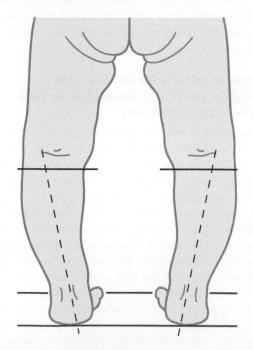

Figure 6.5 Diagram to demonstrate leg position of genu varum in an early walker.

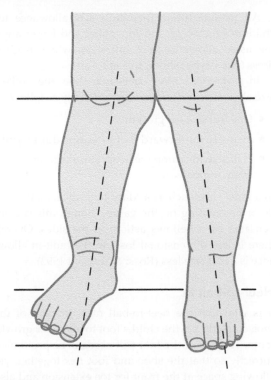

Figure 6.6 Diagram to demonstrate genu valgum. The infant may adopt this position before the legs fully straighten up by age 5 to 6 years.

Toe walking (equinus)

Toe walking is common at the beginning of the walking phase, but within 6 months of walking, heel contact should be developing. If the condition persists, it must be followed up, as a diagnosis should be made as to the cause. It may be simply tight muscles that need exercise to stretch them, or it may be a neurological condition that was not evident before walking started.

In-toe or 'pigeon-toed' child

Toeing-in is not usually a foot-orientated action and is influenced by body and leg actions during movement. It is caused by a rotational force applied to the foot from above, anywhere from pelvis to ankle, which allows the foot to turn inwards.

Anatomical reasons for in-toe can be either simple or very complex. There can be osseous involvement or soft tissue restriction (cartilage, capsule or ligament) around joints, or the positioning of the

limbs may be influenced by inappropriate muscular pull that affects the movement of the lower limb in walking. The condition may be unilateral or bilateral depending on cause.

Out-toed child

This is a less serious problem and is often self-corrected by age 2 years. However, all cases of marked out-toe or in-toe should be treated as soon as possible by a specialist rather than expecting the child to grow out of it. In the meantime, poor postural habits may have become established and the situation is far more difficult to correct.

Treatments include Dennis Brown bars, cable twisters, shoe wedges, angulation of gait plates, reverse-lasted shoes and exercises. These can be used for either condition and are prescribed appropriately.

Pronation

As the toddler begins to walk at the age of about 9 to 12 months, excessive pronation on weight-bearing is common. There is usually a subtalar varus of between 5–10° resulting from the inverted forefoot to rear foot position which is the norm at this stage of development. The forefoot and rear foot varus normally reduces considerably by age 6 years as femoral anteversion and antetorsion occur simultaneously, bringing the knee to the frontal plane. The pronation then evident should not be excessive. Where it is abnormally excessive, diagnosis and treatment should be sought.

The criteria of 'normalcy' in a child's foot and leg varies with different ages and stages of growth and development. The child's foot does not resemble the fully-formed adult foot, being more flexible, soft and mobile in its ranges of motion. The heel-to-toe gait is not adopted until about 3 years, but is rather a plodding or flat-footed action which gradually adopts the heel-to-toe movements.

Measuring children's feet

The foot-measuring procedure is essentially the same as for adults, but with certain considerations:

- Make sure the socks are pulled away from the toes.
- Measure both feet.

- Measure in the position required by the measuring device as this varies, for example seated if using a fitting stool, or standing if the measuring device is designed to take measurements when the foot is fully loaded.

- The size selection is made according to the longest foot and/or the widest foot. Children tend to curl up their toes, so mild pressure with the thumb across the toes will help to get full toe extension when measuring.

- For width measurement, measure across the ball of both feet, but choose the wider fitting if different on each foot.

- Include heel-to-ball measurement as this is vital to the final fitting choice.

- Check the size of the old shoes, as this will give an indication of foot growth since the last pair.

- Feel inside the worn shoe with finger tips and check how much toe nail abrasion has occurred at the toe puff. If a there is a pronounced deep groove, suggest that the parent/carer also feels this. Such a groove can indicate that too long a time gap has been left before the child has been brought in to be remeasured.

- Quickly examine the old shoes for wear patterns including wrinkled linings, severe vamp creases, broken heel counter, excessive turned-up toe end, severe scuff marks, fastenings not being used correctly. An understanding of such wear can help determine the fitting needed and the most suitable style.

Fitting principles

These cover the same areas as adults, but with special consideration for the growing foot that is also very active.

Length fit

Infants' and children's shoes have a built-in length or size allowance incorporated into the last, and this is accounted for by using the specific measuring device produced for the brand concerned. It is therefore inappropriate to measure the child's foot on a device not related to the brand of shoe being purchased as this may not be an accurate size measurement for the shoe produced by a different manufacturer.

All manufacturers include a size allowance for children's footwear, and in smaller and larger boys, the usual allowance is 2 full sizes, while in girls' dress (party type) shoes, this is 1.5 sizes.

In a standard boys' lace-style shoe, the built-in size allowance is divided approximately as follows:

- One full size for growth.
- Half size for forward foot extension during gait.
- Half size for vamp creasing, shrinkage, etc., from original size.

In a girls' shoe such as a Mary Jane style, there is little or no creasing on the vamp, though this is compensated by a bellows action on the sides. Overall there is less dimensional loss, so the built-in allowance is a half size less (Rossi & Tennant 1993).

Heel-to-ball fit

It is vital that the heel-to-ball measurement of the shoe correctly fits the child's foot to allow for growth room. The ball of the foot still needs to be positioned correctly so that the shoe and foot flex together, yet allowing space at the front for toe extension and also providing a small space in the heel fit for rear foot growth. It is important to appreciate that the foot grows throughout, not just in length of toes alone.

The throat/entry

The fit should be such that when the foot is moved forward in the fastened shoe, there is a very small space of 3–5 mm. This space allows for overall growth and foot extension movements. As long as the shoe is *correctly fastened*, the amount of heel slip should be minimal and not cause any discomfort. Care is needed to fit shoes correctly at the entry to prevent excessive vamp creases. Once the heels get higher, 2 cm or more, the creasing is less likely to occur as the toe spring will be increased in the last, but bellowing is likely in the side counters or top line.

Heel fit

Because most young children's shoes have a very low heel height, there will be a large heel lift on walking which requires the shoe to flex and move easily. If the heel fit is too tight, this movement is restricted, causing discomfort and pain at the back of the heel. Generally, less heel irritation is caused by slippage. Mild slippage, especially on firm-soled shoes, is normal and usually disappears after the shoes have been worn a few times, and the sole flexes more easily and the vamp 'creases' appear. If the shoe has adequate width and depth in the counter, it should hold on properly.

Heels of 1–1.5 cm height and above on older children's shoes will affect the tread pattern and vamp creasing may occur as a result of the heel height. The small space at the back of the heel indicates that the shoe has sufficient throat or entry room, but what is important is the presence of a small space in the heel in the initial fitting.

Patterns

The best children's shoes are designed for 'hold-on' ability that ideally keeps the shoe on without interfering with foot function or growth. This applies especially to girls' strap-fastening styles, lace ups and Velcro® styles which should stay on the foot well. If a shoe is cut too low in the counter then more heel slippage is likely to occur, so a style with a deeper counter should hold on better. Slip-on shoes have little 'hold-on' ability and some styles have 'pretend' fastenings that can be slipped over the counter and become decoration rather than functional. These styles do not prevent the foot from slipping forward into the growth space and can severely damage the toes, causing clawing or other toe deformities. Many junior girls' styles mimic adult slip-on styles and these are inappropriate for the young developing foot, as any shoe without proper rear foot control and a functional fastening can cause damage. Add to this scenario the fact that many girls desire the increase in heel height. This is obligingly offered by children's shoe designers and many pairs are sold, but many feet are potentially damaged by it. The old idea of the school insisting on proper lace-up shoes as part of the school uniform was, in fact, far more beneficial for the pupils' foot health than was ever given credit.

Width fit

In testing width fit, pinch the shoe behind the joints and over the widest part of the foot. There should be about 5 mm of ease in the vamp leather. Also check the depth over the large toe joint, as this can be variable. The shoe must also be wide enough to accommodate the joint adequately. Tread width should be checked so that the foot is properly supported by the width of the sole. The upper should not bulge out over the sole.

Counters

In retail shoes, the counter is designed to maintain the shape of the shoe at the heel, and help it to stay on the foot. In the normal foot, juvenile or adult, a moderate amount of pronation is natural on weight-bearing and is part of the body's shock absorbing mechanism. The counter is not designed to lock the heel but to allow a moderate amount of lateral heel movement inside the shoe.

Shoe horns (a note of caution)

Shoe horns are ill-advised when fitting children's shoes. Using one will allow the foot to slip easily into a snug fitting shoe which is not the correct size. A proper shoe size should slip on easily without the aid of a shoe horn.

The ideal shoe

The ideal shoe is very difficult to find and is often a matter of compromise, especially with older children and teenagers who are influenced by peers and fashion dictates. Here is a summary of the main points to consider in choosing children's footwear (Watt 2006) (Fig. 6.7):

- **Adequate length and width**. Children should have both left and right feet measured for both length and width. Ideally children should be taken to a registered footwear retailer with properly trained staff and a choice of footwear in whole and half sizes in up to four width fittings. Many growing pairs of feet are not exactly the same size or width, and care is needed as well as skill to fit both feet adequately.
- **Heel stiffener (counter)**. This is the firm shaped insert in the back of the shoe which helps to keep the shoe securely on the foot and hold it during wear. Combined with a broad base of heel and a fastening, it helps to prevent clawing of the toes which will occur if the shoe is constantly slipping off the heel.
- **Height of heel**. Very young children's shoes should be of very low heel height. This can be gradually increased but ideally should be no

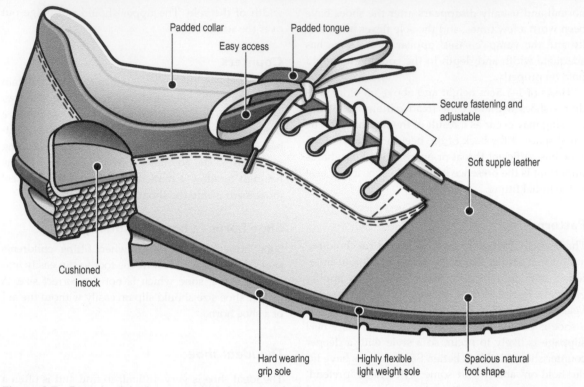

Padded collar

Easy access

Padded tongue

Secure fastening and
adjustable

Soft supple leather

Cushioned
insock

Hard wearing
grip sole

Highly flexible
light weight sole

Spacious natural
foot shape

Figure 6.7 Example of the features to look for in the 'ideal' shoe.

more than 1.5 inches/4 cm as the child reaches teens.

- **Broad base of heel**. The shape of the external heel should be as wide as the seat of the heel, with straight sides rather than being tapered, to give stability. It should ideally be made from a shock-absorbing material.

- **Soling material**. This should be a slip-resistant and shock-absorbing material that retains good flexibility and wear quality.

- **Retaining mechanism (medium)**. This is the term used to describe how the shoe is kept on the foot. Ideally the shoe should be held on by laces, Velcro® or a bar and buckle fastening. A good test of the functional fastening is that the child should not be able to remove the shoe without first undoing it. However, the modern trend of loosely fixing the laces so that they don't have to be retied each time completely defeats their purpose and should be actively discouraged.

- **Upper material**. Ideally this should be leather and have a Gore-tex® type lining if the footwear is likely to be subjected to prolonged wet conditions. Synthetic materials can cause the foot to sweat excessively and consequently increase the risk of fungal infections, verrucae and nail problems.

- **Toe area**. The shape of the toe space should match the outline of the end of the toes and should be rounded rather than pointed. Adequate depth in the shoe is very important to protect the toes and nails from trauma. However, beware of overfitting in length or depth, as too much space can also be harmful, causing deep vamp creasing and improper flexion which can, in turn, also do damage to the developing foot.

Prescription considerations

The commonest problem with shoes for early walkers is that the soles are either too flexible or too rigid.

Shoes that are too flexible in the midfoot region offer nothing to restrict excessive pronation. Footwear that is too rigid hinders natural walking, as the child may not be strong enough to flex the shoe, and hence may prefer to walk without shoes (Thompson & Volpe 2001).

Orthopaedic prescription footwear has:

- A rigid counter to discourage calcaneal eversion
- A rigid shank to limit subtalar and midtarsal joint pronation
- A flexible forefoot to encourage the development of the propulsive phase of gait.

In paediatric orthopaedic shoes, the counters are often very firm indeed to create a support for the foot which is functionally impaired, particularly if the muscle tone is very weak. Long inside counters also are common, again to keep the overpronated foot secure or to aid the function of orthoses.

Ankle–foot orthoses (AFOs)

It is not always necessary to prescribe shoes for AFOs. Many can be accommodated in retail shoes; however, when the AFO is worn unilaterally, poor shoe fitting can result for the 'good foot' if the shoes are oversized to accommodate the AFO.

Prescription footwear to accommodate AFOs is now readily available from surgical footwear manufacturers. This footwear has a deeper counter and lower facings to allow ease of entry. It is important that the footwear prescribed aids the function of the foot, and also allows any orthotics, such as an AFO, to achieve their full potential for the child.

Limb length discrepancy (LLD) is a common condition with children, and adding a raise to their shoes is a simple process as most reasonable quality children's shoes can be adapted. However, where both a shoe raise and callipers are required, prescription footwear is preferable as it is stronger in its construction.

It is the ultimate goal in paediatric cases to minimize the risk of a permanent equinus foot position and encourage full ankle range of motion, especially when the LLD is in the mild to moderate category. To this end, but depending entirely on the diagnosis, prescribing a lower raise than measured and encouraging muscle stretching with regular reviews is a sound clinical plan. The raise prescribed may be half of the measured discrepancy in many instances.

Many children with limb length discrepancy are offered surgical lengthening before they are fully grown to correct any residual discrepancy, thus removing the need for a shoe raise for the rest of their adult lives.

Conclusion

The main purpose of this section was to discuss the properties of footwear and footwear fitting to support healthy, normal development in the child's foot. Pathology in the developing foot is not discussed. As with all patients, no matter what age, it is thoroughly recommended that the multidisciplinary team approach is sought when prescribing footwear and orthoses for the child with multiple pathology states.

Shoes for sporting and leisure activity

When examining its properties, it may be surmised that the trainer is the ideal shoe style for the majority of people. Most people have a pair of trainers in their wardrobe, even though they may not partake in any sporting activity. In essence, trainers are an excellent design but the particulars must be considered. Most trainers are made with numerous seams in the upper and these can irritate the feet when they are placed at vulnerable points, such as over a bony prominence or a joint. The materials included in the upper may not be ideal. They usually comprise of various materials including woven fabrics, plastics and leathers. Generally the soling is made of a flexible and cushioning material and the construction process used (Strobel) means that exact width and girth measurements are not critical and so will fit adequately a variety of foot shapes within a given size. The heel height is usually satisfactory, and the shape of the heel and sole unit and its texture give stability in gait. Trainers and sports shoes have a fashion element, but footwear designed for specific sporting activity does help the feet to function in the most effective way for that activity. All sports footwear has the same basic pattern but the construction technique used in manufacture will vary according to the type of shoe and the rigidity required within it. The properties of materials used in the various

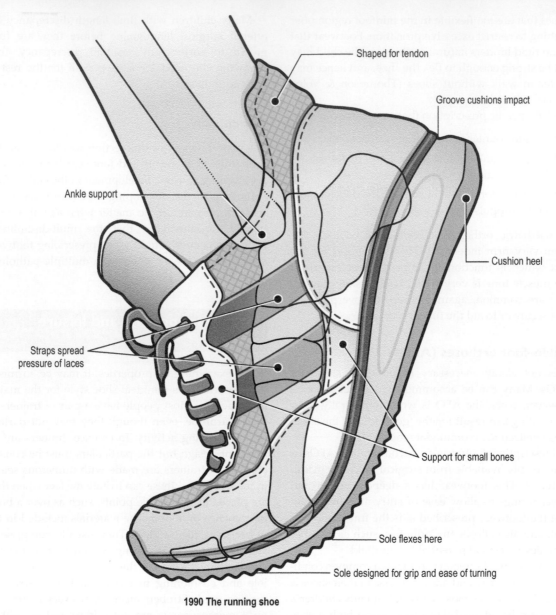

Shaped for tendon

Groove cushions impact

Ankle support

Cushion heel

Straps spread
pressure of laces

Support for small bones

Sole flexes here

Sole designed for grip and ease of turning

1990 The running shoe

Figure 6.8 The first 'trainer shoes' came in about 1990. This diagram demonstrates how the then innovative design worked with the foot structure for support and proper flexion.

parts of the shoe will vary according to the activity required (Fig. 6.8).

In general, where firm footing is required during relatively slow-paced walking-type activity, the footwear will include fairly rigid soles, stiff heel counters and firm toe puffs. This is the case for golf, rambling, hiking and mountaineering. Where walking over rough terrain is involved, such as in hill-walking and

mountaineering, boots are preferred to shoes as they give stability to the ankle joint. The heel counters in such boots will not only be strengthened but will also be extended, both proximally from the malleoli and distally through to the midfoot, in order to give firm control and minimize the likelihood of ankle damage. The outer soling of this footwear will contain a ridged pattern in order to give grip. In the case of golf shoes, the outer soling will contain spikes or dimples in order to hold the feet securely in the turf while the player is taking a shot. Footwear for these activities may also have a selectively permeable lining to allow moisture from the foot to escape while preventing the feet becoming wet from ground conditions and rainfall. The construction methods used in this type of footwear will vary from traditional cemented construction to injection moulding using polyurethane soling materials.

In sports where activity is undertaken at faster speeds, the soling will be more flexible in order to enable the player to move rapidly when necessary. Even footwear for activities such as soccer and rugby will have flexibility in the forefoot. Footwear for rugby still tends to be boot style, with a higher cut to give ankle support. While this style is good for those who rely on lower body strength for power while scrummaging, some players, particularly backs, prefer lower cut soccer-style footwear to give them greater mobility on the pitch. Footwear for soccer is generally low cut with quarter height finishing under the malleoli. All such footwear will have strong heel counters with uppers made either of leather or synthetic material. Leather with its elasticity and plasticity will mould to the foot, but leather uppers can stretch out of shape when worn repeatedly in wet conditions. Synthetic uppers may make the boots lighter and may be cheaper than leather ones. Some manufacturers offer soccer boots with lacing positioned at the side of the boot. This is intended to give a larger top surface area for control of the ball. The outer soling tends to be rigid underneath the heel and midfoot but with flexibility in the forefoot to allow for rapid movement. The soles also contain either screw-in or moulded studs, although boots with soles made up of a series of blades are also available. Blades come in a variety of depths, depending on the model, and some soccer footwear is available with changeable blades. The use of blades is said to make turning easier.

Shoes for racquet sports again need to be flexible but also need to allow for side-to-side sliding while playing. This side-to-side movement is supported by additional stiffening throughout the medial and lateral borders of the shoe. Shoes for tennis are best with additional reinforcement in the toe box to counter the effect of forefoot drag in the serve follow-through. They also feature a herringbone tread in the outer sole to offer greater traction.

Proper shoes are crucial to successful, injury-free aerobics. Impact forces from aerobics can reach up to six times the force of gravity, which is transmitted to each of the 26 bones in the foot. Shoes should provide sufficient cushioning and shock absorption to compensate for pressure on the foot many times greater than that found in walking. The footwear must also have good medial–lateral (side-to-side) stability. Because of the many side-to-side motions undertaken in this activity, shoes need an arch design that will compensate for these forces, and sufficiently thick upper leather or strap support to provide forefoot stability and prevent slippage of the foot and lateral shoe 'breakup'. The shoes should have a toe box that is high enough to prevent irritation of the toes and nails.

The outstanding feature of footwear for faster-paced activities is its light weight. Shoes for sprinters, hurdlers and those who undertake other track activities are generally extremely lightweight and flexible. The forepart of the outer sole will contain spikes in order to maximize performance while running. The spike length may vary according to the activity and the surface on which the athlete is working. Sprint spikes tend to have a slightly stiffer spike plate, distance spikes are more flexible and field spikes are specific to events. For example, high-jump spikes will contain spikes in the heel to ensure traction while planting for the jump. Longer spikes tend to be used when competing on cinder tracks and for cross-country activity, and shorter needle spikes are best for rubber-based track surfaces. The uppers of this footwear will tend to be made of mesh and microfibre for lightness and to allow the evaporation of moisture from the foot.

Shoes for running, training and jogging need to have a comfortably soft upper, provide control and stability in the heel, provide cushioning for the plantar surface of the foot to counter the effects of ground reaction force, have good traction and be lightweight. Within these criteria, patients should choose a shoe which is most compatible with their foot shape and foot type. There will be a wide range of choice available for each activity and foot health professionals should advise their patients on the features of their lower limb biomechanics which should be addressed by the footwear. For example, some running shoes will contain an element to control pronation, and it is helpful for the clinician to become familiar with the features of the various styles available so as to advise patients of the types of shoe to select within the range appropriate for their sport. Needless to say, patients should ensure that the footwear they choose fits them properly following the guidelines for footwear advice included in Chapter 5.

Workplace footwear

Most people today have a footwear wardrobe with shoes for various activities and occasions, and some interchange footwear worn for social or leisure time activity with that which they wear in their place of work. It is quite important that the footwear worn is appropriate for the activity being undertaken wherever that may be. In general, men can wear classic laced-up style shoes for many types of working activity but ladies are expected to wear a very different style for many occupations. The favourite is probably the court shoe and this may be the culprit for many foot lesions and deformities. The fact that it is slipped onto the foot means that it has to be tightly wedged in order for it to stay on the foot during the swing phase of the gait cycle. Its elevated heel means that weight is thrown forward and the toes are compressed into the toe box. The generally slim elevated heel gives a small ground contact point which may lead to instability and an increased incidence of ankle sprains. The heel height can also cause knee, hip and lower back problems. When ladies wear this shoe style throughout the day during their working life, the end result can be deformed toes and painful superficial lesions on toes, the plantar surface of the metatarsophalangeal joints and on the medial and lateral borders of the forefoot. This shoe style is often the one of choice for many social and dancing activities, both of which make heavy demands on foot function.

Ladies whose work involves long hours of standing, such as in the retail environment, should consider carefully the way in which their footwear meets their foot health needs. Clinicians need to consider these effects and be prepared to advise patients appropriately.

Safety, protective and occupational footwear

The inclusion of this section is a first for a therapeutic footwear text and is necessary because we live in an age of health and safety legislation that has become very complex. The requirement for a worker to wear any type of industrial footwear that also needs to address prescriptive issues is becoming a more commonplace situation in footwear clinics and clinicians have a duty to be informed about current legal safety requirements. There are laws governing provision of industrial footwear, and in the European Union, European standards must be adhered to. These laws also apply to bespoke items as the employee will be at risk if the prescribed footwear does not properly protect him as required. In the unfortunate circumstance of an injury being sustained, the fault, if failing footwear protection is implicated, could be found to rest with the prescribing clinician. Therefore, it is strongly recommended that, before an order for any industrial footwear is placed with a supplier, the clinician should establish precisely whether the product will comply with Conformité Européenne (CE) standards. There are also restrictions in place for altering 'off the shelf' safety footwear, as these may compromise the protective qualities already incorporated and tested. Again, seek an assurance from the manufacturer or company undertaking the work that they have any special licences necessary to allow them to alter industrial footwear legally.

Employers have basic duties concerning the provision and use of personal protective equipment (PPE). The main requirement of the PPE at Work Regulations 1992 is that personal protective equipment is to be supplied and used at work wherever there are risks to health and safety that cannot be controlled in other ways. The regulations also require that PPE:

- Is properly assessed before use to ensure it is suitable
- Is maintained and stored properly
- Is provided with instructions on how to use it safely
- Is used correctly by employees (Health and Safety Executive 1992).

Assessing the likely hazards for feet and legs, the following have been identified: wet, electrostatic build-up, slipping, cuts and punctures, falling objects, metal and chemical splash, and abrasion.

Options recommended are: safety boots and shoes with protective toe caps and penetration-resistant midsole, gaiters, leggings or spats.

It is essential that anyone procuring industrial footwear is sure that the chosen item will meet both the product description and the needs of the individual employee. In the therapeutic footwear clinic, it is vital that the assessment for the provision of such specialist footwear is very carefully documented and verified with the employer, so that exactly the right level of footwear provision is achieved. There are three categories of industrial footwear to choose from. In some instances, the need for industrial footwear is not vital to the job but is given routinely by the employer, or it may be the personal choice of the individual involved. These situations allow the clinician some discretion in prescribing the best available for that patient rather than what is required by law.

Manufacturers and suppliers of industrial footwear have a legal duty to provide accurate descriptions of their products. The safety features of footwear are tested according to a set of European test standards written into EN ISO 20344:2004 (www.hse.gov.uk).

The original performance specifications of 1992 are given in an associated set of standards as follows:

EN 345-1:1992 for safety footwear

Basic requirements: safety footwear must have a 200J toecap. Other properties that may be included:

- P: penetration resistance
- C: conductive
- A: antistatic
- HI: insulating against heat
- CI: insulating against cold
- E: energy-absorbing seat region
- WRU: uppers resistant to water penetration/absorption
- HRO: outer sole resistant to hot contact.

The footwear then has a classification number, either I or II:

- I: made from all leather and other materials, but not rubber or polymeric types, as follows:

  SB: basic requirements for safety footwear met
  S1: basic requirements plus closed and energy-absorbing seat region, and antistatic
  S2: as S1 plus water penetration and absorption
  S3: as S2 plus penetration resistance and cleated sole.

- II: made from all rubber or polymeric types:

  SB: basic requirements for safety footwear met
  S4: basic requirements plus energy-absorbing seat region, antistatic
  S5: as S4 plus penetration resistance and cleated sole.

Additional specifications (1996):

- WR: water resistance for classification I
- Chain-saw footwear pictogram (shield enclosing chain saw)
- Firefighting footwear pictogram (a man with a fire hose aimed at a small fire with a strip beneath bearing one of the following):
  F: basic requirements met
  FP: basic requirements plus penetration resistance
  FA: basic requirements plus antistatic
  FPA: basic requirements plus penetration resistance and antistatic.
- Metatarsal protection (M): basic requirements plus metatarsal protection
- Cut resistance (CR): basic requirements plus cut resistance

EN 346 for protective footwear

Basic requirements: protective footwear must have a 100J toe cap. Other markings are as for EN 345-1 and classification numbers are preceded by a 'P'.

EN 347 for occupational footwear

Occupational footwear is not required to have a protective toe cap. Other markings are as for EN 345-1 and classification numbers are preceded with an 'O'. An additional marking is ORO: outer sole resistant to fuel oil.

The footwear products, once tested and certified, are stamped with the CE mark. The manufacturer also provides user information indicating the applications for which the footwear is, or is not, suitable. At present, slip resistance is not included in the EN standards 20344/5/6/7. However, the PPE directive indicates that slip resistance is a 'basic requirement' of all PPE footwear. As such, slip-resistance performance should be tested using European standard BS EN ISO 13287:2004. Note that if industrial footwear is CE marked and claimed to be slip resistant, it must have been tested and the coefficient of friction (CoF) test values must be available. Coefficient of friction values are not generally given in catalogues, but must be provided in the user instructions which can be requested from the manufacturer.

Standards update

The European and international standards for safety footwear published in 2004 have found widespread acceptance and usage, both within the EU and globally. Known as the 20344 series, these documents cover first test methods and then performance requirements for footwear with different levels of toe protection, including shoes without protective cap.

These standards replace the early EN 344, 345 and for CE marking purposes, the conformity of the old standards has effectively been transferred to EN ISO 20345, 6 & 7. [These four standards are subject to possible amendment]. All new footwear styles CE marked for the EU market after August 2005 should have been assessed against the new requirements.

(With kind permission from Turner 2007)

- Resistance to chain-saw cutting: the various test methods in EN ISO 20344 and EN381 part 3 have been merged into EN ISO 20345. Changes include:
  - mandatory 200J toe caps
  - a fourth level (32 m/s) added to the chain speeds given in EN381 to cater for the newer, more powerful machines with longer chains.
- Firefighters' footwear: the Comité Européen de Normalisation (CEN) standard was published mid-2006 as EN15090. It draws on EN ISO 20344, 20345 and adds key properties such as resistance to radiant heat and flame and insulation against heat. New marking symbols have been introduced (H11, H12, H13) to denote three levels of protection.
- Slip resistance: slips and trips are still implicated as the cause of more industrial accidents than any other single cause, and reaching a consensus on the best method to use for measuring the slip properties of safety soles has been difficult. The method defines two key flooring surfaces, steel

and pressed ceramic tile, and two contaminants, glycerol and water plus sodium lauryl sulphate (NaLS), as well as three slip modes. EN ISO 20344 is in the process of being amended and is in the process of being amalgamated into an EN ISO which gives the first internationally agreed method for the slip resistance of safety footwear.

- Toe caps and penetration-resistant inserts: although covered by the EN ISO 20344/5 series, these components have also had their own standards (EN 12568:1998), however constant improvements in materials to replace the heavy steel with composites, like glass-reinforced plastic and heavy textile replacements for steel midsoles, have presented challenges in the way they are assessed, as they behave very differently to metal. EN 12568 is therefore being revised to reflect the changes that have taken place, and different methods for non-metallic caps and inserts are now being considered for the EN ISO 2344/5 standards.
- Motor cycle footwear: the current standard EN 13634:2002 is subject to 5-yearly revision and this will begin shortly.
- Chemical-resistant footwear: a new standard in three parts is currently being progressed and has already been approved by the CEN consultant. The three parts cover terminology, test methods and requirements for various levels of protection against specific groups of chemicals. A PPE standard should soon be published.

PPE footwear standards summary

- EN ISO 20345:2004: PPE test methods for footwear.
- EN ISO 20345:2004: PPE safety footwear.
- EN ISO 20346:2004: PPE protective footwear.
- EN ISO 20347:2004: PPE occupational footwear.
- EN 13287:2004 and ISO 13287:2006: PPE (footwear) test method for slip resistance.
- EN 12568:1998: foot and leg protectors – requirements and test methods for toe caps and metal penetration-resistant inserts.
- EN 15090:2006: footwear for firefighters.
- EN ISO17249:2004 (amended 2006): safety footwear with resistance to chain-saw cutting (see also EN381-3 for test methods).

- prEN 13832 parts 1, 2, 3: dealing with aspects of chemical-resistant footwear.
- ASTM F2412, F2413: effectively replaces ANSI Z-41.

Some of the above information is supplied on the Health and Safety Executive Website and is included here to raise awareness of the symbols and labelling that are currently placed on ready-made industrial items. This may help the clinician to clarify the type of industrial footwear best suited to the specific job of the client. Industrial footwear selection has to take account of several factors such as comfort, durability and any additional safety features such as a steel midsole. The final choice may have to be a compromise, especially when bespoke items are necessary.

Always double check with the employer before going ahead with a prescription for bespoke industrial footwear. Ensure that it will be acceptable for the purpose, meets health and safety requirements for that employer, that funding is available to cover the costs of production and that the footwear will not compromise the employee's insurance cover. If in doubt, search for a ready-made tested item or even suggest that the patient considers changing employment if it becomes impossible to meet these standards satisfactorily without jeopardizing the patient's foot health.

The question of who should fund such a special item also needs to be agreed with the employer at the outset. It is the employer who carries the main responsibility to provide such an item for the working environment, whereas it may be the health service provider who would be responsible for the prescriptive item that is not specifically for industrial work. Footwear manufactures are more than happy to provide an estimate of the cost before the work is started. This can be passed onto the employer for approval.

Point to note: The above information was up-to-date at the time of writing, but as the standards are on a rolling programme of improvements, it remains the responsibility of the clinician to explore the latest standards if and when prescribing safety footwear. As is clear from the above sections, it is a minefield of legislation, hence caution is necessary when getting involved in this highly specialized area.

References

Health and Safety Executive 1992 A short guide to the personal protective equipment at work regulations. (Web-friendly version revised 08/05.) Online. Available: www.hse.gov.uk.

Rossi W, Tennant R 1993 Professional shoe fitting. New York, National Shoe Retailers Association.

Thomson P, Volpe R 2001 Introduction to podopaediatrics, 2nd edn. Edinburgh, Churchill Livingstone.

Turner R 2007 Safety footwear standards update. World Footwear Publication. Jan/Feb 21(1):19–21.

Watt G 2006 Looking out for children's feet. London, Society of Chiropodists and Podiatrists. Online. Available: www.feetforlife.org

World Footwear Publication 2005 Guidelines for children's footwear and patterns (editorial). World Footwear Publication Sept/Oct 19(5):17–19.

Internet articles

American Podiatric Medical Association: 'Children's feet': http://www.apma.org.

Children's Foot Health Register: http://www.shoe-shop.org.uk.

Health and Safety Executive. Role of manufacturers and suppliers of footwear: http://www.hse.gov.uk/slips/manufactfoot.htm.

Health and Safety Executive. LAC number 68–7: Standards for personal protective equipment: http://www.hse.gov.uk/lau/lacs/68–7.htm.

Health and Safety Executive. Slips and trips – relevant laws and standards: http://www.hse.gov.uk/slips/law.htm.

Footwear and orthoses

When prescribing orthoses, the footwear in which the devices are to be worn must be one of the major considerations. If the footwear is unsuitable then the prescription will fail in its therapeutic aim. It is absolutely essential that orthoses and footwear are considered as a single therapeutic entity. The footwear chosen should not only fit adequately when the orthotic is in place, but should also enhance the function of the orthotic and should not hamper its effectiveness in any way. All too often orthotics are prescribed without fully considering the implications of the effect of footwear. Frequently it is assumed that accommodation is the only important factor, and while this is a significant consideration, the shoe can do so much more to contribute to the effectiveness of the orthotic prescription. The shoe and the orthotic must complement each other and must function as a unit. The orthoses are only as functional as the shoes in which they are worn (Michaud 1997).

Before prescribing orthoses, it may be worthwhile considering whether footwear alone might address the patient's foot health needs. In such cases, an orthotic device would not be needed, and a developing knowledge of shoe components, the properties of materials used in footwear manufacture and shoe construction techniques will help the practitioner make an informed choice about the most effective therapy for their patient. For example:

- Would the gait modification and pressure redistribution achieved by a rocker sole address metatarsal head overloading? Rocker soles with their axis placed at about 55% of the shoe length will eliminate dorsiflexion at the metatarso-phalangeal joints and thus maximally reduce pressure beneath them (White 1994).

- Would increasing the width of the heel of the shoe help to control a rear foot varus condition, either obviating the need for an additional orthosis or enhancing the function of a prescribed orthotic device (see Ch. 9)?

- Might a metatarsal bar placed externally on the outer sole of the shoes proximal to the metatarsal heads reduce metatarsal weight-bearing more effectively than orthoses (Janisse et al 1995)?

- Where hyperpronatory and supinatory syndromes need to be addressed, other external shoe modifications can be helpful. A Thomas heel can limit midstance pronation (White 1994), while a reverse Thomas heel, with the anterior extension on the lateral side of the shoe, can limit excessive supination and help in reducing the recurrence of lateral ankle sprains (Black & McCartney 2006).

- The material used in the shoe outer sole can also help in the treatment of certain types of foot pathology. Many new materials used for outer soling, such as the injection-moulded polyurethanes and thermoplastic rubbers, provide excellent shock absorption and can help patients who lack adequate plantar fibro-fatty padding or who have focal high-peak plantar pressures leading to tissue damage and to pain.

The practitioner must determine the prescription on an individual patient basis. There are no hard and fast rules as each patient is different, but modifications to footwear or a combination of footwear and orthoses can successfully address the therapeutic needs of many foot and lower limb pathologies.

Matching the dimensions of the footwear

If the prescription of orthoses is indicated, it is first of all wise to ask the patient to wear, or to bring with them to the consultation, the shoes in which the orthoses will be worn. Before determining the orthotic prescription, consider the footwear. If the footwear is inadequate in length, width, depth or style, or is badly worn, the therapeutic strategy will fail. The first principle of orthotic prescription is that the orthotic is to provide an interface between the foot and the shoe. Therefore the upper surface of the orthotic must match the anatomical profile of the foot, with adaptations as required, and the undersurface must always match the innersole of the shoe.

The orthotic must match the appropriate segment of the shoe in length, so, for example, if the orthotic is full length, its anterior border must end at the front of the inner sole when the orthotic is lying correctly within the heel of the shoe. If the orthotic is three-quarter length, it must end proximal to the shoe flexion point at the tread line. The orthotic must be the same width as the shoe and must reflect the shape of the shoe innersole. The heel, waist and tread line width must match those of the shoe. Similarly the profile of the undersurface of the orthotic must reflect exactly that of the shoe, otherwise the orthotic will not be stable within the shoe and will rock as body mass is transferred through the foot as it moves during gait. Matching the heel pitch of the orthotic to that of the shoe is essential, and information on the height of the heel of the shoe should always be included in any orthotic prescription, so that the manufacturing technician is aware of the degree of pitch required.

If the undersurface of the orthotic fails to match the dimensions and profile of the inner sole of the shoe, it will not fit the shoe and will cause either soft tissue trauma to the wearer's feet or will cause the shoe to become deformed and to function at a disadvantage, again damaging the wearer's foot. For each and every orthotic prescription, a template of the inner sole of the shoe should be available. This template can either be taken from any removable inlay within the shoe or can alternatively be made from an outline of the shoe. To do this, a piece of paper or card larger than the shoe should be placed underneath the sole of the shoe. Draw around the outline of the sole of the shoe onto the card. Remove the shoe and draw another line about 3 mm inside the outline of the shoe. This 3 mm reduction in the perimeter size will allow for the shoe seaming. Form the template by cutting along the inner line and then try it within the shoe for accuracy of fit and adjust it if necessary.

The primary consideration in prescribing an orthotic device is in-shoe accommodation: is there adequate room within the shoe to fit the foot plus the orthotic device? If there is not, do not proceed with the prescription until the patient brings shoes with adequate girth, otherwise it is unlikely that both foot and orthotic together will fit into the shoe. If the patient attempts to wear an inadequate shoe containing the orthosis, they will very likely develop

Figure 7.1 When including an orthotic within footwear, an allowance of twice the depth of the orthotic needs to be added to the girth measurement. In this illustration, the joint girth with the orthotic in place measures 290 mm. Without the orthotic, which is 6 mm in depth, the girth measurement at this point is 278 mm.

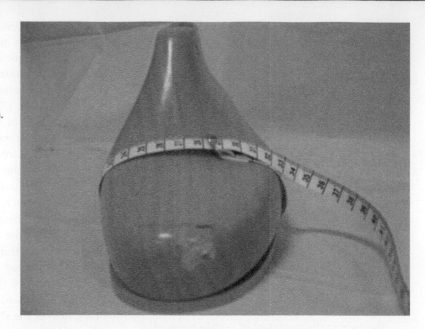

secondary lesions elsewhere as a result – and there is little point in treating one condition and causing another. Shoes to house orthoses will require additional girth at the instep, and across the metatarso-phalangeal joint area will also require greater heel depth. The girth requirement may be calculated by adding twice the depth of the orthotic to the shoe girth allowance. So with an orthotic that is 4 mm deep, the girth of the shoe in which it is to be worn will need to equate to:

$$\text{girth of the foot} + \text{lasting allowance}$$
$$+ 8 \text{ mm for orthotic}$$

The additional heel depth required will equate with the depth of the orthotic (Fig. 7.1).

If the girth and depth allowances are not available, the foot is likely to be damaged by the orthotic and pressure lesions may develop at critical points on the foot, especially over the first and fifth meta-tarso-phalangeal joints and over the toes.

Ideally the shoe should be built around the orthotic prescription. This is quite possible if the patient needs therapeutic footwear. Provided the patient's foot is relatively normal in size and shape, it is also perfectly possible to obtain a retail shoe with features adequate to contain an orthotic. It is important to be able to

recognize the required features in a shoe and to be able to advise patients accordingly so that they may search their wardrobes or purchase specific footwear which will both accommodate an orthotic and enhance the prescription. Many retail shoes contain removable inlays, and additional girth can be gained by removing these before inserting an orthotic. In the case of functional orthoses, inlays should always be removed from shoes and discarded or they may interfere with the prescription. For example, posts may sink into a soft inlay on stance, reducing the therapeutic value of the posting which is designed to function at a very specific angulation (Philps 1995).

Shoe style

The style of the shoe in which the orthoses are to be worn is important. In general, the best shoe is one with an adjustable functional fastening, a fully enclosed heel quarter, a deep waist section, a deep toe box and a low heel height. This is not to say that, in certain circumstances, orthoses may not be prescribed and worn in other styles of shoe, but certain features will need to be addressed and the orthotic manufacturer will need to be given careful and precise instructions about the style of the shoe in which the orthotic is to be fitted and the adjustments which will need to be made to the orthotic pattern.

The heel seat

If orthoses are to be prescribed, the first point to consider is the fit of the devices within the heel seat of the shoe. The heel seat of the shoe must be adequate in width to hold the orthosis, and the shoe heel counter and quarter must be deep enough to accommodate any posting, any required heel raise and the orthotic shell thickness without lifting the foot out of its correct position in the shoe. The back of the shoe quarter is designed to be curved to fit the standard calcaneal profile. If the orthotic causes the foot to be raised too high, the narrow part of the wearer's heel will sit above the coordinating narrow part of the shoe top line, the shoe will not grip the heel adequately and the patient will 'walk out' of the shoe. This is a very common problem and frequently clinicians fail to consider the depth required within the heel of the shoe to accommodate the rear foot orthotic prescription. Careful assessment of the depth available within the heel of the shoe is necessary if the orthotic prescription is to be effective while worn in the shoe. There is a limit to the degree of posting and to the height of elevation which can be effectively included in an orthotic if the shoe in which it is to be worn is to fit adequately. If the raise, posting or shell material is too deep, the orthotic–shoe combination will fail to function.

The base of the heel of the orthotic should match the dimensions of the base of the heel of the inner sole in the shoe. The orthotic base should be flat and not rounded; a rounded base will cause the orthotic to rock within the shoe, the effectiveness of the rear foot prescription will be lost and the foot will be unstable. The orthotic heel base width should match that of the shoe. If it is too narrow, the soft tissue surrounding the heel will be displaced over the edge of the device and the resultant tensile stresses may cause heel callus, fissuring, blister or frank ulcers to develop. If the orthotic heel base is too wide, it may cause the heel counters within the shoe to be deformed, and if the counters are relatively soft, they may stretch apart and splay. This in turn will have a consequential effect throughout the quarters, the top

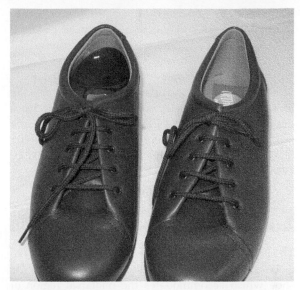

Figure 7.2 Note the difference in the profile of the top line on each of these shoes. The right shoe contains an orthotic which is too wide in the heel seat for the shoe. It is causing the top line to deform.

line of the heel of the shoe will fail to grip the foot and the shoe will slip during the swing phase of the gait cycle. If the orthotic is too wide in the heel seat and it pushes out or breaks down the lower part of the counter, then the top line will be forced in at the centre back because the counter is too strong to be stretched out, putting pressure on the Achilles tendon and forcing the foot forward in the shoe, which in turn affects the flex position and compromises the toe extension space, etc. (Fig. 7.2).

The heel counter

The heel counter within the shoe is extremely important to the functioning of an orthotic where rear foot control is required. The heel counter applies force in a cupping motion to the calcaneus. It can also apply force to the talar head as the foot begins to pronate to prevent the talus from adducting. The amount of force applied by the heel counter depends on how far the foot everts. The further the foot everts, the greater the pressure which can be applied by the medial counter (Fuller 1994). This of course is dependent on the strength of the heel counter. Where shoes are being specially prescribed for a patient, a heel counter reinforcement and, where necessary, heel counter extensions, either medial or lateral, can be prescribed and included in the manufacture of the shoe. A shoe with a firm heel counter also accompanied by a sole with a wide lateral flare or float will cause the foot to pronate faster. A heel counter may decrease the amount of maximal pronation but allow a more rapid pronation on heel strike (see Ch. 9). This is a useful adjunct to an antipronatory orthotic (Fuller 1994).

The waist of the shoe

The dimensions of the waist of the shoe also need to be considered. The waist is the narrowest part of the shoe which accommodates the midtarsal region of the foot, but is the most important area to consider because the arch height of the orthotic requires extra space here. If the orthotic is too deep in this area, the shoe will not fasten properly. If the orthotic is too wide, it will cause the waist of the shoe to splay and will distort the whole of the fastening and the proximal part of the vamp. The consequence of this will be that the shape of the shoe will change. It will become wider and shallower and may cause compression over the dorsum of the foot. It is also important to ensure that the quarters of the shoe are deep enough and substantial enough in this region to hold the orthotic in place. By including an extended medial heel counter, this may help in minimizing any medial

topple in the tarsal area and particularly will control talar head and navicular eversion (Fig. 7.3).

The forepart of the orthotic

The forepart of the orthotic must not cause the toes to be impacted against the toe box of the shoe and must not cause any additional compression, especially over the first and fifth metatarso-phalangeal joints. This may be a particular problem with extrinsic forefoot posts which may well push the foot into the upper of the shoe. The practitioner should be confident that there is adequate depth within the shoe at that point before prescribing extrinsic forefoot posts. In cases of inadequate depth within the forepart of the shoe, intrinsic orthotic posting is the only option.

Where the orthoses need to provide forefoot cushioning, materials which can provide this property while still low in thickness should be considered. The need for full-sock orthoses must also be evaluated. If possible, orthoses which finish proximal to the metatarsal heads or, where plantar metatarsal cushioning is required, just distal to the metatarsal heads, are preferable to those which use under-toe extensions, unless of course the toes are deformed and the apices need palliation. In this case, full-sock orthoses are indicated, but the shoe toe box depth must be adequate to accommodate both the deformed toes plus the orthotic, which can provide plantar cushioning to off-set the effects of ground reaction force on apical tissue which is unable to withstand it.

Figure 7.3 The left shoe contains an orthotic which exceeds the girth available within the shoe. Note how the facings fail to meet properly and are causing compression on the dorsum of the tarsal area. Compare it with the right foot where the shoe fitting is good.

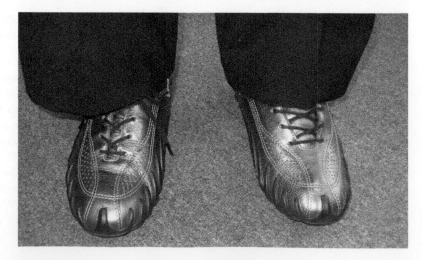

Fitting orthoses into sandals

Sandals do not provide the same degree of stability and control as closed-in footwear, but while closed-in footwear with low heel height and functional fastening is ideal for containing orthoses, this footwear may be impractical during warm weather. During those times, patients who need orthoses may wish to wear them in sandals. In general, sandals are not as effective as shoes in providing the frame which supports the action of an orthotic device, but where closed-in shoes are intolerable, sandals are the only alternative. Where sandals have open sides and open backs, either in the form of mules or sling back, then orthoses cannot be contained within them unless they are adhered in place. The patient may also be concerned about cosmesis as the orthotic device is visible in every area where the normal sandal is open.

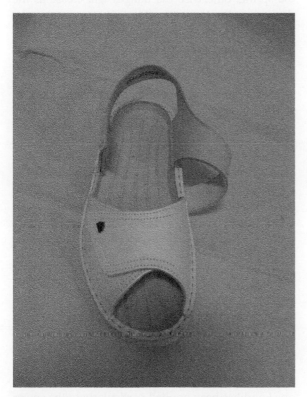

Figure 7.4 This sandal contains a well which can accommodate an orthotic device. Orthotic devices included in wells such as this need to match the dimension of the well and will need to be a full-sock prescription.

Some manufacturers now make sandals with a well which runs throughout the length of the inner-sole in which an orthotic may sit. This well is clearly defined and is effective at holding the orthotic in place. The well system works well for both functional and accommodative orthoses which do not include a prescription for high heel cups or a high valgus support. The orthotic used will need to be full sock and match accurately the dimensions of the well which runs throughout the length of the inner sole. There is, however, a tendency for patients to wear sandals slightly too small, as the foot can easily rest on the borders of the innersole without irritation from the upper – as would be the case in a shoe. It is clearly important that the footwear fits properly so that the functional elements of the orthotic are correctly positioned in relationship to the anatomical landmarks of the foot and the foot segments which they are designed to realign. The clinician will need to ensure that the footwear is of appropriate length and width before proceeding with the orthotic, even when a well is available to accommodate the additional depth required by the device (Fig. 7.4).

Normal sandals are often not available under therapeutic footwear prescription, but healing sandals to accommodate bulky dressings are sometimes available.

Pitching the orthotic

Most shoes and sandals have a raised heel. In a 'flat' shoe, this is usually about 4cm in height or 1.5 inches. There is an established relationship in shoe technology between the heel height and the point on the shoe which corresponds to the flexion of the foot during gait. The shoe flexion point is known as the tread line, which should be in the position of the metatarso-phalangeal joints of the foot. The front part of the shoe will then be elevated from the tread line forwards to the end of the shoe. This elevation is known as toe spring and gives ease of foot flexion immediately prior to toe-off in gait. The relationship between the heel height and the tread line of the shoe is known as the pitch of the shoe. It is essential that orthoses made of rigid material reflect this pitch. Rigid orthoses made without pitch will rock in an anterior–posterior direction when placed in the shoe. The higher the heel of the shoe, the greater the pitch

Figure 7.5 These sandals contain heel pitch. The heel height is 5 cm. The orthoses are unpitched and made of rigid material. Note that when the orthotic sits correctly in the heel, the front portion is elevated, and when the orthotic sits correctly in the forepart, the heel is elevated. A successful orthotic prescription for a rigid orthotic will need to contain heel pitch.

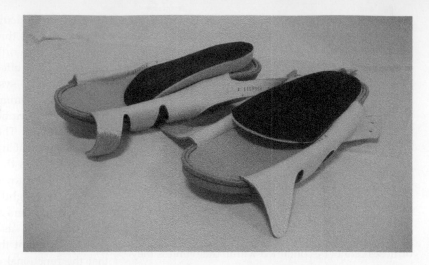

of the shoe, and the greater the potential rock on a non-pitched rigid orthotic placed within it. In the extreme, this could reach the situation where the foot and the orthotic cannot be placed in the shoe together. A non-pitched rigid orthotic will require the foot to be held at 90° to the ankle, and when a non-pitched orthotic is placed within a shoe with high heel pitch, the ankle and forefoot will be unable to plantarflex to gain access into the high-heeled shoe. It is essential that the manufacturer of the orthotic is informed of the shoe size and heel height and is able to pitch the orthotic to match the shoe pitch so that the foot position reflects that of the shoe profile (Fig. 7.5).

Pitching flexible devices is not as important as they can bend to match the shoe pitch. There is, however, one exception to this. This exception is in the case of certain types of devices which have side flanges in the forefoot, maybe to protect the medial side of the first metatarso-phalangeal joint or the lateral side of the fifth metatarso-phalangeal joint. If the device is not pitched, the material used in these flanges will crease and the creases will irritate the foot. These creases will occur at points where the foot flexes, and will irritate the soft tissue and cause superficial lesion development.

Where devices are full sock and extend to the toe area, they will need to be made not only with heel pitch but also with toe spring to match that of the shoe. This again is particularly important in the rare case where a rigid orthotic device is made full length. Flexible full-length devices will acquire toe spring in wear, but if they are made with medial or lateral flanges which cup the medial and lateral borders of the foot, they should also be made with toe spring, otherwise the flanges will crease as the device acquires toe spring (Fig. 7.6).

Orthoses in sports shoes

A proportion of patients requiring orthoses may be sports enthusiasts or may be wearing sports type shoes or trainers. These shoes should be carefully checked to identify whether or not they contain any heel pitch. Many have no pitch and so rigid orthoses without pitch may fit them well. However, careful examination of the shoe in which the orthotic is to be used is necessary. It is not only pitch that should be considered. Many running shoes contain antipronator control units and these may make it difficult to fit an orthotic device into a shoe. If the antipronatory unit is fixed as part of the heel counter and arch design of the shoe itself rather than in a removable insole, orthoses should not be used within the shoe. The necessary flat inner sole base against which to place the orthosis will not be available and no orthosis will sit comfortably and effectively against a permanently contoured inner sole.

In recent years, materials technology has developed and has been applied particularly to the sports shoe market. Many shoes, particularly those in the upper price bracket, contain complex combinations of materials now lighter in weight and offering a blend of durable cushioning and stability. Flexibility

Figure 7.6 This flexible orthotic has side flanges to protect the medial aspect of the first and lateral aspect of the fifth metatarso-phalangeal joints. As it bends (as it will do to acquire heel pitch and toe spring), the sides crease and these can irritate the foot. Any flexible device with side flanges should be made with heel pitch and toe spring to avoid such creasing.

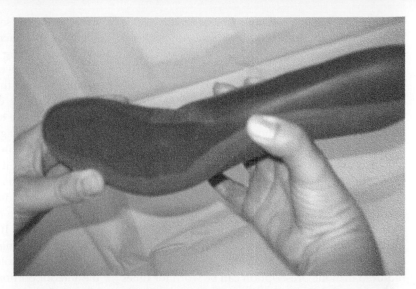

has evolved and is placed in the most appropriate position to satisfy biomechanical needs. This is achieved by the use of a combination of careful placement of materials and flexion grooves. It is important that the orthotic does not inadvertently jeopardize this flexibility. Most sports shoes, particularly those used for activities where fast movement and agility are required, have flexible sole units, and the anterior border of a rigid functional orthosis should be placed proximal to the foot flexion point at the metatarso-phalangeal joints, otherwise it will impair flexibility and activity. Any forward extension of the orthotic will have an effect on the shoe function and should be carefully considered as the orthotic will need to be fabricated with an appropriate degree of toe spring to match the elevation at the front of the shoe. Certain sports, usually those requiring slower, more sustained activity such as rambling or golf, use rigid soles. Orthoses made of rigid materials for those shoes should reflect the pitch of the shoe, and where the orthoses are designed to extend distal to the metatarso-phalangeal joints, they should also accurately reflect the toe spring of the shoe. Instructions to the laboratory manufacturing the orthoses should indicate the degree of pitch and the degree of toe spring required. The laboratory will need to know the height of the heel of the shoe and a measurement of the elevation of the end of the toe of the shoe when the shoe is standing correctly on its tread line.

Orthoses in fashion shoes

Historically, patients wearing fashion shoes, especially court-style shoes (pumps), were denied orthoses by healthcare practitioners. It now seems that practitioners understand that many people need to wear such footwear as part of a uniform or indeed may wish to wear it for fashion alone. For example, air cabin crew need to wear fashion footwear and are on their feet for many hours, especially during long-haul flights. Where foot pathologies exist, an appropriate orthotic within the uniform shoes will certainly assist in improving foot health and well-being. Many in the retail trade also stand for long hours and are required to wear footwear which is less than ideal for foot health. Such patients should not be denied the therapy they need, and because of advances in materials technology, it is possible to manufacture small, slim functional devices to fit within such footwear. These devices may range from small silicone half insoles placed under the metatarsal area or heel pads to semi-rigid devices with posting for functional control. Functional devices are often 'S' shaped with a valgus support and heel periphery extension into which a post is combined. Such devices are discreet and work well within the limited accommodation offered by a court shoe.

The treatment of forefoot functional anomalies within such footwear is, however, difficult. Because of the small toe box which is characteristic of this style of shoe, there is very little space in which a functional orthotic, or even a post alone, can be accommodated. Where forefoot pathologies are present and are symptomatic, it is advisable to try to discuss footwear options with the patient. A shoe of similar size and style, but of a different width fitting, may contain just enough room to include the required posting. A post alone, rather than one fitted onto an orthotic shell, may fit into the shoe if the post is made from prefabricated posting strips containing a preset degree of posting. This posting strip may be trimmed to match the inner sole of the shoe and the resultant post adhered in place to the existing shoe inner sole. Alternatively it may be that footwear capable of accommodating the required orthotic prescription can be worn for times other than when the patient is obliged to wear court shoes. Although this is not ideal, it is a compromise which gives the best available therapy to the patient while continuing to allow the required footwear to be worn to work.

Wearing orthoses within court shoes usually offers only limited therapeutic effect, and patients who need to wear this type of footwear to work should be advised to consider wearing less restrictive footwear which will enhance orthotic function at times when they are not in work. Separate orthoses will need to be manufactured for each shoe type, as those for court shoes will not fit other styles.

Fitting ankle–foot orthoses within footwear

Patients with conditions such as adult acquired flat foot secondary to posterior tibial tendon dysfunction, peroneal nerve damage and drop foot, old poliomyelitis and cerebrovascular accidents may be prescribed ankle–foot orthoses (AFOs). Ankle–foot orthoses may be fitted into shoes or boots which contain a functional fastening and which meet the criteria for the ideal shoe identified in previous chapters. Ankle–foot orthoses require additional room within footwear in length as well as in width and girth. The element of the AFO at the back of the heel requires additional shoe length, and it may also require the shoe to contain additional girth around the top line and in the long and short heel circumference

measurements (see Ch. 5) to ensure that there is adequate girth across the instep and to ensure that the shoe fastening position is correct.

The foot plate of the AFO is usually flat and may not fit the foot, the shoe inner sole or both. Ankle–foot orthoses are usually off-the-shelf devices rather than being made to measure, and if the patient's foot is not to be damaged by the AFO, it is first advisable to ensure that the foot plate matches the patient's foot in length if it is a full-sock plate, or in the case of a three-quarter plate, that its anterior border is placed just proximal to the metatarsal heads. The AFO should also match the dimensions of the inner sole of the shoe. If the AFO is too wide for the shoe, it will cause damage to the upper where it overlaps the shoe inner sole. If it is too long, it will damage the anterior portion of the vamp and will push the toe box and toe puff forward. This in turn will have the effect of making the shoe longer and wider but also shallower. The foot plate of the AFO can be trimmed to fit the shoe, but ensure that the finished edges are bevelled and are smooth so as not to cause any damage to the foot or to the fabric of the shoe.

The fact that the AFO footplate is completely flat, containing no pitch and no toe spring makes functioning within the shoe difficult. However, AFOs are usually made of thermoplastic material and, on receipt from the supplier, can be easily moulded by using a heat gun on the appropriate part of the foot plate. When warm, the part can be held at the required angle to obtain heel pitch and then allowed to cool when it will hold the new shape. To acquire heel pitch, the central portion of the plate will need to be heated and moulded so that the rear part remains at a height above the forepart which corresponds to the heel height of the shoe. To acquire toe spring, the area which corresponds to the tread line and the metatarso-phalangeal joints will need to be curved upwards to correspond with the toe spring angle of the shoe. These simple modifications will not only aid the fit of the device into the shoe, but will also facilitate the patient's gait. Alternatively the supplier may be requested to do this, but many are solely suppliers with no laboratory facilities available to them. In these cases, practitioners may have no alternative but to undertake the modification themselves.

Patients wearing AFOs may still need additional orthotic therapy to address foot function or accommodate foot anomalies. Where orthoses are needed, they should sit next to the foot on top of the AFO foot plate. Footwear should be large enough to hold both the AFO and the orthotic when the foot is comfortably in place. The additional girth requirements of twice the depth of the orthotic plus the additional requirement for the AFO must both be met. The orthotic heel pitch and toe spring should also match that of the shoe and the AFO, satisfying the same criteria detailed above, as if there was no AFO in place.

In many instances, only one limb requires the AFO, and this causes major issues for the patient in purchasing retail footwear due to the increase in length and girth needed for the AFO. Many patients using AFOs will require modified stock orthopaedic footwear to ensure that both feet are correctly and safely fitted.

Using blocks

Some patients will have undergone partial foot amputation. Unless the amputation is at a very minor level (for example, a fifth toe only), the effect on footwear fit may be considerable. Where the upper of the shoe is not filled by the foot, it will collapse if it is not stiffened or blocked in some way. This collapse will be accompanied by creasing and possibly bending in the affected part and also in the area of the shoe which surrounds it. This creasing and change in shape may have an irritant effect on tissues immediately adjacent to the amputation site. Blocks are a useful tool to fill in the part of the shoe which corresponds to the amputated site and so reduce any creasing or collapse of the shoe. They may be separate units which fit into the appropriate part of the shoe or they may be included as part of an orthosis. The block itself should be of semirigid material, such as ethylene vinyl acetate (EVA; shore 60 and above) or high-density plastazote, and should fit the depth, length and width of the shoe in the place where tissue has been amputated. The positioning of the block should allow for slight extension and forward movement of the foot, and the area of the block which is to be placed adjacent to the foot should contain an area of softer material capable of cushioning. This will lessen the impact of any movement of the foot against the block. This is especially necessary in the case of neuropathic feet where any damage sustained may not be felt by the patient.

Cradles (or compensating corks)

Cradles are the equivalent of total contact insoles but with the upper surface made to reflect the shape of the last on which the shoe is made and the undersurface made to reflect the inner sole of the shoe. They may be included in a prescription for bespoke footwear and are useful aids to the management of foot problems when the foot is unable to function from a fully plantargrade position. For example, if the patient has an extreme fixed ankle equinus or has a foot fixed in inversion, the cradle will hold and support the foot in its fixed deformity while allowing the shoe to function with its outer sole fully plantargrade. Cradles may be made of cork, EVA or high-density plastazote with a softer top covering over the cradle surface which is next to the foot.

A cradle can only be made accurately if a plaster of Paris cast of the foot is provided, as this captures the shape and angle of the fixed position (see Ch. 11) and forms the negative shell from which the last is then produced, usually using a liquid plastic foam material rather than the traditional wood or plastic form. Cradles very often include a raise as well which is described as an internal cork raise (Fig. 7.7).

Footwear and orthoses – combined therapy

For many patients, either footwear alone or orthoses placed within specially selected standard footwear provides an effective therapy in addressing a wide range of foot conditions. However, footwear with special prescription features together with bespoke orthoses, combined and operating as a single therapeutic entity, form an invaluable management tool for a large number of foot conditions. Table 7.1 suggests prescription choices for some common foot disorders where elements of therapy need to be derived from both footwear and orthoses.

Problem solving

No matter how experienced the practitioner, there may be cases where orthotic therapy fails to be 100% successful. Many problems may be footwear related

Figure 7.7 This cradle (compensating cork) fits within a bespoke shoe and contains a heel raise for a patient with a fixed equinus position of 25° (5 cm heel raise). It allows the foot to function with the heel making contact with the ground via the raise.

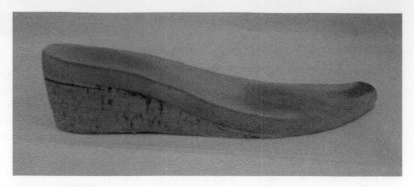

Table 7.1 Suggested prescription choices for some common foot disorders where elements of therapy need to be derived from both footwear and orthoses

Foot condition	Features of orthotic therapy	Special footwear features
Hallux valgus syndrome	Orthotic with rearfoot control and valgus support and, if necessary, cushioning under metatarsal heads.	Footwear with additional girth for broadened forefoot, with a rim toe puff and deep vamp over toes. Ensure adequate heel-to-ball length.
Plantar fasciitis	Orthotic with valgus support, deep heel cup with base excavated and replaced with cushioning material.	Effective heel counter and waist.
Achilles tendonitis	Heel raise, gradually reducing in height as condition improves.	Shoe with deep heel seat to accommodate raise. Possibly a padded collar.
Interdigital neuroma	Rear-foot post to control pronation and forefoot component to off-load metatarsals adjacent to neuroma.	Forepart of shoe wide enough to accommodate all metatarsal heads and digits without compression. Low heel height, ensure functional fastening to minimize compaction of forefoot into the front of the vamp.
Pes cavus	Total contact insole with reinforced valgus area.	Reinforced heel counter, adequate girth in tarsal region and adequate depth over toes. Lateral flare if necessary and consider rocker soles. Facings with 4–6 eyelets or more allow easier entry for the high instep. Padded tongue to reduce pressure on dorsum.
Pes planus	Total contact orthosis.	Strong heel counter with extension along medial side of midfoot. Medial flare if necessary.
Rheumatoid foot	Orthotic with rear-foot control, posteriorly placed metatarsal bar and valgus filler. Cushioning under metatarsal heads.	Determine gait pattern. Where gait is totally apropulsive, maybe rocker soles, but in the majority of cases, use flexible soling with adequate cushioning properties. Minimal seams in the forepart and deep vamp with rim toe puff to minimize trauma to deformed toes are indicated. Padded collar.

(Continued)

Table 7.1 Continued

Foot condition	Features of orthotic therapy	Special footwear features
Diabetic foot at risk	Total contact insole to equalize plantar pressures, laminated with firm base and cushioning top layer.	Shoe with rim toe puff. Deep vamp. Soft upper material containing no seams. Alternatively, very soft, seam-free full leather linings with a firmer upper material allow more control and reduce torsion that can occur if shoe is too soft. In all cases, a firm sole but not rigid with a rocker if required rather than too flexible to complement the orthotics.
Charcot deformity	Total contact insole with firm valgus control, but cushioned foot contact.	Preferably boots with reinforced heel counters extended medially into waist area. Rocker soles.
Charcot rocker bottom foot	Total contact insole.	Preferably boots with reinforced heel counters extended medially into waist area. Rocker soles.
Partial foot amputation	Total contact insole with block for amputated area.	May need shoe which extends high up the foot, or alternatively a boot. Ensure that the tread line of the shoe or boot is in the optimal position for gait – in the case of forefoot amputation, this may be within the blocked area of the footwear (consider the original shoe size before surgery). Rocker sole.
Posterior tibial tendon dysfunction	Orthotic with valgus support, and posting for any associated forefoot varus.	Firm heel counter extended medially. In extreme cases, consider medial flare.
Posterior tibial tendon rupture	AFO and orthotic to support medial segment of the foot.	Footwear with adequate girth to accommodate AFO and orthotics. 4–6 eyelets for easier access with the AFO in position.

Table 7.2 Common footwear-associated problems when wearing orthoses

Problem	Cause	Solution
Pressure or pinching is felt around the heel seat of the orthosis.	Heel seat of the orthosis is too narrow and tissue is displaced over the edge of the orthosis and into the heel seat of the shoe.	Remake orthoses with correct width heel seat.
Heel lifts out of the shoe when walking.	Orthotic shell material is too thick.	Reduce thickness or remake orthotic using a more rigid material at a lower thickness.
	Rear foot post is too thick.	If possible, reduce post thickness without losing the post angle. If not possible, change footwear to a shoe with deeper heel counters and quarters.

(Continued)

Table 7.2 Continued

Problem	Cause	Solution
	Raise is too great.	Check that raise is of the required height. If too high, reduce it.
	Orthotic is too wide and is causing the heel counter within the shoe to splay.	Reduce width of orthotic at the heel or choose shoe with wider heel seat.
	Height of shoe heel quarter and counter is too low.	Choose shoe with deeper quarters and counters.
The shoe quarter fails to grip the heel.	Heel base of orthotic is too wide.	Narrow the heel base width of the orthotic.
Orthosis squeaks during walking.	Movement of the orthosis in the shoe causing rubbing against the shoe upper or insole material.	Check the fit of the orthosis and adjust if necessary. If fit is good, sprinkle talcum powder inside shoe.
Foot slides forward on the orthosis.	No functional fastening on the shoe to hold the foot in place.	Advise patients to wear shoes with fastenings, and to ensure that they use the fastening effectively.
	The surface of the orthosis is slippery.	Re-cover the orthosis in a different material.
	The shoe heel height is too high.	Patient to choose shoe with lower heel height, but note that pitch of orthotic will need to be adjusted to match new heel height.
Orthosis slips forward in the shoe.	Orthosis does not fit shoe.	Either adjust or remake orthosis.
	Orthotic has too high a heel pitch for the shoe.	If possible, reduce heel pitch on orthotic by reheating appropriate point of thermoplastic material. Remake orthotic with lower heel pitch.
Orthotic rocks from side to side following on from heel strike.	Base of orthotic is not flat and does not match the surface contour of the shoe inner sole.	Flatten the base of the orthotic.
There is a gap between the patient's heel and the back of the shoe.	Foot sits too far forward on the heel seat of the orthosis because the perimeter of the heel seat of the orthotic is too wide.	Reduce material around the heel seat perimeter of the orthotic.
	The material at the back of the heel of the orthotic has not been under-bevelled and does not match the profile of the heel counter of the shoe.	Adjust bevel.
Top line of counter rubs the Achilles tendon.	Heel seat of orthotic is too wide causing distortion of counter which pulls top line in above the counter.	Reduce material around the heel seat perimeter of the orthotics. Check heel-to-ball length of footwear. If too short, will also cause top line distortion.
Dorsum of the toes rub against the upper of the shoe.	Orthosis is too bulky.	Reduce thickness of orthosis or use footwear with deeper toe box.

(Continued)

Table 7.2 Continued

Problem	Cause	Solution
	Orthotic posting is too severe	Either reduce post if prescription will allow or find footwear with a deeper toe box.
Hallux abducto valgus pain increases with use of orthotic.	Large rear-foot/forefoot varus post lifting the medial aspects of the forefoot into the shoe upper.	Check posting. If possible, reduce the depth of the post and shell without losing the post angle. Stretch the shoe upper. Find footwear with deeper vamp. Check flex point of shoe is correct.
Discomfort on dorsum in region of fifth metatarsal.	Large forefoot valgus post lifting lateral aspect of foot into the shoe.	Check posting. If possible, reduce the depth of the post and shell without losing the post angle. Stretch the shoe upper. Find footwear with deeper vamp.
Interdigital neuritis continues despite use of orthotic.	Patient continues to wear tight-fitting shoes or overly flexible shoes which allow for dorsiflexion of toes that traps interdigital nerve against the transverse ligament.	Use footwear with a wider vamp and stiffer soling to reduce dorsiflexion.
Pain or discomfort around medial or lateral border of the foot.	Orthotic too narrow for footwear and soft tissues are being trapped between orthotic and shoe inner sole.	Remake orthotic to match shoe inner sole.
Lesions develop on medial or lateral side of forefoot flexion point.	Flexible orthotic device made with medial or lateral flange but without heel pitch and toe spring – sides crease.	Remake orthosis with required pitch and spring.
The orthotic is not level within the shoe.	The shoe inner sole may not be flat. Look especially for an arched valgus area.	These shoes are unsuitable for orthoses. Choose different footwear with a flat inner sole. Has the patient placed orthotics into a different shoe?
Amputation stump shows sign of lesion development.	Possible shoe collapse because of absence of effective block.	Insert block of correct size with cushioned area next to foot.
	Block included is too large and is irritating adjacent tissue.	Reduce size of block and ensure that the border which contacts the foot is cushioned.

and Table 7.2 identifies the most common ones and suggests solutions.

References

Black JA, McCartney WJ 2006 Orthoses. In: Lorimer D, French G, O'Donnell M et al (eds) Neale's disorders of the foot. London, Elsevier.

Fuller EA 1994 A review of the biomechanics of shoes. In: Jones LJ (ed) Shoes, orthoses and related biomechanics. Clinics in Podiatric Medicine and Surgery 11(2): 241–258.

Janisse DJ, Wertsch JJ, Del Toro DR 1995 Foot orthoses and prescription shoes. In: Redford JB, Basmajian JV, Trautman P (eds) Orthotics clinical practice and rehabilitation technology. New York, Churchill Livingstone.

Michaud TC 1997 Foot orthoses and other forms of conservative foot care, 2nd edn. Massachusetts, Michaud, Newton.

Philps JW 1995 The functional foot orthosis. New York, Churchill Livingstone.

White JM 1994 Custom shoe therapy. In: Jones LJ (ed) Shoes, orthoses and related biomechanics. Clinics in Podiatric Medicine and Surgery 11(2):259–270.

Prescription footwear

for any orthopaedic, physiotherapy or podiatry need allows the patient to be seen quickly, assessed and referred to the most appropriate clinical specialist. Footwear therapy has often been overlooked or ignored because of the previously complicated and tortuous referral route and also because of long waiting times for appointments, but the triage system has obviated this. There is therefore some merit in providing additional training in basic footwear assessment to enable the triage clinician to become familiar with the most appropriate clinical specialist for the range of foot health conditions. It is in the triage setting that patient evaluation begins.

Indications for prescription footwear

The success of any therapy, and particularly that of therapeutic footwear, is dependent on thorough and accurate patient assessment. The initial footwear assessment should include an evaluation of both foot health and footwear needs. The evaluation of these two inseparable aspects of health should become part of the specialist clinician's assessment strategy and should also become part of the triage procedure, particularly in cases where the patient has been referred for triage by a generalist rather than by another consultant. The recent introduction of triage for referrals

Common conditions likely to benefit from therapeutic footwear

There are many conditions seen regularly in foot clinics which would respond positively to the prescription of therapeutic footwear. They vary from localized pathologies such as digital deformity to multisystem conditions such as diabetes mellitus. A diagnosis of pathology does not necessarily indicate therapeutic footwear prescription, but often the extent and severity of the condition will be a guide which infers that footwear would provide a useful tool in the therapeutic armoury available for the patient.

However, footwear as a therapy often seems far from the clinician's thought. A combination of lack of footwear knowledge, inaccessible referral routes and restricted budgets for therapeutic footwear may often leave patients faced with either no offer of help or perhaps given advice they either cannot afford to implement or find impossible to achieve. By improving the triage process to include footwear assessment at the initial appointment, and only referring those patients in obvious need and who indicate concordance, time will be saved and inappropriate prescribing avoided, and the budget will be used more effectively.

The types of condition commonly seen in foot clinics include (Figs 8.1–8.4):

- All types of arthritis, from generalized osteoarthrosis in small joints to rheumatoid disease: in such cases, joint function may be impaired and foot shape may be abnormal. Patients will have difficulty in fitting their feet into retail footwear without sustaining pain and damage. Carefully prescribed orthopaedic footwear can do much to improve mobility and joint function and aid the healing of superficial lesions.

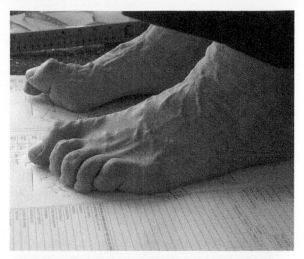

Figure 8.2 Example of severe toe deformities, right retracted trigger toe, lesser toes clawed and visible prominent superficial veins.

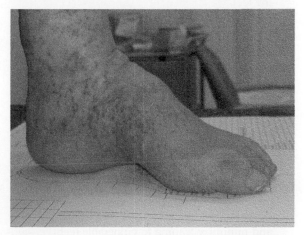

Figure 8.3 Example of a classic pes cavus foot shape.

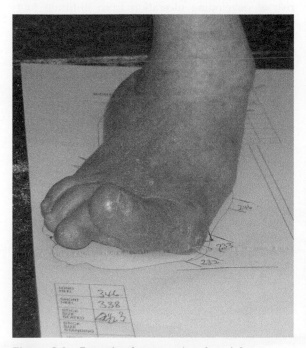

Figure 8.1 Example of severe valgus foot deformity with hallux valgus complicated by osteoarthritis.

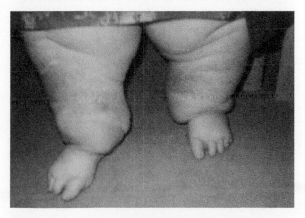

Figure 8.4 Example of bilateral lymph oedema.

- Cases where there have been orthopaedic interventions/surgery as a result of accidents and injuries affecting the lower limbs and feet: in such cases, the biomechanics of the foot may have changed. The use of features such as sole modifications can be helpful in overcoming any gait anomalies which may develop.

- Patients who have suffered scarring as a result of burns, tissue grafts and muscle flap repairs to debriding injuries: these patients may develop contractures and thus may have an altered gait pattern. Prescription footwear can help ease any discomfort from inappropriately fitting shoes and can improve gait.

- Cases of diabetes: where the complications of the disease have affected the feet, footwear may be used to redistribute any areas of high plantar pressure and provide a non-irritant housing for the feet.

- Patients with leg ulcers who may have suffered contractures or may need to wear heavy dressings to treat their leg wounds.

- Lower limb or foot oedema: this can lead to considerable difficulty in finding footwear which fits and protects the feet. Patients may be unable to fit their feet into normal retail footwear and may benefit from the additional width and depth available in therapeutic footwear.

- Peripheral vascular disease: this may lead to atrophy of the skin and nails of the foot, and may cause severe pain. Appropriately prescribed footwear can help to insulate the foot and minimize trauma to vulnerable feet.

- Conditions where gait is abnormal and mobility is difficult: these include pathologies such as multiple sclerosis and cerebral palsy which may be helped considerably by the careful prescription of therapeutic footwear.

- Severe dermatological conditions such as psoriasis, epidemolysis bullosa, eczema: these lead to poor quality of skin on the feet and may be helped by therapeutic footwear designed not to irritate the affected parts.

- Common foot pathologies such as hallux valgus syndrome, hallux rigidus, pes cavus, triggered, hammered and severely clawed toes: such cases may benefit from the prescription of footwear which accommodates the deformity.

- Patients who have an allergy to leather, chrome tanning, adhesives and dyes commonly used in footwear manufacture: the footwear specialist can help by prescribing footwear which avoids the use of these irritants

The 'at risk' foot

There are many systemic conditions which have an impact on foot health. Either the condition or perhaps the treatment prescribed for it may have an adverse effect on healing. Some conditions carry with them complications which directly affect the feet, including poor peripheral circulation, sensory neuropathy, reduced motor function or poor proprioceptive ability. Seemingly unrelated conditions such as reduced visual acuity or special educational needs may also indicate that patients are unable to adequately care for themselves and that their foot health is at risk. A carefully prescribed therapeutic package including orthopaedic/therapeutic footwear may provide a useful prophylactic aid.

In diabetes mellitus, patients may have sensory, autonomic and motor neuropathy as well as peripheral ischaemia affecting their feet. They may be at risk of developing ulceration from ill-fitting footwear or may have a changed foot shape which leads to areas of high plantar pressure and this may need redistributive orthoses. Such orthoses may not be accommodated within retail footwear and therapeutic footwear may provide a workable solution, saving ulceration and surgical intervention (Fig. 8.5).

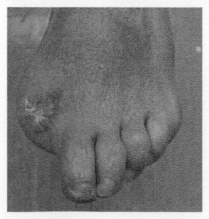

Figure 8.5 Example of a neuropathic diabetic foot after first toe amputation.

Where patients have renal disease or a condition where liver function is affected, any traumatic foot lesions, perhaps caused by poorly fitting footwear, may fail to heal. Patients with renal impairment may also display oedema with variation in foot size from day to day. Therapeutic footwear may be prescribed to address the oedema and also as a prophylactic measure to reduce the risk of trauma from ill-fitting footwear.

In connective tissue disorders and autoimmune diseases such as rheumatoid arthritis, lupus erythematosus and scleroderma, the foot may be affected by joint destruction, soft tissue changes and circulatory impairment. The patient may be in considerable discomfort, may have painful superficial lesions and have impaired gait. All such symptoms can be improved with the use of appropriate therapeutic footwear strategies.

The foot is at the end of the circulatory tree and any impairment in the circulatory status is likely to have an effect at this level. Footwear designed to thermally insulate the foot and provide a protective covering can help considerably in reducing the effects of the symptoms of peripheral vascular disease, of congestive heart disease and of conditions that involve Raynaud's phenomenon as well as Raynaud's disease.

Conditions such as anaemia also have an effect on the quality of the nutrition reaching the tissues in the foot. While all anaemias can have an effect on foot health, in cases of pernicious anaemia, there may also be a sensory loss and patients may be unaware of damage to their feet and may be at risk of developing ulcers.

Patients with conditions such as multiple sclerosis, post polio syndrome and cerebral palsy may have severe gait difficulties which could be improved with the use of specialist footwear and orthoses. Therapeutic footwear will be indicated for the mechanical properties it can include, such as specialist soling, but also for the additional accommodation it can offer for prescribed orthoses.

Limb length discrepancy

The human body is designed to be symmetrical and any condition which causes either an anatomical or a functional limb length discrepancy will lead to impaired mobility and frank discomfort. Limb length discrepancy is best treated by the use of therapeutic footwear which includes a carefully measured raise or elevation. Detail of evaluating and prescribing elevations can be found in Chapters 11 and 13.

Limb length discrepancy can arise from any of a number of conditions including:

- Epiphyseal growth dysfunction
- Fractures
- Poliomyelitis
- Juvenile rheumatoid arthritis
- Adult arthritic conditions
- Hyperpronatory syndromes of the foot
- Surgical procedures such as knee arthrodesis and hip arthroplasty
- Congenital disorders such as congenital dislocation of the hip and spina bifida (Fig. 8.6).

In cases such as those described, footwear may be considered an expensive option. However, the implications of failing to address the patient's footwear needs can have more costly, unfortunate consequences. The cost may not only be financial, but may affect mobility and quality of life, restricting activity levels and causing patients to become less independent. Prophylactic footwear prescription can prove to be a cost-effective clinical approach and can

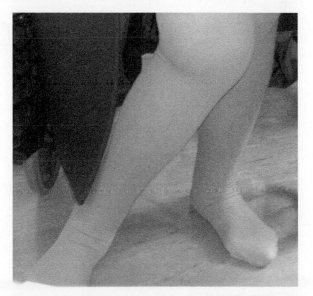

Figure 8.6 Example of long-term, untreated limb length discrepancy causing permanent knee flexion to right leg.

reduce the incidence of foot infection, ulceration and amputation.

Footwear features

In order to minimize the risks of damage from footwear and maximize patient recovery and comfort, certain features which can be included in therapeutic footwear may be helpful. They include:

- Minimal toe puffs and heel stiffeners
- Soft leather uppers
- Extra depth either at toe box only or throughout the full length of the shoe to accommodate orthoses, cradles or moulded inserts
- Stable, broad-based heel shape of suitable height (too low can be unsuitable for patients who have a degree of ankle equinus)
- Padded collar to avoid any irritation at malleolar level or retrocalcaneally
- Custom inlay/orthotic
- An acceptable means of fastening, either laced or Velcro® if patients have difficulty with bending or are unable to use their hands to fasten shoe laces
- Appropriate sole modifications
- Acceptable style
- Seam-free vamp with minimal stitching or pattern
- Padded tongue
- Light weight.

All of these features can be found throughout the range of stock prescription shoes. They are readily accessible and available within short delivery times.

Therapeutic footwear is not the universal panacea. It is designed for specific purposes and will not be able to address every foot condition. Shoes are prescribed and designed to:

- Accommodate a disability or deformity
- Be available in a design and finish which is acceptable to the patient
- Provide protection from damaging external surfaces, from the extremes of heat and cold and from the wet
- Not irritate the foot in any way

- Be safe for walking on a variety of surfaces in all conditions
- Reduce pain and control foot movement, particularly after injury/surgery
- Allow normal day-to-day activity
- Accommodate orthotics, insoles or partial foot prostheses
- Provide a functional solution to complex problems.

Patients frequently find that styling is an issue for them as therapeutic footwear is limited to low-heeled, laced or Velcro®-fastened styles, although colour ranges and decoration may be added to enhance the overall appearance. Some patients will find this footwear unacceptable, and it is advisable to discuss the need for footwear with them and to reach an understanding either to provide the shoes with the agreement that they will wear them or alternatively that footwear will not be provided. It is wasteful of resources to provide footwear which will not be worn.

Each patient's perspective on footwear is unique. On occasion, a patient may find difficulty in relating this to a clinician. Developing empathy with patients and learning to interpret their attitudes and opinions can be very helpful. Footwear provides a means of facilitating mobility by providing foot comfort and enhancing foot function, and can improve quality of life by enabling the patient to better undertake the activities of daily living.

In cases where patients meet the criteria for footwear referral, where footwear prescription is likely to be able to address their foot health needs, where footwear is the optimal prophylaxis and where the financial implications of footwear provision are balanced in favour of preventing further foot damage, all clinicians should seriously consider referral for therapeutic footwear.

Assessment

Competent assessment of the patient is paramount in the triage process (Fig. 8.7). Adopting a systematic approach to assessment and having a clear method saves time and ensures that the assessment is comprehensive. The following provides a guide on which an assessment tool might be based.

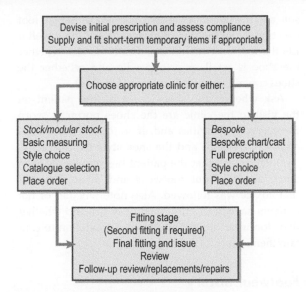

Figure 8.7 Assessment/triage flow chart.

Referral form

Read thoroughly the initial information included on the referral form received and note any particular requests (for example, stock orthopaedic shoes (Fig. 8.8) or boots), letters from other clinical departments, any additional appointments with consultants, planned surgery or any other procedures which might have a bearing on relevant underlying systemic pathologies, foot health and foot shape, and which might inform the prescription or the decision to go ahead with a prescription for therapeutic footwear.

Medical conditions

Take a full history, including details of current medication. Note the existence of any medical conditions which might have an impact on foot health. In particular, note the existence of conditions such as diabetes, any conditions which might give rise to lower limb and foot oedema, and any planned surgical procedures, especially those involving orthopaedics.

Podiatric condition

Identify the contributory factors which may have led to the development of any presented foot lesions. Take a full podiatric history, paying particular note to any previous episodes of ulceration, other significant foot conditions or previous foot lesions. Undertake a full foot examination of dermatological, circulatory, neurological and biomechanical systems and note all relevant findings. It is often helpful to photograph conditions so that progress may be monitored (Fig. 8.9).

Existing footwear/orthotics

Existing footwear can provide an insight into foot function. It will reflect foot action in the dynamic situation and is an invaluable aid to diagnosis. Worn footwear shows what the foot is doing when the patient is mobile, which is usually when foot damage occurs. It is advisable to check the wear marks on the

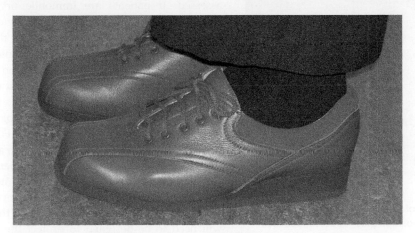

Figure 8.8 Example of well-fitting stock depth shoes with orthotics.

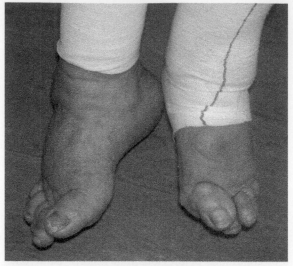

(a)

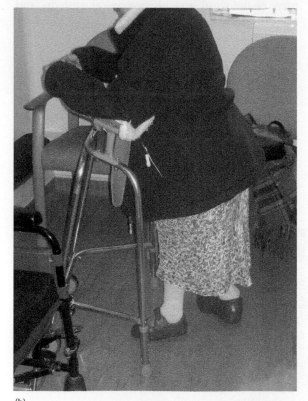

(b)

Figure 8.9 Example of multiple pathology footwear. (a) Right equinus foot position plus retracted first toes and oedema. (b) Same patient wearing bespoke footwear for the equinus helps to level the limbs sufficiently to manage some walking with the aid of a frame.

sole and the upper of the shoe and relate them to foot function. Note the size of each shoe and how well it fits the foot on which it is worn. Note also whether the shoe is retail or orthopaedic and whether the shoes contain any modifications (Fig. 8.10).

Ask whether the shoes worn by the patient on the visit to the clinic are the shoes normally worn for everyday activities and, if so, consider the suitability of the shoe and the shoe style for that activity. Identify whether the patient has previously been given advice about footwear and, if so, whether that advice was followed. Also note whether or not patients have been prescribed orthotics and whether their footwear has sufficient accommodation to contain them.

Footwear history

A footwear history can provide information on a patient's footwear preferences. It is useful to consider these, as a patient may have a justifiable reason for choosing the preferred style. If the patient has previously been fitted with orthopaedic footwear but has found it unsuccessful, it is useful to identify the cause of the lack of success to ensure that this failure is not repeated in a further prescription.

Occupation, activities and mobility

It is helpful to gain an insight into the daily lives of patients so that their footwear needs may be fully assessed. If patients are immobile or wheelchair bound, their footwear will need to provide a protective covering for their feet and support them during transfer from wheelchair to chair. Those who use walking aids will need to have soling on their shoes which facilitates the slower shuffling gait which often accompanies the incapacity which leads to the need for the walking aid. If a patient is in employment, the activity level needs to be considered. For example, the footwear needs of sedentary workers are different from those of manual workers. The patient's hobbies and activities also need to be factored into the equation. If a patient enjoys walking in the countryside, and regularly crosses uneven terrain, the footwear will need to be designed to protect the feet in this environment.

Consideration also needs to be given to the patient's visual acuity, which may govern the type

Figure 8.10 Patient fitted with the same style as previously, but the new shoes have a longer heel-to-ball fitting. Note vamp creases on the old shoes where heel-to-ball length was too short.

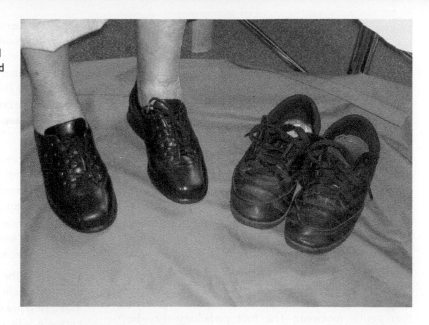

of shoe fastening that can best be coped with. The optimal shoe fastening may also be determined by the ability to bend to reach the feet, and the degree of flexibility a patient has in the hands. In some instances, Velcro® fastenings may be much easier to cope with than laces.

Factors which may affect concordance

While the practitioner may feel that a suitable footwear prescription has been devised for the patient, the shoes may not be successful unless the prescription has taken into account several issues personal to the shoe wearer. Patients will evaluate the footwear in the light of self-image. They may have expectations of the footwear function and appearance which do not match the footwear prescribed. They may feel that the footwear is designed for individuals much older than they are, that the footwear appears 'heavy', or is unsuitable for their wardrobe. The style which is acceptable to the patient, and particularly the fact that orthopaedic footwear needs to be fastened

onto the foot, is often a stumbling block. The patient needs to be fully aware of the aim of the footwear and what it can be expected to achieve.

Difficulties can arise with certain patient groups and it is important to have an advocate present in situations where the patient has learning difficulties. If the patient is from a different background to that of the clinician, there may be language barriers. Even when the patient's first language is English, regional variations in terminology can lead to misunderstandings. Where the patient's first language is not English, an interpreter may be able to help. Ethnicity is often important in making footwear choices, especially about style, component materials and the environments in which footwear is unacceptable.

Finally the clinician needs to evaluate overall patient concordance and give the patient the option of whether or not to proceed with the footwear prescription.

Cost-effectiveness

Orthopaedic footwear is an expensive commodity. Stock footwear can cost from £90 (approximately

US$180 at the time of writing) per pair while the fully bespoke option can range from £350 (US$700) to £500 (US$1000). These costs have to be borne by various bodies. In the UK, the NHS has a budget for such services which must be adhered to. Patients may wish to fund the cost of purchase themselves, while others, particularly in the USA, may be covered by Medicare or other insurance services.

While the cost of therapeutic footwear is high, this must be counterbalanced by the possible costs of not providing footwear. For example, where patients are at risk of foot ulceration, the costs of treating ulcers which may develop are far in excess of providing the footwear. If footwear keeps patients mobile and enables them to maintain employment, the footwear costs are far less than the costs to social services of supporting an unemployed person.

Not all patients who have foot problems need therapeutic footwear. The foot pathology may be adequately addressed by wearing specific types of shoes available from retail outlets. It is important that the clinician is aware of what is available and can advise the patient of what to buy and where to buy it. A selection of illustrated manufacturers' catalogues and a list of retail sources or Web sites for footwear are useful to keep in the clinic.

All these factors should be borne in mind in making the decision whether or not to prescribe therapeutic footwear, but before the final decision is made, consider too the implications of not prescribing footwear.

Clinical approach to prescribing

- Assess the immediate need. Is it urgent, high risk or non-urgent?

- Urgent or high-risk patients need immediate action if possible, and it may be best to prescribe a healing shoe, sandal or bootee initially.

- Choose a temporary short-term solution or long-term option if appropriate. For example, where a patient is wearing four-layer bandages, ulcer dressings or postoperative dressings, footwear will need to be prescribed and available immediately if the patient is to be mobile. Immobility may well have detrimental effects on a patient's healing capacity and may prolong recovery.

- Where a patient is prescribed temporary footwear, ensure that reassessment is carried out at an appropriate time for permanent footwear and ensure that a sufficient appointment time is given for the full assessment and measurement process to be completed. A general guideline is that temporary footwear is used for up to 12 weeks.

- Regular reviews are essential for all footwear patients. Temporary footwear is often worn for overlong periods of time. This can be depressing for patients and can contribute to low self-esteem and lead to a lack of motivation to get better. Long-term patients also need annual review for repairs/replacements.

- Ensure that the patient is referred to the most appropriate clinic, especially if there are different types of clinic on separate days. For example, where there are varying skill levels among staff, it may be that certain clinics are retained for the fully bespoke footwear service, while the stock orthopaedic footwear service is available on other days.

Decision criteria for stock, modified stock (modular) or bespoke options

In the triage process, knowing whether the client requires stock or bespoke footwear is very helpful as these may be supplied in different clinics or there may be only one clinician who can deal with full bespoke work. Making an informed decision at this point makes the whole process more efficient for the patient as well as saving clinical time.

A high percentage of feet needing orthopaedic footwear will be accommodated in stock or modified (modular) stock, which are available in a large selection of sizes and fittings. However, there are some very obvious foot shapes that will require a bespoke last. Table 8.1 makes a comparison of the foot shape variations and a guide to choosing stock or bespoke. An understanding of these decision criteria will aid the triage process considerably.

Point to note: As a rule of thumb, if it is necessary to modify a stock item with three or more changes, then choose bespoke.

Table 8.1   Stock versus bespoke: indications for choosing footwear

Indications for stock	Indications for bespoke
'Forefoot' only deformity. (If the foot has a 'normal' heel fit, there are lasts for this type of foot now.)	Rear-foot deformity of ankle or heel (varus, valgus or equinus) requires a special last and cast.
Forefoot and moderate instep deformity, i.e. correctable valgus or high arch.	Extreme forefoot deformity, i.e. gross hallux abducto valgus, over-riding toes.
Foot needs more depth or width than retail footwear allows.	Where measurements deviate from typical proportions, i.e. long heel-to-ball, short digits.
Orthotic prescription needs extra depth and retail footwear has been exhausted.	Orthotic or levelling cradle combined with other prescriptive features that may make modified stock inappropriate.
Cost-effective first choice, particularly if compliance is a concern, provided there is no 'major' deformity.	Major deformity, i.e. pes cavus, fixed valgus deformity.
Good temporary options available for immediate use over bandages, casts, dressings or for oedema.	At risk skin/ulcer areas requiring special padding, linings, etc.
Accommodating splints/AFO, especially if unilateral. Split sizes are often available. Calliper adaptations can be added.	Bespoke is occasionally required for AFOs or callipers when combined with other pathologies.
'Raise' where deformity or limited range of motion is also involved below 5 cm.	Raises 5 cm or higher require a bespoke item as they need to be constructed into the body of the shoe.
Sole or heel adaptations, i.e. rockers, floats.	Bespoke should not be required for simple sole or heel adaptations.
Split fittings in width and/or length.	Bespoke was traditionally offered for large size discrepancies but is not the only choice now.
One foot needs a modification only, i.e. unilateral hallux abducto valgus.	Major bone deformity anywhere on the foot or heel that changes the upper shape more than the 9–12 mm allowance on modified stock.
Single digit amputation but excellent fit must be achieved.	Major amputation requiring partial foot prosthesis/cradle.

Footwear sole and heel units

Chapter contents

Footwear can protect the feet from potentially harmful environmental factors, but one of its most important features is its role as the interface between the body and ground during gait. Footwear outer soles and heels can alter the mechanical load on the lower limb during the stance phase of gait (Mundermann 2004) and can affect biomechanical function during the various components of the dynamic phases of gait. The outer sole shape and grip are extremely important for effective gait. While the shoe upper and insole are primarily responsible for the fit between the foot and the shoe, the outer sole is responsible not only for traction between the shoe and the ground but also for ameliorating the effect of ground reaction force on the foot and for modifying foot function and ensuring postural stability. The properties of the shoe outer sole will also have an effect on the function of any orthosis which is used within the shoe, and it is essential when prescribing footwear that sufficient consideration is given to selecting the most appropriate materials, style and profile for the outer sole and heel units for each patient on an individual basis. The patient's complete biomechanical profile and the spectrum of therapies which may be used to treat any anomalies must inform the prescription. It is important to remember that the patient is the infinite variable and that each patient is unique.

Soles

Outer sole material

Historically, outer soles and heel units were made of leather. In most parts of the world, leather was the most suitable of the available materials for shoe outer sole use. Indeed leather has become synonymous with quality footwear and leather outer sole and heel units tend to be hard wearing and durable. However, leather has some disadvantages. It has poor slip resistance, especially in wet conditions, tends to have little effect in reducing the magnitude of ground reaction force against the foot (Perry 1995) and will absorb and retain water when underfoot conditions are wet. Advances in technology have made available a range of materials more suitable for outer sole units, many with varying properties which are specifically indicated for certain types of activity. Modern soling materials include polymers, most commonly polyurethane, thermoplastic rubber and ethylene vinyl acetate (EVA). The construction of these materials makes them particularly good at shock absorption. This is obtained via air flow through interconnecting air cells within the materials. These materials have visco-elasticity, but the overall effectiveness in reducing plantar pressure is dependent on the thickness of the material, the durability of its elasticity and the speed of recovery of the outer sole following deformation under body weight during gait (Even-Tzur et al 2006). Both viscosity and elasticity are important factors in reducing the magnitude of ground reaction force against the foot. A highly elastic interface will return stored energy to the foot, generally resulting in an increased force between the foot and the ground, whereas a highly viscous interface will absorb most of the energy of the impact caused by the foot hitting the ground. However, if a material were to be viscous without also possessing the property of elasticity, it would fail to recover its previous shape after impact and would remain flattened and so would be ineffective during subsequent strides. Thus an element of elasticity is required in soling material to promote material recovery before the next step is taken (Whittle 1999). A guide to identifying the properties of the range of soling materials can be found in Table 1.3.

All soling materials should prevent the foot from becoming wet, should tolerate the range of external temperatures which the patient is likely to experience, should be durable and possess a coefficient of friction high enough to prevent slippage, but low enough to allow movement across the ground surface without any adherence to it. This coefficient of friction of the outer sole material is important. It should be at a level sufficient to allow the foot to move easily across the surface without slipping, but also without gripping too firmly to the ground surface when the body's momentum is likely to cause the body to continue to move forward while the feet stay still, thus causing a fall.

The suitability and therefore the success of the footwear prescription will depend largely upon the choice of sole material and its appropriateness for the environmental conditions in which it is to be worn. When prescribing, it is essential to be aware of

the type of activities that the patient regularly undertakes, and in particular, to take note of the patient's occupation, bearing in mind that some patients may report themselves as retired while still working part time. Of the many others in work, it is important to remember that some may have more than one job and that all working environments in which the footwear is likely to be used should be considered in devising the outer sole prescription. It is extremely important to establish the types of surfaces on which the footwear being prescribed will be worn and the prevailing conditions which may affect its function.

Studies on safety footwear (Rowland et al 1996) show that the wear characteristics of the floor/sole combination must be considered in addition to the materials with which the sole unit will come into contact during wear. Certain chemicals will react with soling materials and will alter their characteristics. Some chemicals may even act as a solvent, completely altering the state and texture of the sole unit. The footwear requirements of patients with foot pathologies who need therapeutic footwear and who work in such industrial environments should be carefully considered. There are established legal criteria which such footwear must meet for health and safety purposes, and links with suppliers of such footwear should be firmly established to ensure that patients' foot health needs and the safety needs of the working environment are both fully met (see Ch. 6).

All materials identified for use as shoe outer soling are subjected to vigorous laboratory examination as laid down by the British Standards Agency (BS 5131), which tests the suitability of the material for this specific use and evaluates its wear characteristics.

Outer sole profile

The pattern and profile of the outer sole material can be helpful in ensuring stability. Footwear can help in facilitating a wide range of activities, for example the risk of slips and falls in icy conditions can be dramatically reduced by the use of appropriate outer sole material with a surface pattern, and people who walk over muddy terrain will benefit from wearing footwear with soles which have a deep tread groove design. Experiencing muddy terrain can vary in situation and in extent, for example from walking for leisure in the countryside to working on building sites. For all patients, the need to consider the grip offered by the soling material is paramount, as slips, trips and falls on level ground account for a large number of injuries. In the UK alone, it is estimated that about 35 000 industrial injuries related to slipping occur annually (Health and Safety Executive 2004), and up to one million injuries caused by slipping need hospital treatment annually in the population at large (Menz & Lord 1999). Many of these hospital treated injuries may have occurred in the older age groups, and a careful balance needs to be secured between soling with a pattern which will not allow adequate facility of movement over surfaces and gives too strong a grip on the floor, in comparison with footwear which gives insufficient grip, as both scenarios may cause falls. This is particularly significant when considering the changes in gait which occur with age and the more shuffling gait adopted by elderly folk who have a degree of postural instability.

It is not only health and safety issues which need to be considered. Sole pattern can do more than just ensure that we do not slip or trip on the floor surface. Sports shoes are often designed so that outer sole grooves promote foot flexion at appropriate points (Pribut & Richie 2004) and, of course, sports shoes for various activities will contain specific features in the outer sole pattern. Soccer boots, for example, may contain studs for grip on turf or cleats designed to maximize traction, speed and acceleration. Golf shoes contain studs or regular nodes which will give grip and allow rotational foot motion while keeping the player stable. While this footwear is not necessarily therapeutic, the principles used in outer sole design of sports footwear can be applied to therapeutic footwear. Tread groove design is very common in footwear outer soles and generally it has been found that wider sole tread grooves result in better grip on most surfaces (Li & Chen 2004). However, it is not only the outer sole tread pattern that is significant in minimizing the risk of falls, but other factors including the heel height, the size of the sole contact area, sole thickness and sole flexibility all contribute to gait stability (Tencer et al 2004). Outer sole patterns vary considerably between shoes and will range from 'commando' type units through to almost entirely smooth outer sole profiles that are seen on slippers and house shoes.

Outer sole flexibility and cushioning capability

When prescribing shoe sole units, the degree of flexibility required should be considered. In general, if the joints of the foot have near-normal ranges of motion and there are no foot pathologies which require specific outer sole prescription, flexible sole units are preferred for general activities. The shod foot will never be as flexible as the unshod foot, and flexible soled shoes are best for everyday activity and for specialist activities requiring relatively rapid motion. More rigid units with a rocker element are suitable for slower, sustained activity such as rambling. Rigid soling units are also useful in pathologies where joint motion is limited, as gait changes minimize the requirement for high propulsive phase activity. Rigid soles are also useful in patients where load transfer from the metatarsal heads is indicated (see section on rocker soles, p. 133). Certain shoes may have outer soles where the flexibility of the sole varies from one part to another. This offers blends of flexibility and stability. Most work on combination flexibility/rigidity has been done in developing trainers, and a 'force flow/flexion' combination has been achieved by using firmer material at the rear of the shoe and using a more flexible material in the forefoot, allowing a natural degree of flexion at the metatarso-phalangeal joints assisted by the use of grooves and notches in the outer sole profile towards the tread line of the shoe.

A well-designed shoe can alter the centre of pressure during gait and can have an effect on foot motion. Softer materials will improve shock absorption while firmer ones will more effectively control motion. Manufacturers will sometimes include a combination of materials in midsole units. The chosen placement of the varying density materials will have an effect on controlling foot motion. Duodensity midsoles often have softer material on the lateral side to temper impact forces and decrease the velocity of pronation, and firmer material on the medial side to counter excessive pronation.

The cushioning capacity of heel and sole units can be a positive or a negative influence on foot function. Too high a degree of cushioning may cause increased rear foot pronation when compared with more rigid, firmer shoes (Prilbut & Richie 2004). Care needs to be taken in prescribing cushioning in the soles of shoes worn by elderly people, and certain studies have identified that a high degree of cushioning can result in falls as proprioceptive function, which declines with age, is impaired by the cushioning. Some researchers have suggested that the use of thick, soft materials in footwear soles can cause instability and falls, as this material induces a state of 'sensory insulation' thereby reducing afferent input to the brain regarding foot position (Robbins et al 1992) and this may be the case with elderly folk.

Heels

Heel height

The height of the heel of a shoe is measured from the point vertically beneath the lateral malleolus. The heel height relates to the elevation of the heel above the level of the metatarsal heads and so the depth of shoe sole material running throughout the shoe, including the area underneath the heel, should be excluded from the measurement of the height of the heel. To assess the heel height, the total heel height should be measured and the depth of the sole unit running through the entire length of the shoe should be subtracted from it.

It has long been understood that there is a relationship between forefoot loading and heel height. The higher the heel, the greater is the forefoot loading and the lighter the heel loading. We need to bear this in mind when considering therapeutic footwear for the treatment of foot pathologies (Broch et al 2004). Normal heel height for therapeutic footwear is between 2 cm and 3 cm and averages at 2.5 cm (1 inch). Certain pathological states will require the prescription of a higher than normal heel height. When prescribing the height of a heel required on a shoe, bear in mind the range of motion at the ankle joint. This is especially the case where there has been surgical intervention. Where the ankle joint has been fixed, the fixation may vary from the normal 90° and the required heel height for this patient will be determined by the actual angle of fixation. If an ankle is fixed at 90°, the heel of the shoe should be absolutely flat and should contain no added heel height. Fixation at other angles will require careful measurement of the heel elevation required to ensure that no additional stress is placed on the ankle and the forefoot. Modifications such as this would require a bespoke shoe because altering the heel pitch significantly alters the last and toe spring (see Ch. 3). Detail of how to prescribe such modification is included in Chapter 11.

Ordinarily, shoe pitch is set in favour of the heel with a difference in sole and heel height of approximately 2.5 cm ($\approx$1 inch). Increasing heel height increases forefoot loading (Broch et al 2004; Gastwirth 1991). Negative heels pitch the heel lower than the forefoot, shifting the body's centre of gravity posteriorly. This reduces forefoot loading, redistributing to the mid and rear foot. Shifting the centre of gravity posteriorly requires greater core musculature stability and contraction of muscle groups in the abdomen, while walking with a negative heel requires increased muscular activity in the gluteal region, the back of the thigh and in the posterior muscle compartment of the leg. Adequate ankle joint mobility must also be available as negative heel pitch requires additional dorsiflexion of the foot at the ankle and extension of the Achilles tendon about the calcaneus. While negative heel users may benefit from improvements in core stability, they might experience discomfort or damage in the associated soft tissue changes required to walk effectively while wearing this footwear.

High heels directly alter the alignment of the joints of the foot (Menz & Lord 1999), cause increased forefoot loading, alteration in the function of the first metatarso-phalangeal joint during the propulsive phase of gait, increased arch height, alterations in the articulation of the knees and ankles, a reduction in lumbar lordosis and decreased stride length. These factors lead to a reduction in subtalar joint motion during gait, and an increase in the supination angle of the foot at heel strike. Studies on balance testing indicate that increased heel height results in increased postural sway, reduced stability and increased risk of falling. It should also be borne in mind that some female patients who have worn high-heeled shoes over many years develop altered lower limb posture, and these patients may have a less stable posture and gait when they change to wearing low-heeled shoes. Where a low-heeled shoe prescription is indicated in patients who have a history of habitual high-heeled shoe wear, the heel height should be reduced gradually over time to allow compensatory lengthening of appropriate muscle groups, particularly in the muscles of the posterior muscle compartment of the leg.

During normal gait, the heel is the first part of the shoe to come into ground contact, and a wide heel base with top-piece material with an effective coefficient of friction leads to greater stability than a narrow heel (Rubenstein et al 1988). Wedged heels offer even more stability.

It is possible to increase whole foot stability during gait by increasing the surface of the entire outer sole unit in several ways. The combined sole and heel unit can be wedged so that the sole and heel unit are one single pitched run through from heel to toe, with no separate heel entity, and floats or flares may be used on heels or on combined heels and soles, as may other adaptations detailed below.

Adaptations to heel and sole units

While the outer sole material, profile, flexibility and cushioning are significant factors which need to be considered in all footwear, certain adaptations can be included during manufacture of boots or shoes, or may be added to the sole units of existing footwear. Such modifications can be used to address the needs of a range of foot pathologies. Adaptations are commonly made to the outer sole and heel units to accommodate fixed deformity and improve stability of the foot (Tollafield & Merriman 1997). Historically, orthopaedic footwear adaptations were made to the midsole (between the insole and outer sole). These included bars and wedges to help control tri-planar movement. With modern technology and the wide range of materials available, modifications are now more usually made to the outer sole itself.

The aim of the adaptation is to enable the patient to walk more efficiently and painlessly, and can help in the treatment of a range of conditions. For example, in rheumatoid arthritis or patients with diabetic neuropathy, pressure redistribution may be required and rocker soles may help. In cases where the medial side of the foot is required to take more load, varus wedging can help and will cause magnification of peak pressure, maximal loading rate at the medial forefoot and rear foot and a medial shift in the centre of pressure. The inverse will occur with valgus in-shoe wedging (Gheluwe & Dananberg 2004). Limb length discrepancy can have serious consequences for patient mobility, and shoe raises prescribed after careful examination can restore relatively normal function,

reduce trauma on the knees, hips and lower spine and can have a dramatic effect by improving mobility and having a positive effect on quality of life.

The sole and heel units cannot be effective without appropriately phased contact with the foot's plantar surfaces. Footwear must be well-fitted and adequately secured. In situations where the foot has an extreme deformity, for example a fixed inversion deformity or classic midfoot Charcot with rocker bottom profile, a cradle may be used to fill in the gap between the foot and the inner sole of the shoe when the foot is in its optimal position for function. Such cradles are made to fit within the shoe so that the foot is held in its adopted position, and the outer sole of the shoe meets the ground in a full plantargrade position. Cradles, usually made of cork, plastazote or EVA, can bring the ground into contact with the plantar surface of feet with marked deformity. Such cradles are made on bespoke lasts and usually accompany bespoke shoes. For further details on cradles, please see the chapters on bespoke footwear and the case studies. In cases of minor foot deformity, improvements can be made in the foot–sole interface by the use of total contact insoles made from impressions of the foot taken either using phenolic foam or plaster of Paris. These impressions must then be married up with the inner sole of the shoe so that the upper surface of the insole matches the plantar contours of the foot and captures any minor biomechanical adjustment required, while the undersurface matches the inner sole of the shoe. In recent years, computerized milling of these devices has become possible with use of computer-aided design/computer-aided manufacturing (CAD/CAM) foot and impression scanning technology.

Heel modifications

Solid ankle cushion heel (SACH) or buffer heel

The SACH is a heel where a portion of the heel material is removed and replaced with compressible material beneath the outer heel top piece (Fig. 9.1b). The traditional SACH places the softer material posteriorly and this helps absorb shock at heel contact, reducing muscular effort required for dorsiflexion of the foot (Münzenberg 1985). The traditional SACH or buffer heel is indicated whenever impact energy on heel strike needs to be converted into deformation energy, for example in painful heel strike,

Adaptations to shoe outer soles and heels	Function
1. External metatarsal support bar	1. To provide external pressure relief to the metatarsal heads where there is no room inside the shoe for an internal metatarsal support inlay.
2. Wedges 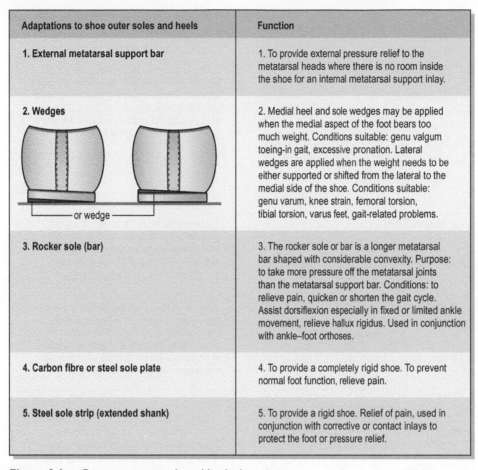 or wedge	2. Medial heel and sole wedges may be applied when the medial aspect of the foot bears too much weight. Conditions suitable: genu valgum toeing-in gait, excessive pronation. Lateral wedges are applied when the weight needs to be either supported or shifted from the lateral to the medial side of the shoe. Conditions suitable: genu varum, knee strain, femoral torsion, tibial torsion, varus feet, gait-related problems.
3. Rocker sole (bar)	3. The rocker sole or bar is a longer metatarsal bar shaped with considerable convexity. Purpose: to take more pressure off the metatarsal joints than the metatarsal support bar. Conditions: to relieve pain, quicken or shorten the gait cycle. Assist dorsiflexion especially in fixed or limited ankle movement, relieve hallux rigidus. Used in conjunction with ankle–foot orthoses.
4. Carbon fibre or steel sole plate	4. To provide a completely rigid shoe. To prevent normal foot function, relieve pain.
5. Steel sole strip (extended shank)	5. To provide a rigid shoe. Relief of pain, used in conjunction with corrective or contact inlays to protect the foot or pressure relief.

Figure 9.1a Footwear outer sole and heel adaptations.

degenerative and painful changes in the knee and hip joints and in weakness of the dorsiflexor muscles to facilitate roll over. The traditional SACH may also be used to compensate for reduced ankle joint motion (Wu et al 2004).

Where the softer element of the heel is placed posteriolaterally, the foot becomes inverted at heel contact, and this may be used to reduce excessive pronation in young adults. A lateral SACH (lateral portion of the heel is softer) is sometimes used to help bring the subtalar joint to neutral in cases of hyperpronation, particularly in adolescents.

Rounded heel (or round-edged heel)

The posterior portion of the heel is tapered off to encourage smooth heel contact, promoting loading and progression. This adaptation is useful for relieving conditions where there is painful heel strike and proximal joint pain.

Thomas heel

The Thomas heel has an anterior medial extension of half an inch which may be applied medially or laterally using a small distal extension to the anterior heel base. The traditional Thomas heel is applied medially and is designed to give additional support to the sustentaculum tali and medial longitudinal arch.

A lateral or reverse Thomas heel, with the extension applied to the lateral side of the shoe, will support the cuboid and tend to rotate the foot externally. Thomas heels reinforce the waist of the shoe and stabilize the shoe waist in the area where it is anticipated

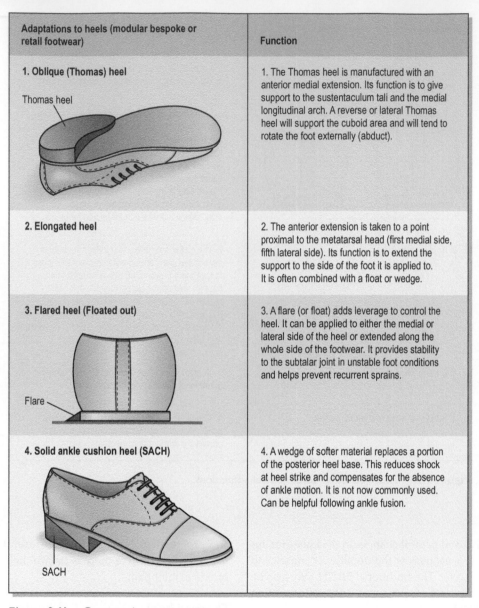

Adaptations to heels (modular bespoke or retail footwear)	Function
1. Oblique (Thomas) heel Thomas heel	1. The Thomas heel is manufactured with an anterior medial extension. Its function is to give support to the sustentaculum tali and the medial longitudinal arch. A reverse or lateral Thomas heel will support the cuboid area and will tend to rotate the foot externally (abduct).
2. Elongated heel	2. The anterior extension is taken to a point proximal to the metatarsal head (first medial side, fifth lateral side). Its function is to extend the support to the side of the foot it is applied to. It is often combined with a float or wedge.
3. Flared heel (Floated out) Flare	3. A flare (or float) adds leverage to control the heel. It can be applied to either the medial or lateral side of the heel or extended along the whole side of the footwear. It provides stability to the subtalar joint in unstable foot conditions and helps prevent recurrent sprains.
4. Solid ankle cushion heel (SACH) SACH	4. A wedge of softer material replaces a portion of the posterior heel base. This reduces shock at heel strike and compensates for the absence of ankle motion. It is not now commonly used. Can be helpful following ankle fusion.

Figure 9.1b Continued.

that collapse might occur due to increased stress from foot action.

Flared heels (floats)

A flared heel will add leverage to control the heel and increase the base of support. If the patient has a grossly inverted heel strike, a lateral flare may help in stabilizing the ankle joint. Similarly a medial heel flare will help if the strike is too everted.

Flares help correct foot motion at foot contact. They do not alter the resting position of the foot. Heel flares provide a correctional moment of force at the heel when the heel makes contact with the ground. This is achieved by the additional width of the flare moving the point of foot contact either medially (for a medial flare) or laterally (for a lateral flare). The moment created by the ground reaction force opposes the deforming moment.

Adaptations to accommodate callipers (modular, bespoke or retail footwear)	Function
1. Sockets a) Round - ask for spur ends, back straps prevent plantarflexion	Sockets are metal tubes and come in a variety of sizes according to the weight and diagnosis of the individual. It is important that you state the size and shape of the socket you require. They are embedded into the heel in line with the malleoli. Purpose: to allow the attachment of the calliper to the footwear.
b) Rectangle	
c) Spring-loaded callipers	Spring loading: allows ankle movement in dorsiflexion only. Can be adjusted to individual needs. Used for foot drop.
d) With backstop	Backstop: allows dorsiflexion only, or restricts ankle movement where there is limited function.
e) Medial (inside), lateral (outside) or double sockets	Sockets are only applied to the side required to hold the calliper arm. Callipers are either single or double supports. It is necessary to state which side the single socket is to be applied. Where double arm callipers are used, inform the shoe maker that this is the case.
2. 'T' Straps	'T' straps are leather additions with a buckle or Velcro® fastening that attaches around the ankle to hold the calliper securely to the lower leg. It helps prevent it from 'springing out' on weight-bearing. Double decker 'T' straps have two straps above the ankle. They are usually placed on the opposite side to the socket except where there is a double socket.
3. Stirrup strap	This is a less obtrusive strap and buckle that is attached to the side of the heel counter above the socket to hold the bottom of the calliper firmly to the shoe.

Figure 9.1c Continued.

Combined heel and sole modifications

Flares (floats)

A flare or float (Fig. 9.2) may be added to the heel of the shoe or to both heel and sole. It extends to the heel or heel and sole either laterally, medially or both, and increases the surface area available. Extending this contact base in stance improves stability, and increases the coefficient of friction. By increasing the total contact area of the foot, it reduces overall pressure.

A medial flare will result in a correctional moment being produced by ground reaction forces which will oppose deforming moments (Tollafield & Merriman 1997). This creates either inversion of the foot, so resisting pronation when applied medially, or when applied laterally, will create eversion which resists supination. Posterior placement of a flare creates an extension moment at the knee, and is sometimes used to supplement weak quadriceps musculature. Posterior flares also cause rapid 'foot-slapping'

Figure 9.2 Heel floats (flares).

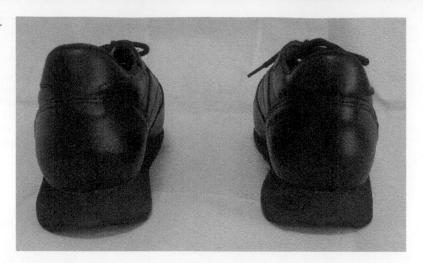

plantar flexion. They are not commonly used and best avoided unless extreme pathology dictates their use.

Negative posterior heel flares will shorten the lever arm between the ankle joint axis and the ground and will alter the velocity and range of initial ankle joint motion during heel strike by increasing the amount of dorsiflexion required. It is suggested (Michaud 1997) that such a modification should be considered in competitive walkers as a method of reducing strain on the anterior compartment musculature.

These flares may be extended along the entire length of the sole and heel unit, but in order to achieve this, a wedged sole and heel unit is preferred (see below). These combined sole and heel flares are useful if the foot is excessively inverting (lateral flare) or everting (medial flare). They increase the ground surface contact area and stabilize the foot.

Buttress heels

Buttress heels are an extreme type of float or flare and serve to reinforce the heel counter of the shoe as well as extending the surface contact area of the sole (Figs 9.3 and 9.4).

Wedges

Medial heel and sole wedges may be prescribed when the medial aspect of the foot bears too much weight, and may be considered in cases of hyperpronation or depression of the medial longitudinal arch.

Lateral heel wedges with anterior extensions will transfer weight off the fifth metatarsal shaft.

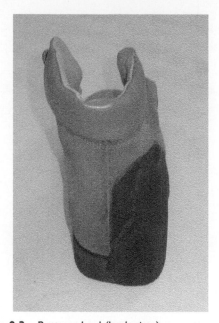

Figure 9.3 Buttress heel (back view).

The apex of lateral heel and sole wedges should not extend beyond the fifth metatarsal head as this will stiffen the shoe and cause two main problems:

1. In time, the toe will curl upwards causing the foot to roll more to the lateral side.
2. The stiffness of the shoe encourages the shoe to slip off the heel when the patient is walking.

Wedges can be applied to either side of the heel, over the whole length of the sole or used on a localized

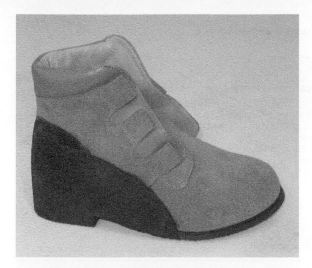

Figure 9.4 Buttress heel (side view).

area of the sole. Sole and heel wedges are used to tilt the footwear relative to the ground and may reflect the varus or valgus foot type. Four millimetres is a typical height; any higher values would tend to cause the foot to slide down the incline. For wedges to be effective, there must be appropriate range of joint motion available. Wedges can be useful in managing cases of pes planovalgus (medial heel wedge) and pes cavus (lateral heel and sole wedges). They promote inversion or eversion of the foot.

Contralateral wedging

This includes a medial heel extension or wedge and a lateral forefoot wedge. This combination was traditionally used to reduce pronation.

Through sole and heel wedging

This wedging gives greater stability in gait. The shoe remains flexible, but the ground surface contact area is increased and the central portion of the shoe is strengthened. People who play bowls will request this adaptation because they are not allowed on bowling greens in footwear with separate sole and heel units.

Sole modifications

Lateral sole wedges

These may be used when weight needs to be transferred from the lateral to the medial side of the shoe.

Medial toe wedges

These will discourage in-toeing, but should be used with caution as they will have an effect throughout the kinetic chain.

Bars

Metatarsal bars may be added posterior to the metatarsal heads on the outer sole of shoes in a line which reflects the angle between the first and fifth metatarsals. They help in off-loading the metatarsal heads. The effect is in fact to move the tread line more proximally.

A Jones bar can be placed between the shoe inner sole and outer sole. It is of the same shape as the metatarsal bar. It must be cemented in place and requires the shoe outer sole to be removed and then replaced on top of the bar.

Rocker soles (roller soles)

The prescription of rocker or roller soles requires careful consideration. Rocker soles are rigid with a pivotal point placed strategically from which the foot rocks or rolls forward. They remove the propulsive phase of gait (Fuller et al 2001). The basic clinical function of the rocker sole is that of 'rocking' the foot from heel strike to toe-off, thus altering both motion and force distribution patterns (Myers et al 2005). In gait, the body pivots over this central axis when the centre of gravity is displaced beyond the axis, rocking or rolling from the posterior to anterior sole. Rocker soles are used to restore sagittal plane movement, limit painful movement, aid progression, redistribute pressure and reduce loading time over sites vulnerable to excessive pressure. However, while pressure may be removed from one site, it will be added to another elsewhere on the foot and it is important to consider whether the site on which the additional load is placed can tolerate it without itself becoming damaged. Note that in some rocker-soled, below-knee walkers used in the treatment of foot ulcers, some load may be transferred from the foot to the leg of the walker.

The rocker shoe is characterized by a rigid sole that restricts movement at the joints of the foot, particularly dorsiflexion of the metatarso-phalangeal joints. The limitation of movement at these joints is believed to decrease plantar pressure by preventing anterior displacement of the submetatarsal head soft

Table 9.1 Table of summary findings of percentage load change at each of seven sensor positions for three types of rocker sole

	Hallux	First metatarsal head	Second metatarsal head	Third/fourth metatarsal heads	Fifth metatarsal head	Fifth metatarsal base	Heel
Toe-only rocker	−89%	−10%	−42%	−43%	+18%	+48%	−36%
Negative heel rocker	−44%	−7%	−36%	−36%	−5%	+23%	−34%
Double rocker	−87%	−7%	−30%	−24%	−7%	−4%	−25%

tissue cushioning and by distributing forefoot load over a larger area (van Schie et al 2000). Walking in the rigid shoe is possible because the shoe tips forward when the centre of pressure moves distal to the rocker fulcrum.

Schaff & Cavanagh (1990) suggest that the mechanism of unloading in the rocker-soled shoe may be some combination of the following effects:

- A redistribution of load over a larger area.
- An increase in the loading time for the regions of the foot in contact with the rigid sole.
- A change in the function of the foot due to the restriction of motion, particularly at the metatarso-phalangeal joints.
- A change in the patterns of motion of the lower extremity due to the altered geometry and rigidity of the shoe.
- A reduction in shear pressure on the plantar surface.

They further suggest that rocker soles reduce peak plantar pressures over the medial and middle plantar metatarsal areas but increase it over the lateral forefoot, midfoot and heel (Tables 9.1 and 9.2).

There are various types of rockers (Fig. 9.5). The toe-only rocker is the traditional rocker sole unit which is added across the tread line of the shoe. If it is added to an existing shoe, it will alter the heel pitch/toe spring relationship. The normal height of these toe-only rockers is about 12 mm, and to maintain the balance of the shoe, an additional 12 mm in height should be added to the heel height of the shoe. The toe-only rocker may be inserted onto the sole unit at the tread line or may be included in a wedged sole and heel unit.

Table 9.2 Rocker sole styles and description of use

Rocker style	Description of use
Toe-only rocker	Loads weight-bearing area of the foot proximal to the metatarsal heads.
The rocker bar	Effectively repositions joint line to reduce pressure at metatarsal heads – stiff soling is needed to prevent bar sinking into shoe.
Mild rocker sole	To reduce effort of walking, assist gait with increased propulsion and provide metatarsal pressure relief.
Heel-to-toe rocker	Decreases pressure at heel strike, increases toe-off propulsion, shortens stride length and increases motion.
Negative heel rocker sole	Redistribute load from the forefoot to the rear and midfoot, accommodate fixed dorsiflexion.
Double rocker sole	Relieve midfoot pressure, decrease heel strike, increase motion and propulsion at toe-off.

The toe-only rocker includes only a simple anterior curve and provides a fulcrum from the mid to late stance phase to limit unwanted motion. The rocker should be sufficiently thick to stiffen the sole unit, otherwise the effect will be minimal. Adding an effective rocker to a shoe decreases the functional length of the sole of the shoe while allowing the metatarsals to move through a lessened range of motion

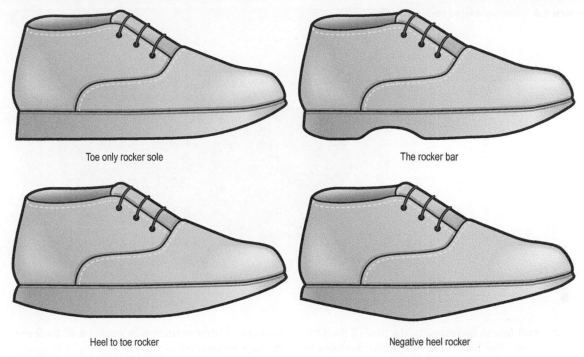

Toe only rocker sole

The rocker bar

Heel to toe rocker

Negative heel rocker

Figure 9.5 Types of rocker soles.

during the propulsive phase of gait (Michaud 1997). Toe-only rockers are useful where reduction in the amount of dorsiflexion by the metatarso-phalangeal joints is required, for example in hallux rigidus and rheumatoid arthritis.

Where the rocker element is added but no compensatory raise is added to the heel, the result will be a negative heel rocker.

The double rocker contains two curves: one curve at the heel and one near the tread line (this is also sometimes known as the heel rocker). This profile is useful where a reduction in midfoot pressure is required as in midfoot Charcot neuroarthropathy. However, it should be noted that the central off-loading effect will be reduced if a wedged sole is used. Where central off-loading is required, a separate, traditional sole and heel unit should be prescribed.

Some rocker soles actually include a three-curve profile, all of which have a separate radius. They will include one curve at the heel, another in the midfoot and another at the tread line position. Such triple curve rockers are always in wedged sole form and are those traditionally used in diabetic footwear.

Traditional rockers are curved, but it is possible to have a sharply-angled rocker (Fig. 9.6). Rockers of this design, where the fulcrum is placed immediately proximal to the metatarsal heads, will totally eliminate dorsiflexion of the metatarso-phalangeal joints and lead to a more rapid forward progression at the end of the gait cycle.

Many practitioners and orthopaedists choose varying placement of the fulcrum of the rocker to suit specific foot pathologies, for example the Lisfranc rocker has its fulcrum positioned at a point corresponding to the base of the first metatarsal. This reduces propulsive force to the midfoot. It is helpful in treating midtarsal arthritic conditions and midfoot collapse.

Brown et al (2004) examined the effects of rocker soles on 40 patients without health problems. They examined patients wearing normal shoes and three types of rocker soles. These were toe-only rockers, negative heel rockers and double rockers. They investigated their effect on peak plantar pressures and pressure/time integrals. They placed sensors at seven points on the feet of their sample: the hallux (first toe), first, second and fifth metatarsals, between

Figure 9.6 Sharply-angled rocker sole.

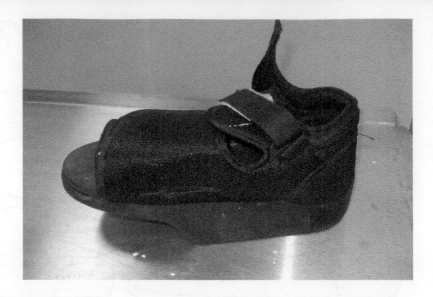

the third and fourth metatarsals, the base of the fifth metatarsal and the heel. They measured the sample first wearing normal shoes and then in shoes of the same internal and external upper design but with a variety of rockers added to the sole unit.

They found that toe-only rockers reduced pressure and the pressure/time integral at the heel, the first toe (hallux), and the first and second metatarsal heads, and between the third and fourth metatarsal heads. They loaded the base of the fifth metatarsal, increased mid-stance time and loaded the midfoot. The reduction in pressure at the heel was thought to be due to the lack of a walking heel on the shoe, which may have increased foot slap shortly after heel contact (in other words, the heel was quickly off-loaded and the midfoot then hit the ground quickly causing a slapping-like action – and maybe a slapping sound).

The negative heel rocker moves weight-bearing posteriorly, back towards the heel. This is only useful in patients who have adequate ankle joint dorsiflexion. It achieved results similar to the toe-only rocker but with the addition of the feeling of stability in patients who wore it. Two patients complained of cramps in the back of their legs.

The double rocker achieved reduction in peak pressure and pressure/time integral at the heel, under the first toe, under the first and second and between the third and fourth metatarsal heads. There

was also a little reduction in pressure at the base of the fifth metatarsal.

Reduction in pressure with rocker soles

Walking foot pressures vary with velocity and body mass. The reduction in pressure with rocker soles depends on the angle of the tibia to the ground and the available range of ankle motion. These two factors are related to the individual's stride length (Fuller et al 2001). If an individual chooses to take long strides, the entire angle of the rocker may be used and it is possible to roll off the tip of the shoe and create high pressures under the hallux. With shorter stride lengths, the rocker makes it more difficult for the individual to achieve high pressures under the hallux. Therefore it is not the rocker alone that reduces plantar pressures, but a combination of the individual gait style and the rocker angle. It is easier to get the tip of the shoe to touch the ground with a smaller rocker angle. Where the tip does touch the ground, the force from the ground can be transmitted to the distal aspect of the foot. High pressures have been found under the hallux in shoes with a smaller rocker angle.

It has also been found that the more rigid the rocker sole, the better the metatarsal head off-loading, but again this protection may be lost under the toes if the toes touch the ground during gait. It is also important that the shoe has a well-functioning fastening and the heel is held into the shoe if the rocker is to achieve its aim of forefoot off-loading.

Certain studies have identified that patients wearing rocker-soled shoes reduce their cadence and velocity, but Hsi et al (2004) found this not to be the case. The implication of this finding for weight transfer and the overall effectiveness of the rocker in treating conditions where lesions affect digits should be evaluated.

Positioning of the rocker

Rockers should be positioned perpendicular to the line of progression. Therefore, a wider angle of gait requires more angled sole to the midline of the shoe (White 1994). In some cases of out-toeing, this in itself can cause an inefficient gait, and a motion akin to the gait style adopted when ice skating will need to be adopted by the patient.

Van Schie et al (2000) identified that the positioning of the rocker is critical in off-loading pressure. They identified four criteria and inter-related design variables which need to be considered in the design of the rocker shoe:

1. The rocker angle (angle in the front part of the shoe to the ground).
2. The shoe height.
3. The rocker axis position (A-P location).
4. The rocker axis angle with respect to the long axis of the shoe.

The best position for redistribution of load from the metatarsal heads is generally about 55–60% of shoe length (measured from heel to toe) and for off-loading the hallux 65% of shoe length (Fig. 9.7). The axis position for optimal placement is variable between subjects and no single optimal position for particular pathologies was identified. In general, the axis angle should follow the metatarsal formula and should be placed posterior to the metatarsal heads. Where there is an acute metatarsal angle and the fifth metatarsal head is very much more proximal than the head of the first metatarsal, the danger in using standard rocker axis angles is that the load will be redistributed to the fifth metatarsal, causing damage to the soft tissue in that area.

In a study undertaken by Stacpoole-Shea et al (1999) the peak pressure reduction using rocker soles was found to be markedly variable between

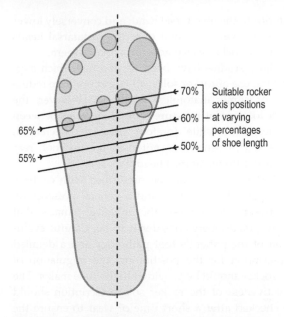

Figure 9.7 Choosing the rocker axis position. The most distal (top) line indicates a position at 70% of the shoe length; the second at 65% of the shoe length; the third at 60% of the shoe length; the fourth at 55% of the shoe length; the most proximal (bottom) line showing the position at 50% of the shoe length.

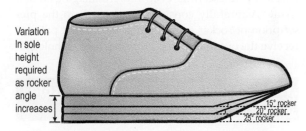

Figure 9.8 Rocker angles. Increasing the angle of the rocker will require additional height throughout the remainder of the sole and heel of the shoe.

individuals. The effect of the rocker was shown to be different at different locations of the foot. The first metatarso-phalangeal joint pressure was highest in a 15° rocker and lowest in a 25° rocker. However, to increase the angle of the rocker, the height of the sole has to be increased, and patient tolerance of height must be considered before prescription (Fig. 9.8).

Higher pressures in the metatarso-phalangeal joint areas were recorded when the rocker was placed anterior to the metatarsal head, and conversely lower pressures were recorded over the metatarsal heads when the rocker was placed proximal to them.

Many studies have been carried out which support the use of rocker soles; all report pressure reduction at some anatomical locations. However, the exact location of pressure reduction varies between studies, and while forefoot pressures decreased, increased pressure was noted in the midfoot, rear foot and fifth metatarsal head.

Rocker soles should be prescribed with caution. Each patient is different and a general prescription of 'rocker sole' is rarely the universal panacea that many practitioners consider it to be. Careful evaluation of the patient's foot pathology and a detailed prescription for the positioning and angulation of the rocker should be provided to the shoe maker. The effectiveness of the rocker sole prescription should be checked after a short time of wear to ensure the desired effect is being achieved. It should be noted that the decrease in pressure in one part of the foot is always accompanied by an increase in pressure elsewhere and the pressure/time integral may be more important than peak pressure alone. It is not only high plantar pressure which leads to damage. Quite frequently, a lower pressure applied for a longer period of time can be even more damaging to soft tissue. A carefully considered approach to the prescription of rocker soles should ensure that patients receive the optimal therapy for their foot pathology.

Raises (elevations) to heel and sole units

Leg length discrepancies are often treated with a shoe raise. In such cases, a raised sole on the shorter limb can be used to ensure that the limbs function at the same length and the pelvis is level (Alexander & Goldberg 2004). For relatively small limb length discrepancies between 5 mm and 9 mm, a heel lift only can be considered, either applied internally to the heel seat of the shoe or onto an orthotic (see Ch. 13 for further explanation on internal heel lifts), or it can be applied externally to the heel of the shoe (see points to note, below).

The choice of positioning will depend on the height of the raise required and the preference of the patient. The consensus in the literature is that internal

heel raises within shoes, and therefore not visible externally, can be given for heights up to 1 cm, although there appears to be little research to support this figure. However, the style, size and heel height of the shoe are limiting factors. Care needs to be taken when prescribing an internal heel raise that the heel-to-ball ratio of the shoe is not affected, thereby influencing the position of the tread line and reducing toe spring.

Points to note:

- Additional consideration should be given to the fact that increasing heel height has been shown to increase pressure under the forefoot (Broch et al 2004), and if the patient has a forefoot pathology, this may be an undesirable effect. For cosmetic reasons, some patients find only internal raises acceptable, but patients who have a large variance in the length of their limbs should be encouraged to consider external modification applied to the entire length of the outer sole of the shoe.

- External heel raises can be added to many different types of footwear, including commercially available footwear, providing the sole and heel material is such that the raise can be successfully bonded to it. However, the addition of a heel raise only is not ideal as it will impair effective shoe function. A heel raise reduces the mechanical length of the foot and causes a shorter stride length (Münzenberg 1985). It also puts additional stress on the metatarsal heads and affects the functioning of the shoe. Since it causes the existing toe spring to disappear, the shoe will then acquire additional toe spring and the upper will crease accordingly, causing potential damage to the dorsal surface of the foot in the metatarsal joint area (Fig. 9.9).

For differences greater than 1 cm, it is recognized that modification is required both to the heel and sole which will raise the foot as a whole unit, thus lengthening the shorter leg. If a solid piece of material is applied along the whole length of the shoe, the shoe will not bend when or where it needs to, and the heel will slip off as the foot begins to enter the propulsive phase of gait (Levine 2004). In order to assist forward progression, a rocker is often incorporated into the raise. The raise requires that extra material

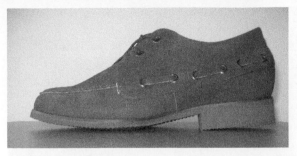
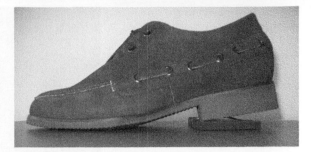

Figure 9.9 Elevating the heel only will alter the relationship between the heel height and toe spring. It will depress the toe spring and the shoe will no longer function correctly on its tread line.

is incorporated into the shoe and this will obviously increase the weight of the shoe. Care then needs to be taken to ensure that the weight does not become a limiting factor. The material used in the raise needs to be carefully chosen for its lightweight property. For example, high-density plastazote is much lighter than cork or micro-soling material, although it is more expensive. Manufacturers do, however, have preferences for certain materials and may not be so willing to offer all the types now available unless specifically requested.

Identifying any leg length inequality is vital in the prescription of outer soles and heels (White 1994). Several methods are used for evaluation. The assessment must consider whether the leg length discrepancy is anatomical or functional (see Ch. 13 for more detail). If the limb length discrepancy is functional then orthotic therapy should be considered. It may be that orthotic therapy alone will address the limb length discrepancy or that a raise is required in addition to the orthotic. The possibility that either functional or compensated anatomical limb length discrepancy has led to permanent contractures must be considered and, if so, the effect of such contracture will need to be included in calculating the raise required. Remember also that, in certain cases, patients require a limb length inequality to allow progression of the swing limb.

There are, of course, many causes of limb length discrepancy including congenital anomalies, traumatic injuries, nerve and muscular damage. Following careful measurement of both limbs, the extent of the limb length discrepancy should be established.

Accurate measurement of each limb is required. With the patient supine, measurements of each limb

should be taken from the anterior superior iliac crest to the medial malleolus. Additional measurements should be taken from the ziphoid process of the sternum to the medial malleolus of each limb. These measurements should be used as a guide. To determine the height of the actual raise, a full biomechanical examination should be performed, paying particular note to several other significant features. First, check hip flexibility, then knee flexion and also the range of motion available at the ankle. Any hip or knee flexion deformity will affect functional limb length as will any degree of ankle equinus. These factors can have an effect on functional limb length and need to be factored into the final calculation of the raise required.

Patients with longstanding limb length discrepancy may use specific coping strategies to improve ambulation. Commonly they may:

- Flex the knee of the longer limb
- Rotate the pelvis to shorten the longer limb
- Pronate the foot of the longer limb and supinate the foot of the shorter limb (Fig. 9.10).

Where such compensation is evident, care should be taken not to assume that the actions involved are reversible. The changes in gait which have resulted from them may be permanent and, for example, the patient may no longer be able to straighten a flexed knee. It is important that the range of motion within joints is evaluated before the height of the raise is decided.

To confirm the raise required, blocks of material equating in height to the estimated difference in limb lengths may be placed under the shorter limb. A pelvic level measurement tool can be used to evaluate the symmetry of the limbs (Fig. 9.11).

139

Figure 9.10 Limb length discrepancy. Note pronation of the foot of the longer limb and supination of the foot of the shorter limb.

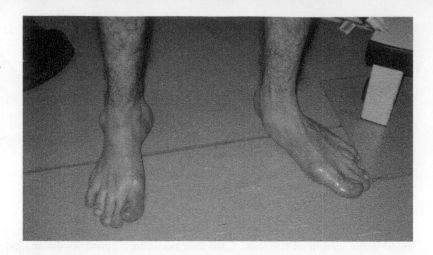

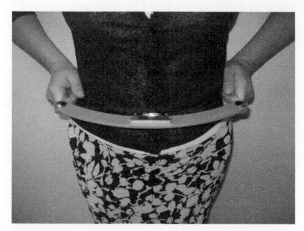

Figure 9.11 Using a pelvic level. The instrument contains a spirit level in the central band, and with its arms placed on each anterior superior iliac crest, the equality of limb lengths can be evaluated by checking the position via the spirit level.

Establish whether the patient is comfortable with the height adjustment with the blocks in place and readjust if necessary. Patients often find it more acceptable to use a raise slightly lower than the measurement indicated, as the compensatory strategies they have undertaken previously are not easily overcome and tend to remain as a feature of gait.

If the patient has previously been prescribed and has worn a satisfactory elevation, measurements may be taken from that. If possible, access the previous prescription for detail.

Measurements for the actual raise to be applied to the shoe need to be taken from specific points. Heel raises must be measured at malleolar level in the sagittal plane. They need to be taken from the side of the foot, directly under the malleolus at the centre of the base of the heel and not from the extreme back of the heel (see also Ch. 4).

Raises over 1 cm in height (just less than half an inch) should be tapered and extended through the remainder of the shoe sole to prevent excessive unilateral pelvic tilt. The ratio of the gradation through the sole should be:

- Heel raise = 1 unit
- Raise at metatarso-phalangeal joints = 0.5 unit
- Raise at toe = 0.25 or 0 unit.

So, using this formula, if the raise required is 3 cm, then:

- Heel raise = 3 cm
- Raise at metatarso-phalangeal joints = 1.5 cm
- Raise at toe = 0.75 cm or 0 cm.

In cases where there is joint rigidity at the ankle, it is unwise to use a tapered raise. In such cases, maintain the calculated height at the ankle through to the metatarso-phalangeal joints and then taper at the toes with a rocker. Joint measurements should be taken from a point directly under the metatarsal heads.

In cases where the leg lengths are equal, but a fixed equinus results in the forefoot extending beyond the foot of the normal leg, it will be necessary to raise the normal side in order to level the pelvis.

Types of shoe elevation

Internal elevations

It is not possible to use a through elevation inside footwear without having the footwear specially made. If a shoe is either a normal retail shoe or an orthopaedic (surgical) shoe made without a raise, to include a raise within the forefoot would cause an unacceptable reduction in the available girth and the shoe would be too shallow for the foot. However, heel elevations only may be included within footwear if the elevation is lower than 1 cm. Where the elevation is higher than this will cause the foot to be lifted out of the shoe, will damage the heel height/toe spring relationship and will affect the tread line as described above. External elevations may be used for raises over 1 cm, but it is possible to use a combination of internal and external raises, thus splitting the raise into two parts, to improve the overall appearance of the footwear.

In the case of internal elevations, the raise will be applied to the heel seat of the shoe, and in retail footwear, the maximum available allowance might be as little as 5 mm because of the design of the shoe and the retro-calcaneal profile of the heel counter. In many cases, the foot will be lifted out of the shoe if the raise is greater than 5 mm. In general, patients requiring raises above 5 mm but no greater than 1 cm will either need to be prescribed surgical footwear or else purchase retail footwear which has deep quarters. The internal raise may be made of cork, EVA of 70 shore or materials of similar density and shore value, and may be:

- Included in an insole (e.g. heel lift)
- Made as an internal cradle (e.g. for fixed equinus)
- Included in a moulded total contact inlay incorporating an elevation (raise).

Internal raises are cosmetically more acceptable as they are disguised within the shoe (Fig. 9.12). If the raise cannot wholly be accommodated within the shoe, it is possible to split the raise using between 5 mm and 1 cm within the shoe (depending on quarter height) and the remainder as an external elevation (see also Ch. 13).

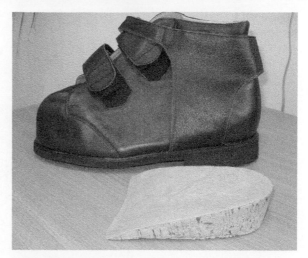

Figure 9.12 An example of an internal heel raise contained within a bespoke shoe.

External elevations

External elevations are more commonly used than internal elevations and can be used on retail footwear. The raise itself can be made of lightweight material and may be covered with the same material as the upper of the shoe, when it is known as a randed raise, or can remain uncovered to appear as part of the sole unit (Figs 9.13 and 9.14). The external raise can be:

- Inserted into the existing sole. Here the outer sole is removed, the raise is adhered to the bottom of the shoe and the outer sole replaced over it.
- Stuck on to the existing sole.
- Made from cork, high-density plastazote, micro-soling material.
- Uncovered (material exposed).
- Leather covered to match the shoe (randed raise).

The form which the external raise takes can be either as a tapered elevation, as a solid wedge or as a bridge raise where a gap is made in the area which corresponds to the waist of the shoe.

In selecting the form of the raise, consider the weight of the shoe plus raise, remembering that plastazote is the lightest material and that less material will be necessary if a bridge raise is used. Consider also patient concordance and how the addition of the raise

Figure 9.13 Shoe with an external through wedged tapered elevation which is made of micro-soling material.

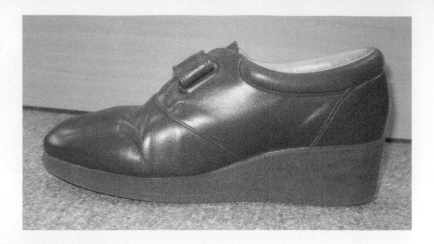

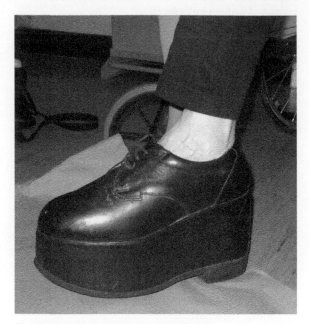

Figure 9.14 An external randed raise.

will affect the appearance of the shoe. Many patients prefer a randed raise when the outer sole appears the same on both shoes thus improving aesthetics.

For a comparison of internal and external elevations, see Table 9.3.

The use of callipers

Where a patient has been prescribed callipers, they will need to be inserted into the heel unit of the shoe,

immediately inferior to the malleolus. The calliper may have a unilateral arm, in which case an entry socket will need to be included on the appropriate side of the shoe heel, or bilateral arms, in which case sockets on both sides of the shoe heel will be needed. Calliper end rods may be circular or flat ended. With circular end rods, the diameter of the entry socket may be either $\frac{5}{8}$ or $\frac{1}{4}$ inch. Flat end rods may require entry sockets of $\frac{9}{16}$ by $\frac{3}{16}$ or $\frac{3}{16}$ squared or $\frac{1}{2}$ by $\frac{1}{8}$ inch. It is important that the prescription also states the required position of the entry socket in the heel or raise. T straps or Y straps inserted between the shoe upper and heel unit will be necessary to hold the calliper arms and prevent any possibility of the calliper springing open, out of the heel placement. T straps are usually attached to the opposite side of the shoe to the calliper arm; Y straps are used for callipers with bilateral arms and are often positioned at the back of the heel, again inserted between the shoe upper and heel unit. They will encircle both calliper arms and fasten at a chosen point over the calliper with either a buckle or Velcro® fastening.

The calliper entry socket may also be accompanied by a metal backstop to prevent excessive plantarflexion (Fig. 9.15). This is a small, flat piece of metal attached directly behind the calliper entry socket that prevents backward movement of the calliper, which would be required for more than a small degree of plantarflexion of the foot. Where dorsiflexion is required to be limited, a similar block may be placed in front of the calliper. Where firm control of

Table 9.3 Comparison of external and internal raise options

External raises may be:	Internal raises may be:
Inserted into the existing sole (by splitting the sole open and re-gluing).	Added to an inlay (e.g. heel lift).
Uncovered (material exposed).	An inside levelling cork, e.g. equinus.
Tapered (reducing in height towards the toe end).	A moulded contact inlay incorporating an elevation (raise).
Made from cork, high-density plastazote, micro-soling material, EVA.	Split in height with a combination of outside and inside raises to lessen the obvious external appearance.
Leather covered to match the shoe.	Limited in use with retail footwear due to limited height of back quarters.
Full length (no taper at toe).	
Stuck on to the existing sole.	Cosmetically more acceptable.
A bridge shape (cut out through the centre).	Part of a prosthetic foot.
A heel raise only (not recommended as toe spring is lost).	

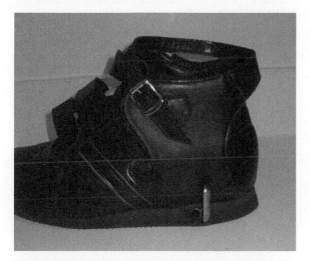

Figure 9.15 Calliper entry socket in heel of shoe with backstop to prevent plantarflexion of the foot.

both dorsiflexion and plantarflexion are required, both stops may be used.

The use of any sole material or adaptation must be specifically designed to met the needs of the individual patient, be it their medical or lifestyle needs. Appropriately prescribed sole and heel units should be part of the process in prescribing footwear suitable for purpose. Outer sole and heel modifications can have a significant effect on modifying foot function, in minimizing the effect of a range of foot-related sagittal plane pathologies and in reducing pain and discomfort. When carefully prescribed, they can have a dramatic effect on patient mobility and can help in improving quality of life, enabling patients to undertake more fully the activities of daily living. When considering the prescription, remember that a three-component system exists: the patient, the footwear outer sole and heel units, and the ground surface. The requirements of all three need to be evaluated and considered if the footwear prescription is to be successful.

References

Alexander N, Goldberg A 2004 Gait disorders: search for multiple causes. Cleve Clin J Med 72(7):586–600.

Broch NL, Wyller T, Steen H 2004 Effects of heel height and shoe shape on the compressive load between foot and base. JAMPA 94(5):461–469.

Brown D, Wertsch JJ, Harris GF et al 2004 Effect of rocker soles on plantar pressures. Arch Phys Med Rehabil 84:81–86.

Even-Tzur N, Weisz E, Hirsch-Falk Y, Gefen A 2006 Role of EVA viscoelastic properties in the protective performance of a sports shoe: computational studies. Biomed Mater Eng 16(5):289–299.

Fuller E, Schroeder S, Edwards J 2001 Reduction of peak pressure on the forefoot with a rigid rocker-bottom postoperative shoe. JAPMA 91(10):501–507.

Gastwirth BW 1991 An electrodynamic study of foot function in shoes of varying heel heights. JAPMA 81:463–472.

Gheluwe B, Dananberg H 2004 Changes in plantar foot pressure with in-shoe varus or valgus wedging. JAPMA 94(1):1–11.

Health and Safety Executive 2004 The assessment of slip risk. London, Health and Safety Executive.

His WL, Chai HM, Lai JS 2004 Evaluation of rocker soles by pressure-time curves in insensate forefoot during gait. Am J Phys Med Rehabil 83:500–506.

Levine D 2004 Inside insights on shoewear modifications. Podiatry Today 17(9):60–66.

Li KW, Chen CJ 2004 The effect of shoe soling tread groove width on the coefficient of friction with different sole materials, floors and contaminants. Appl Ergon 35(6):499–507.

Menz H, Lord S 1999 Footwear and postural stability in older people. JAPMA 89(7):346–357.

Michaud TC 1997 Foot orthoses and other forms of conservative foot care. Massachusetts, Michaud.

Mundermann A 2004 Long term effects of footwear on gait may be most critical. Biomechanics March Issue.

Münzenberg KJ 1985 The orthopaedic shoe: indications and prescription. Weinheim, VCH Verlagsgesellschaft.

Myers KA, Long JT, Klein JP et al 2005 Biomechanical implications of the negative heel rocker sole shoe. Gait kinematics and kinetics. Gait Posture 24(3):323–330.

Perry JE 1995 The use of running shoes to reduce plantar pressures in patients who have diabetes. J Bone Joint Surg 77(12):1819–1828.

Pribut S, Richie D 2004 Separating the buzz from the biomechanics: a guide to athletic shoe trends and innovations. Podiatry Management October:85–97.

Robbins SE, Gouw GJ, McClaran J 1992 Shoe sole thickness and hardness influence balance in older men.

J Am Geriatr Soc 40:1089. (cited by Menz H, Lord S 1999 Footwear and postural stability in older people, JAPMA 89(7):346–357.

Rowland FJ, Jones C, Manning DP 1996 Surface roughness of footwear soling materials: relevance to slip resistance. Journal of Testing and Evaluation 24:6.

Rubenstein L, Robbins A, Schulman B et al 1988 Falls and instability in the elderly. J Am Geriatr Soc 36:266–278.

Schaff P, Cavanagh P 1990 Shoes for the insensitive foot: the effect of a 'rocker bottom' shoe modification on plantar pressure distribution. Foot Ankle 11(3):129–140.

Stacpoole-Shea SJ, Shea GA, Armstrong DG, Lavery LA 1999 Do rocker soles reduce plantar pressure in persons at risk for diabetic neuropathic ulceration? Proceedings of the Foot Pressure Interest Group, Leeds.

Tencer AF, Koepsell TD, Wolf ME et al 2004 Biomechanical properties of shoes and risk of falls in older adults. J Am Geriatr Soc 52(11):1840–1846.

Tollafield DR, Merriman LM 1997 Clinical skills in treating the foot. Edinburgh, Churchill Livingstone.

Van Schie C, Ulbrecht JS, Becker MB, Cavanagh PR 2000 Design criteria for rigid rocker shoes. Foot Ankle Int 21(10):833–844.

White J 1994 Custom shoe therapy. Current concepts, designs, and special considerations. Clin Podiatr Med Surg 11(2):259–269.

Whittle MW 1999 Generation and attenuation of transient impulsive forces beneath the foot: a review. Gait Posture 10:264–275.

Wu WL, Rosenbaum D, Su FC 2004 The effects of rocker sole and SACH heel on kinematics in gait. Med Eng Phys 26:639–646.

Stock and modular footwear

Chapter contents

Since the 1960s, the introduction of 'stock' or 'ready-made' therapeutic footwear into the healthcare system has transformed the whole provision of prescription footwear. It has proven to be cost-effective, and combines rapid delivery with a wide range of fitting options. These early ranges have been expanded and updated to include more 'retail' or modern high street styles, which allow patients to have depth footwear that imitates current footwear fashion. Hence this has led to improved concordance.

The further addition of then offering a 'modular' option is the ultimate, as this gives the clinician the opportunity to slightly modify the footwear because rarely do a single individual's non-pathological feet match in width or length, let alone those feet that become damaged or diseased.

Alongside the rapidly developing stock ranges there has also been considerable progress in orthopaedic

procedures, especially for congenital defects, which has the long-term benefit of restoring optimal foot shape and function thus reducing the long-term requirement for so many bespoke items. The older generation of patients that did not benefit in this way are members of a diminishing population whose feet are often severely deformed and who provided a great challenge to all who prescribed their footwear. There is a definite improvement in the clinical outcome of treatments available for such challenging foot conditions today, and with this, the traditional skills required to provide bespoke footwear for such deformities are also gradually dying out. This directly affects the profile of orthopaedic footwear manufacture and the market for bespoke footwear manufacture has dropped in percentage terms to a very low figure while the use and supply of stock items and modular footwear has risen correspondingly. This is good news for the patient, for the suppliers of stock orthopaedic footwear and for the budget gatekeeper, as generally these items are about one-third of the cost of fully bespoke footwear.

Ranges available

The range of stock footwear available has improved vastly over recent years and covers all adult shoes, boots and indoor items such as healing sandals, cast walkers and safe 'indoor' shoes. Children's shoes, accommodating ankle–foot orthoses (AFOs) and/ or orthotics and a high degree of ankle support, set these shoes apart from anything available from retail outlets. In addition, orthopaedic sports footwear, such as golf shoes and orthopaedic work wear, such as protective safety boots, are also available.

Apart from the wide range of styles available for both men and women, there are also choices of sole finishes, varying from very light and flexible to heavy-duty commando type material. Some variation in sole design is also available and this includes features such as wedge soles, smart leather covered heels and regular non-slip cushion sole units. As technology advances and becomes more affordable, manufacturers are able to introduce injection-moulded soles for the first time. These sole units vastly improve the appearance and performance of the footwear. All such features can be selected from a catalogue, but it is very useful to have samples in the clinic for trial fitting and to give patients some idea of what they are to receive.

As mentioned earlier, modular footwear options are also easily obtained from many of these manufacturers. In essence, this means that the existing last dimensions can be altered to accommodate a deformity more satisfactorily. The majority of makers give clear guidelines in their catalogue as to how and where to measure the various last changes they can offer. The degree of modification is also frequently stipulated and the catalogue information will identify a maximum limit in centimetres. In practice, however, this means that the clinician needs plenty of experience in fitting skills in order to prescribe modifications to a shoe or its last to achieve the required end result.

Case study example

Task: evaluate the client's footwear needs and, from a choice of stock ranges, select the most suitable footwear while being sensitive to the patient's wishes.

As the patient walks from the waiting area into the clinic, the evaluation process starts by observing stance, type of gait, whether aids are used, the quality of mobility and the condition of the current footwear.

The assessment needs to be detailed to discover what demands patients will place on their footwear during daily wear in addition to any particular prescription requests. It is essential to know the medical background to establish how this will affect footwear needs. For example, conditions such as diabetes, peripheral vascular disease and oedema will have a major impact on optimal footwear design.

It is essential to find out what patients want or prefer to wear, their lifestyle, daily activities, any help with dressing, etc. It is very important to explain the basic requirements of prescription footwear, for example the need for a strong fastening, so that the patient is willing and able to accept what is proposed.

In offering patients a choice of suitable footwear, narrow down the options of what is required before looking through the catalogues to find examples to show them.

For example, a lady in her early sixties had been referred originally for an orthotic device to relieve a painful metatarsal and instep problem. The orthotic had been made and advice given regarding footwear to accommodate it. On review, the patient had not been able to wear the orthotic in her shoes so it was arranged to see her again with her shoes in the clinic. The following week, the patient attended with three pairs of shoes and it was agreed that the orthotic would fit none of them as each was too shallow in the vamp area to accommodate both foot and orthotic. The shoes were the preferred styles; two were lace ups, one a trainer type. Having established that she was doing her best to wear the correct type of shoe, but noting that the foot condition had got worse because of the lack of comfortable shoes to wear with the orthotics, the referring consultant had written again to ask for help with footwear. (As a general rule, shoes are not supplied to accommodate orthotics alone until we are very sure retail footwear has been thoroughly explored.)

The feet were measured for overall length, joint girth and instep circumference and, knowing that a basic lace-up style would be acceptable as she had purchased this style before, the measurements were compared in the size charts of the manufacturers' catalogues to establish the closest match. A size 5 medium fitting with good depth to accommodate the orthotic was decided on.

The client wanted a smart looking shoe that was lightweight, easy to fasten and which appeared similar in style to a high street shoe.

- Choice 1: considered 'smart' with a patent inset vamp, but she did not like these, although the fit was quite good.

- Choice 2: these did not fit in the heel-to-ball and the toe shape was wrong for the foot (Fig. 10.1).

- Choice 3: these were too narrow and tight over the toes and again she did not like the look of them as they were very plain (Fig. 10.2).

- Choice 4: a shoe with a padded vamp and a lower opening lace (similar style as found in retail outlets). This was received with more interest, and fitted very well. The orthotic fitted the shoe shape and the lower opening lace allowed for easy adjustment over the instep. The toe box depth was sufficient with the orthotic inside and there was no pressure on the toes. The heel-to-ball was correct and the shoe flexed nicely on walking with no heel slip. The heel counter gripped around the heel properly and was deep enough with the orthotic inside. The shoe was light and comfortable to walk in and the patient was very pleased with the overall look of the shoe and its comfort (Fig. 10.3).

The fourth shoe matched the patient's wishes for something easy to fasten, lightweight and which did not look 'orthopaedic'. The shoe accommodated the foot and orthotic properly, allowed good walking function and a good overall fit had been achieved. It was helpful that the shoes were available from stock held in the clinic and the patient was able to take them with her that same day, as she was due back to the referring clinic within a few days for evaluation of the effect on gait of the footwear and the orthotic.

The patient was very pleased with the outcome of the fitting session and left wearing the new shoes and orthotics, thanking us for the trouble we had gone to in helping her. A high level of compliance was achieved by taking time to ensure that the footwear met not only the therapeutic criteria, but also met the needs of the patient's self-image.

Similar styles to this are offered by several manufacturers, however each will have a different last design, therefore fitting the same style from more than one brand helps to find the best possible fit, and having samples of these shoes available at all times is invaluable.

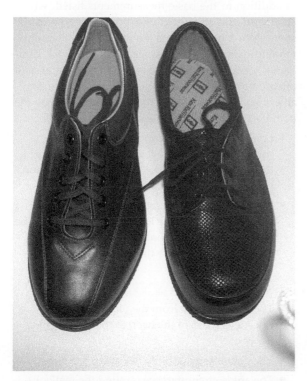

Figure 10.1 Examples of stock shoes offered. The left shoe was the wrong shape; the right shoe was a good fit but disliked by the patient. (Reproduced with permission of Mile End Hospital Footwear Centre.)

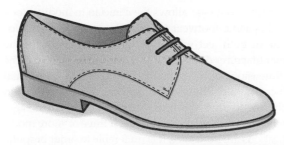

Figure 10.2 A classic Gibson lace shoe style rejected as old looking.

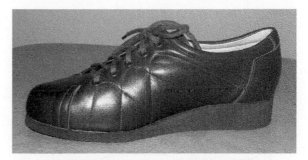

Figure 10.3 The stock shoe style that met the patient's needs, imitating a similar high street style, was acceptable. (Reproduced with permission of Mile End Hospital Footwear Centre.)

Measuring for stock footwear

Measurements of the foot need to be taken in order to establish a size and fitting. These are basic and will need to be taken for all types of orthopaedic footwear. There are no official guidelines set out for basic measuring, but the more complex measurements required, in addition to these for the prescription of bespoke therapeutic footwear, are detailed in Chapter 11.

To measure for footwear, a flexible tape measure (preferably 1 cm in width), a standard measuring stick or a measuring gauge are needed.

The basic measurements which need to be taken for stock orthopaedic footwear are (Fig. 10.4):

- **Joint circumference**: place the flexible tape measure around the widest part of the foot, encompassing the first metatarsal phalangeal joint, and measure all round the foot. In addition, it can be useful to measure the joint width by placing the size stick across the width and measuring the gap with a tape measure.
- **Waist**: place the tape immediately behind the metatarsal joints to measure the reduction in circumference from the joint measure.
- **Instep**: the tape should be placed distal to the tuberosity of navicular where the top line of the facings should be positioned. If placed too high on the dorsum (proximal to the tuberosity), this can be misleading and cause the measurement taken to be inaccurate.
- **Toe depth** (if excessive): measure the height of clawed or damaged toes. The majority of depth footwear will accommodate 35 mm without any change being needed.

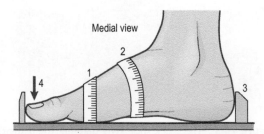

Figure 10.4 Basic measurement positions: 1. joint circumference; 2. instep circumference; 3. size stick length measure; 4. toe depth.

- **Overall length**: using a standard size stick or any measuring device available, measure the length of both feet from the back of the heel to the longest toe. Convert to the shoe size convenient to you (UK English or Continental; the US scale is different to the UK scale).

Modular footwear measurements

In addition to the basic measurements listed, where an alteration is requested or if boots are to be made, some extra measurements are required to ensure the modification is done accurately. All the stock catalogues include the necessary instructions and will often give maximum millimetres of allowance available for specific areas of the shoe. Ensure that the manufacturers' guidelines are followed (Fig. 10.5):

- **Long heel**: place the tape measure around the back of the heel at the lowest point and bring the tape around the foot to meet on the dorsum where the instep measurement was taken.
- **Short heel**: place the tape measure around the back of the heel at the lowest point and bring the tape around to the front of the ankle as high as possible, making sure the tape is laying flat to the foot.

Boots also require:

- The upper height from the plantar border of the calcaneus (base of the heel) to the top height of the boot.
- The circumference of the leg at the top height.
- The ankle circumference (around the malleoli), especially if this differs from left to right.

Modifications available

Modular footwear allows the clinician to modify stock orthopaedic footwear in order to improve the fit for one or both feet where the dimensions listed by the manufacturer do not appear to be sufficient to meet the dimensions of the patient's feet. This may be a small increase in depth or circumference, or a major pattern change to alter the upper from its standard design. It is worth noting, however, that if three or more modifications are necessary, it is preferable to order bespoke instead, as each modification will be charged and too many make the overall cost very high.

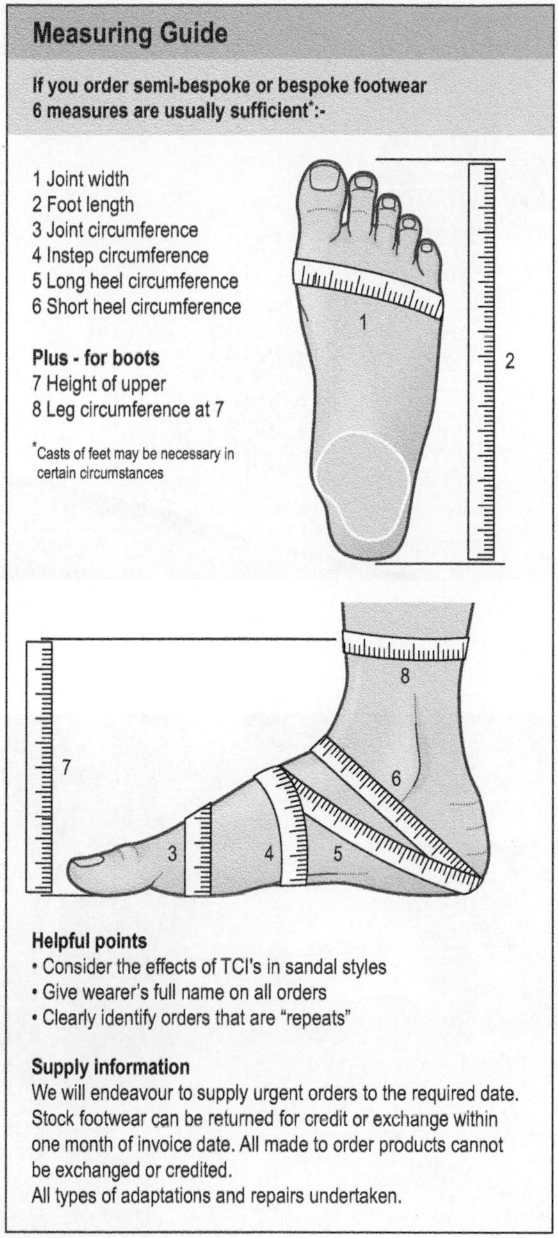

require pattern piece changes unless plenty of allowance is available on the existing patterns. Last modifications that can be achieved are:

- Back curve shape
- Medial or lateral ankle width or depth
- Extra depth or width of heel seat
- Extra depth of instep
- Extra depth of fore part
- Bunion pocket to the first metatarsal head (medial side) or fifth metatarsal head (lateral side)
- Extra depth or width at toe end only.

2. **Pattern modifications**: this means that the initial style pattern has to be changed before the leather is cut, to incorporate the alterations requested. This then becomes a one-off personalized item and usually the special pattern is filed away for future use on repeat items. Pattern changes that can be achieved are (Figs 10.7 and 10.8):

- Raising or lowering of back height or top line
- Repositioning of seams to avoid problem areas on foot
- Opening or closing of lace gap
- Changing fastening method
- Shortening or lengthening of Velcro® straps
- Moving tab position to assist entry (low entry)
- Bellows tongue
- Increasing top height above standard
- Adding/removing a padded collar.

3. **Sole modifications**: this means that the changes will only affect the sole/heel of the shoe and not the upper or the last. Sometimes a sole modification is combined with an upper or last modification, but be aware of the costs. Sometimes it is better to choose the bespoke option from the outset. Sole modifications that can be achieved are:

- External compensating raises made of high-density plastazote or leather covered cork
- Colour-matched 'Micro' soling for elongated heels, float heels, sole and heel wedges

Measuring Guide

If you order semi-bespoke or bespoke footwear 6 measures are usually sufficient*:-

1 Joint width
2 Foot length
3 Joint circumference
4 Instep circumference
5 Long heel circumference
6 Short heel circumference

Plus - for boots
7 Height of upper
8 Leg circumference at 7

*Casts of feet may be necessary in certain circumstances

Helpful points
- Consider the effects of TCI's in sandal styles
- Give wearer's full name on all orders
- Clearly identify orders that are "repeats"

Supply information
We will endeavour to supply urgent orders to the required date. Stock footwear can be returned for credit or exchange within one month of invoice date. All made to order products cannot be exchanged or credited.
All types of adaptations and repairs undertaken.

Figure 10.5 Example of measuring guide, with thanks to Gilbert and Mellish manufacturers.

Modifications can be divided into three sections:

1. **Last modifications**: this means that extra material such as cork is added to the last to physically alter its dimensions before the upper is cut and made up (Fig. 10.6). It may also

Figure 10.6 Example of a plastic last modified with cork additions to match measurements supplied. (Reproduced with permission of Jane Saunders and Manning.)

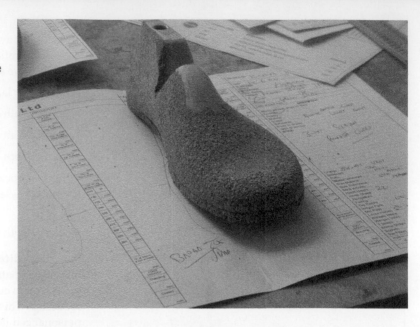

Figure 10.7 Pattern of vamp being altered. (Reproduced with permission of TayCare Medical Ltd.)

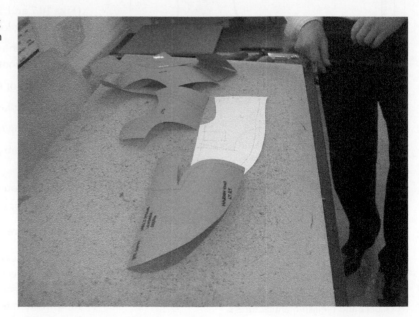

- Rocker soles with/without compensating heel piece
- Calliper sockets
- 'T' or 'Y' straps

- Commando soles and heels
- Leather soles and/or heels
- Hard-wearing soles and/or heel top pieces (neolite, heavy ribbed).

Figure 10.8 Shoe pattern being adjusted before clicking. (Reproduced with permission of TayCare Medical Ltd.)

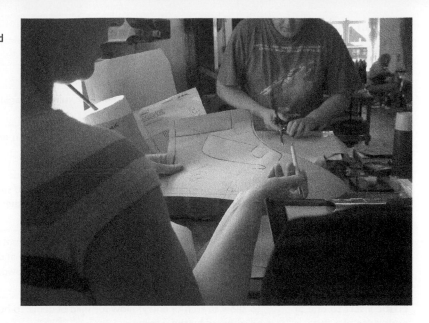

Accessories and adaptations

In addition to the above listed changes, there are other items which may be required that can also be added during the manufacturing process (Table 10.1). Examples of these are:

- Casted total contact inlays to rectified specification
- Metatarsal and valgus inlays
- Full leather, plush or wool linings
- Extended or high stiffeners
- Ski hooks or D-ring fastening to replace eyelets
- Half and split sizes
- Diabetic specifications (i.e. soft leather uppers, full leather seam-free linings, low stiffeners and wall toe puffs, rocker soles)
- Scuff guards to protect from toe dragging or wheelchair wear
- Ankle or toe retaining straps (children's shoes) (Fig. 10.9).

Fitting modular footwear

In most instances, a modified shoe will be sent through at rough fit stage, allowing the clinician to check the progress and accuracy of the modifications. This is important to the successful outcome of the footwear but causes delay in supplying the items to the patient. Experienced clinicians can make simple changes with confidence, avoiding the rough fit stage and receiving the shoe fully completed. Where a modular footwear prescription has previously been successful, further pairs of shoes made to the same prescription can be ordered without the necessity for a fitting (provided the manufacturer has kept proper records). In some instances, these items may also be slightly cheaper as no extra work has had to be done in preparing the patterns and modifying the lasts.

How and when to modify after a fitting can be confusing, but the detail of fitting procedures and the fitting solutions table contained in Chapter 12 will be helpful.

In essence, the modular shoe should only need one fitting as the modifications should not be complex. Where the stock version of the shoe has already been tried, a fitting stage may be unnecessary provided the exact changes required have been clearly requested, using the correct terminology to describe the parts of the shoe to be changed (Fig. 10.10).

It is essential to ensure that the shoe chosen is suitable for the situations in which it will be worn (e.g. indoor or wheelchair use or a walking boot).

Table 10.1 Summary of the many adaptations possible

Additions to uppers (semi-bespoke or bespoke)	Purpose
Padding between upper and lining.	Protection of any bony prominence or vulnerable area, e.g. scar tissue.
Metal valgus or varus steel insert between upper and lining. Rigid or jointed.	Internal ankle support, possibly as a substitute to an external support such as a calliper.
High stiffener, one or both sides, to either boots or shoes.	Internal support for ankle. Can be shaped to a cast to support and protect bony prominence. May be single or double layer of material (usually leather). Thermo-plastics are also used.
High uppers.	In adult footwear, high uppers start at a point 150 mm above the heel insole or a compensating raise where fitted. This is an additional charge to the normal charge and is applied per 25 mm of extra height. Purpose: To provide extra support and protection to lower leg and ankle; to go over a cosmetic calliper.
Elastic insert to one or both sides of a shoe.	To allow stretch of entry; allow for mild oedema; to help where normal fastenings cannot be managed by the wearer.
Heel retaining strap.	To provide extra grip around the ankle, particularly where AFOs are worn.
Balloon patch.	A hole cut in the upper to be filled with a larger, softer leather patch, to relieve pressure over a prominence.
Fastenings: laces can be converted to Velcro® straps. Extra buckles and straps can be applied.	To improve the method of fastening or the management of the fastening.
Reinforced toe caps.	Can be added to footwear to protect the toe area from excessive wear where there is a gait difficulty. Made from either matching leather or a synthetic material such as neolite or textured rubber.
Tongue pads.	Extra cushioning can be added to the tongue to protect the dorsum of the foot; to decrease the girth of the shoe over the instep; to stiffen the tongue to stop it creasing, especially if in a high boot.
Tongue slots.	Vertical slits cut into the tongue to allow the laces to be threaded through to keep the tongue in correct position.
Stitched-down tongue.	The tongue can be stitched down to the upper on either the medial or lateral side at the top of the facing or all the way down one side. This is often useful where the wearer has poor hand control and finds the tongue gets twisted or rucked up when putting on the footwear, or finds that it constantly slides around the foot into an uncomfortable position.
Pull tabs.	A strong cotton loop attached to the back of the heel counter to help assist the wearer to pull on the boot.

Table 10.1 Continued

Additions to soles (modular; bespoke or retail footwear)	Purpose
Outside metatarsal support bar.	To provide external pressure relief to the metatarsal heads where there is no room inside the shoe for an internal metatarsal support inlay.
Wedge: sole, heel or full length.	Medial heel and sole wedges may be applied when the medial aspect of the foot bears too much weight. Conditions suitable: genu valgum, toeing-in gait, excessive pronation. Lateral wedges are applied when the weight needs to be either supported or shifted from the lateral to the medial side of the shoe. Conditions suitable: genu varum, knee strain, femoral torsion, tibial torsion, varus feet, gait-related problems.
Rocker sole (bar).	The rocker sole or bar is a longer metatarsal bar shaped with considerable convexity. Purpose: to take more pressure off the metatarsal joints than the metatarsal support bar. Conditions: to relieve pain, quicken or shorten the gait cycle. Assists dorsiflexion especially in fixed or limited ankle movement, relieves hallux rigidus. Used in conjunction with AFOs.
Steel sole plate.	To provide a completely rigid shoe. To prevent normal foot function, relieve pain.
Steel sole strip (extended shank).	To provide a rigid shoe. Relief of pain, used in conjunction with corrective or contact inlays to protect the foot or pressure relief.

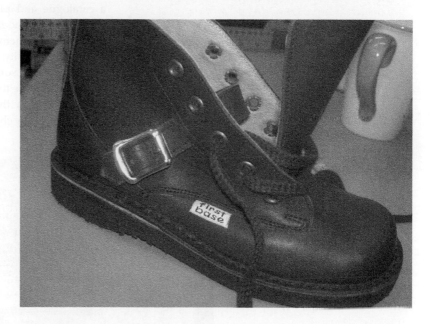

Figure 10.9 Example of an ankle retaining strap in a child's therapeutic shoe. (The source, First Base, is no longer available.)

The choice of construction method and materials selected in stock therapeutic footwear often makes the shoes suitable only for lighter use. For very heavy-duty wear, stronger leather uppers as well as hard-wearing soles may be needed. These might be available on request but very specific instructions are needed to ensure that durability and wear properties are ensured.

The quality of footwear components varies considerably from one manufacturer to another. Therefore, knowing the brands, the construction techniques and the quality of materials used can influence

153

initial choice. Knowledge of the weight and wear properties needed for an individual prescription will determine the most suitable manufacturer. Again, having consignment stock available is very helpful for a comparison of the materials, overall finish and wear quality (in addition to checking on the fitting), and will ensure that the most suitable product is selected.

Many manufacturers make similar styles, but the quality of components will vary slightly. Having a good knowledge of the products available is invaluable and this can only be gained by doing some research. Trial and review will soon help to evaluate

how well the item wears, retains its shape and serves the purpose for which it was selected. It is so important to follow up patients to gain knowledge of the functionality of the product and to evaluate the outcomes. This experience may prove invaluable in selecting footwear for similar future cases. Practitioners at the early stages of their footwear career may find it beneficial to follow up every patient and to learn from the best and the worst features of each footwear prescription and product chosen. It is advisable for all practitioners to become familiar with new products, to evaluate them and to increase the range and knowledge of prescription choices available to meet the therapeutic footwear needs of patients.

Costs and cost implications

Inevitably, the cost of prescribing footwear comes into any decision that is ultimately made, however it should not be the prime factor in determining whether or not to prescribe. Every supplier produces a catalogue and price list. This list will also contain details of modifications and the costs incurred in prescribing them. A comparison of prices can be useful, but quality, reliability and fit must also be considered, and sometimes the cheaper option does not always prove to be the most cost-effective. Stock items are exactly that; identical and mass produced and therefore the cheapest option (Fig. 10.11).

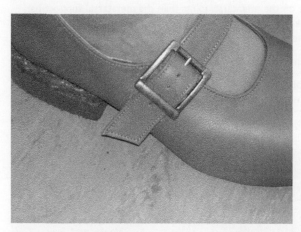

Figure 10.10 Modular fitting stage with temporary heel and no sole.

Figure 10.11 Mass production of stock shoes: uppers ready for lasting. (Reproduced with permission of Klaveness Portugal.)

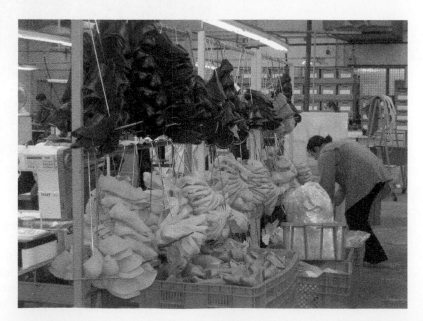

If a pattern or last modification is needed, it will attract extra charges as each change has to be done individually by hand and then checked. Every change requested is an extra, so too many changes to a stock item can become uneconomic. It is so tempting to overuse the modular option and, unless the costs of the modifications are discussed with the manufacturer before the order is sent, the final cost may come as an unwelcome surprise (Fig. 10.12).

Read the directions in the catalogues very carefully, to gain an awareness of the charges likely to be incurred in meeting your prescription requirements. For example, some manufacturers supply trial/rough fit stage free of charge and some do not. Some will always send the trial/rough fit; others only when requested to do so. Some stock and modular shoe makers do not provide a full bespoke service, and if the modifications requested are beyond what can be done effectively, the result can be disastrous. Therefore, select the manufacturer with care and use ones whose work best meets your needs. Developing a rapport with manufacturers and ensuring that their staff are accessible for discussion about orders is helpful. A direct conversation with the member of staff undertaking the work is most useful when complications arise, to clarify what exactly needs doing, how it can be achieved and how to request it correctly. This saves time, effort, unnecessary frustration and money.

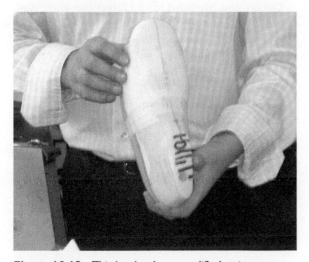

Figure 10.12 This last has been modified to increase depth with a full-length orthotic allowance last addition. (Reproduced with permission of TayCare Medical Ltd.)

Subjective views

The patients' viewpoints cannot be ignored when it comes to what they will or will not wear on their feet. Much of what patients say is related to tightness and discomfort, to fashion and to what others might think about their appearance in certain shoes. Many orthopaedic footwear patients have poor superficial sensation, and as sensory impairment can develop gradually, patients may not fully appreciate how little they really feel of their feet. This factor impacts on the practitioner to make sure the shoes fit very well and to protect the feet of this vulnerable group.

Superimposed on this is often the added problem of concordance. Patients may have difficulty accepting the need for change in the type and shape of their footwear. Many practitioners have heard it said that patients prefer their shoes to be of a certain heel height, toe shape or slip-on for ease of dressing. All of these areas are personal to the patient and very often conflict with prescription footwear. Because these features are subjective, it is challenging to make changes that are acceptable to the patient and appropriate to the prescription. To achieve a satisfactory outcome, time needs to be taken to explain the benefits of deeper/wider shoes, more support, etc. so that patients are able to understand the aims of the prescription so that they may in turn make informed objective decisions based on facts, not feelings.

Clinicians expect a patient to wear what is suitable, but unless the patient actually wishes to wear the footwear prescribed, the therapy will be pointless and the clinician can do nothing until a change of attitude is volunteered by the patient and both parties agree with the final choice of the proposed footwear. Experience has shown that this affects a very small number of patients referred, but they often prove to be the most challenging and time consuming (see section on patient concordance in Ch. 2).

It would seem that footwear patients bring along with them complex feelings about their situation which are often not resolved in the first visit to the footwear clinic. There is much concern over wasted items and non-compliance, however a person cannot be forced into compliance, and failure to recognize this has led to the failure of many prescriptions in the past. The clinician may know what is required in terms of prescription, may complete the order and obtain the footwear, without properly involving the patient in the decision process. If the patient is struggling to accept the needs of the prescription and is not ready to make the change, the footwear will not be accepted despite the fact that it may work if worn. Many of these newly referred patients need time and empathy from the clinician before footwear is prescribed. Simply being understanding and allaying fears about the colour and styles available, showing examples and allowing time to make choices ultimately saves more than just the budget, even though an additional return visit may be necessary.

Point to note: The definition of disability given by the Disabled Living Foundation is 'a physical or mental impairment which has a substantial and long-term adverse effect on a person's ability to carry out normal day-to-day activities'. It is useful to include this definition here because as much as we may have misgivings over prescribing footwear to some non-concordant patients, we still have a duty of care and cannot discriminate against them, especially if they are disabled. However, we may be able to involve an advocate or family member in order to reduce the risks of poor outcomes rather than waste resources on prescribing items which we know will otherwise not be accepted.

Today's working environment is very time focused, and the pressure put onto clinics to perform so many contacts and to achieve performance-related outcomes does not sit comfortably with this particular patient group, who need time, understanding and a real sense that they are listened to and understood before the prescription is decided upon. The multidisciplinary approach has been proven to work best here, as it reduces the pressure on one individual to sort all the complexities. The combined experience and skills often saves initial mistakes which can be damaging to the final outcome. Compliance depends on building up confidence in the clinician and understanding what the aims may be. Supplying poorly fitting items does nothing for the patient's confidence in either the clinic or in the items being supplied.

Stock items may be held in a clinic or may be available for delivery in anything from 48 hours to a couple of weeks, and this can make a vast difference to the concordance issue. Providing the footwear quickly and efficiently may suggest to the patient that the footwear prescription is simpler than imagined, and leaving the clinic in comfortable shoes gives a similar feeling as leaving the shoe shop. This is a vital component of normality of experience which lessens the gap in patients' subconscience mind of 'being different'. Many patients have left the footwear clinic with a completely different opinion of prescribed footwear to what they imagined. The converse of this attitude is that patients may devalue the time, care and expertise which is necessary to ensure that their footwear prescription is effective.

An example worthy of mention is that of a patient re-referred after 10 years, having initially refused any orthopaedic footwear. The consultant persuaded her to come back and see what was now available as she desperately needed better footwear. When the lady attended, she was honest in saying she was not hopeful that her footwear needs could be met, but having gone through the whole assessment procedure and looked at the many ranges available, suitable footwear was provided. This patient was open to change and willing to wear special footwear despite the 'orthopaedic' label. This was a satisfactory outcome and her view of the service was changed for the better.

Acknowledgements

We give thanks to the following:

Gilbert and Mellish Ltd, 3 Lightening Way, West Heath, Birmingham B31 3PH, UK.

Jane Saunders and Manning, 1070–1072 London Road, Thornton Heath, Surrey CR4 7ND, UK.

Klaveness UK, 14 Woodland Avenue, Narborough, Leicester LE19 3FF, UK.

Mile End Hospital Footwear Centre, Bancroft Road, London E1 4DG, UK.

TayCare Medical Ltd, Swallow House, Tong Road, Leeds LS12 4QG, UK.

Reference

Disabled Living Foundation, 380–384 Harrow Road, London W9 2HU, UK; tel (switchboard): +44 (0)207 289 6111; e-mail: advice@dlf.org.uk; Web site: www.dlf.org.uk.

Measurements for bespoke footwear

Chapter contents

Patients whose feet are not normal in shape may need to have their footwear made on an individual last which is specially designed for them. Footwear made on these individual lasts is known as bespoke. The factor which determines whether or not the patient needs bespoke footwear is whether a last exists which closely matches the shape of the shoe needed, or whether a last needs to be made specifically in order to manufacture a shoe which fits the patient's feet. The accuracy of the last is

the key to obtaining footwear of a satisfactory fit (Fig. 11.1).

Unusual foot shape may be due to an anatomical variation, to pathological changes or just to the fact that the patient has feet which are larger than the normal size range. Even when the feet appear to be abnormal in shape, bespoke footwear may not be necessary. For example, the footwear needs of patients who have undergone partial foot amputation may be adequately met by using stock or modular surgical footwear if the shape of the remaining foot segment is relatively normal. In such cases, a block may be used to fill the part of the shoe which corresponds with the amputated part of the foot. In all cases, it is important to ensure that the shoe can be adequately fastened onto the foot and is securely held in position.

Where the foot is just outside the range of available lasts, it is possible to have existing lasts modified to meet a variety of minor changes in foot shape, and an allowance of up to about 2 cm in additional girth can be added to existing lasts, thus saving on the cost of having a new individual last made for a patient.

Modular footwear can be made to a fitting stage where the shoe is available to try on the patient without the final outer sole in place. It is preferable to obtain modular footwear at a fitting stage where the upper is completed and is attached to a temporary

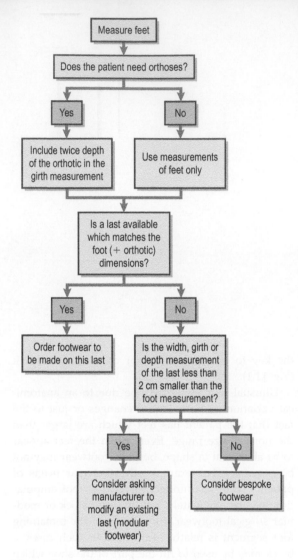

Figure 11.1 Which type of orthopaedic footwear does the patient need?

inner sole. It is possible to try it on the patient's foot at this stage before it is completely finished, as adjustments cannot be made once the shoe is completed and the outer sole is attached. Chapter 10 gives further detail on this. It is worth bearing in mind that when modular footwear is made to a fitting stage, any adjustments made following the fitting will usually attract an extra charge. So when ordering modular footwear, be aware that the charges for the modifications, fitting, any further modifications and secondary fitting may eventually amount to more than the cost of bespoke footwear, where fitting and

adjustment charges are usually included in the overall price quoted. Footwear manufacturers are very helpful and will usually indicate the most economical approach. So if they receive a prescription for modular footwear which includes several modifications to the last, they will usually advise if ordering footwear using a bespoke last would be less costly overall.

Assessing the patient for bespoke footwear

British Standard 5943 provides an extremely useful measurement system for all involved in the prescription and manufacture of bespoke footwear. However, it is necessary to assess footwear needs thoroughly before deciding whether or not bespoke footwear is necessary to meet the needs of each patient's foot and limb pathologies. This is probably best done by observing the patient's gait, identifying the possibility of limb length discrepancy, taking a medical history and evaluating biomechanical status. If the result of each of these evaluations indicates that bespoke footwear may not be necessary, then a less detailed measurement process may be undertaken.

Footwear manufacturers use a range of standard lasts and give details of the dimensions of specific parts of the foot which their lasts are designed to fit. They provide length sizes, usually in the English size system; the width of the foot at the metatarso-phalangeal joints (joint width), usually in millimetres, but sometimes in inches; and fittings relating to girth at the metatarso-phalangeal joints (joint circumference) and at the tarsus (instep circumference). These latter girth measurements are usually given in millimetres. Girth measurements also usually indicate an allowance for insoles or orthoses and these need to be considered when prescribing footwear. Standard lasts will also be made with standard heel height and toe spring relationships. If the patient needs a heel height which is either higher or lower than the standard height – which is usually 2.4 cm or 1 inch – then a bespoke last will need to be made.

A large number of patients requiring surgical footwear may be accommodated within the stock last range, but by using this basic measurement system it is possible to have satisfactory modular footwear made. If, for example, the forefoot measurements appear to match accurately but the tarsal area requires a greater girth than that indicated, the manufacturer will make shoes on a last to which the specified additional girth has been added in the areas indicated by the clinician. Similarly, for example, additional toe depth may be added, quarter heights adjusted or pockets for hallux valgus deformities added to the existing last. The footwear made on this last will include extra depth, width or girth to accommodate those specific features. However, there are limits outside which it is necessary to make specific lasts for patients, and in these cases, the British Standard system is extremely useful. Such limits usually amount to about 2 cm (0.75 inch) in additional girth and about 6 mm (0.25 inch) in depth to various areas of the last.

The footwear styling also needs to be considered. The upper and soling material must be specified and the choice of lining material also needs to be indicated to the manufacturer. It almost goes without saying that the footwear must be strapped or laced in style in order to ensure that the shoes or boots will stay on the foot while accommodating adequate length, width and girth for the foot. A slip-on style would need to be wedged onto the foot to ensure that it stayed on during the swing phase of gait. It would then necessarily be too small during the stance phase when the foot is fully loaded. The fastening type chosen should be one which the patient can do up and undo easily. Some patients will require footwear which is capable of being opened to a greater extent than is normal, and special low openings can be requested for patients who may lack the necessary mobility within their foot to enable them to get the shoe on easily. The height of the heel required on the shoe needs also to be established at the outset, whether or not any heel raise is required. This will determine the profile of the last and cannot be altered once the last is made.

In patients who have a limb length discrepancy and who require a very high raise under the heel, it is probably best to prescribe a boot to ensure sufficient purchase on the leg and foot so that the feet are held adequately within the footwear. It may be that the patient with a large limb length discrepancy who may have spina bifida, post polio syndrome, fixed equinus or various other conditions will also require callipers. If this is the case, any T-straps and calliper entry sockets will need to be included in instructions to the shoe maker. The shoe maker will need to be advised of the shape and positioning of the T-strap,

the length of the fastening strap and number and positioning of buckles or Velcro® required to fasten it. The size and position of calliper entry sockets will also need to be included in instructions. Details of the size of calliper entry sockets are included in Chapter 9.

Taking measurements using the British Standard system may in any case be useful for the manufacturer if the practitioner is undecided as to whether fully bespoke footwear is required. Good relationships with manufacturers will ensure that they advise when fully bespoke footwear is not required. They will be quite prepared to modify an existing last and to supply less costly modular footwear which will meet the needs of the patient. This may be produced to a fitting stage to ensure that the fit is satisfactory before the shoe is finished by the addition of the outer sole.

Patients who need bespoke footwear include those with Charcot deformity, post polio syndrome, rheumatoid arthritis, spina bifida, gross oedema, severe fixed ankle equinus and other fixed deformities. This list is far from exhaustive, and in determining whether or not to prescribe bespoke footwear, the clinician may need to be guided by first measuring the patient's feet, identifying the dimensions of existing lasts used by a range of manufacturers and evaluating how well the dimensions of the patient's feet match those of the lasts. Secondly, they may wish to consider styling. For example, a patient with a forefoot amputation may have difficulty in wearing a stock orthopaedic shoe, but may find a stock orthopaedic boot quite acceptable as the boot has a more proximal fastening, enabling it to stay on the foot without any additional muscular effort from the patient.

Once it has been decided to proceed with bespoke footwear, measurements should be taken using a process which provides all the necessary information and detail required by both the last maker and the shoe maker to enable them to make a pair of shoes that meet the needs of the patient. British Standard 5943 provides a useful and detailed measurement system allowing the clinician to record comprehensive details of the dimensions of each of a patient's feet and to transmit them in a standard format to the last maker and shoe maker. These measurements may also be supplemented by a plaster of Paris impression of each foot also taken in a standard position, although these impressions are not always necessary.

It may also be useful to include a phenolic foam box impression of the plantar surface of the patient's foot as this will provide a greater degree of detail than the plaster of Paris impression. It is essential to follow the British Standard system, or one similar to it, for the satisfactory production of bespoke footwear. It is a useful means of communication between the clinician taking the measurements and the last maker and shoe manufacturer.

British Standard system of measurement for orthopaedic footwear

The British Standard 5943 specifies the basic methods for the taking and recording of all details of the feet necessary for the manufacture of orthopaedic footwear. It provides an extremely useful guide for all involved both in the prescription and in the manufacture of footwear.

The system suggests that before taking measurements, a note is made of brief particulars of the patient including age, shoe-wearing environment and occupation, an evaluation of body mass, diagnosis of the patient's condition, whether the patient's feet and/or ankles are oedematous and, if so, whether the swelling was present at the time of measurement, and how much swelling occurs as the day wears on. The clinician should also assess the patient's peripheral circulatory status, and note the existence of any allergies (particularly to materials used in shoe manufacture), the quality of the skin, the presence of any ulceration, the neurological status and the existence of any significant biomechanical anomalies.

The patient's gait pattern needs to be evaluated and any feature relevant to the footwear prescription should be recorded. It is also useful to note any points of unusual wear on existing footwear, or any other problems such as difficulty in getting shoes on or off, or with securing fastenings.

After evaluating the type of hosiery normally worn by the patient, socks, stockings or tights need to be removed and the feet carefully examined. The last maker needs to have a general description of the feet and needs to be aware of significant features, including the presence of deformities and the existence of any painful lesions, and a description of the overall foot shape indicating whether the feet are short, long, wide, thin, plump or bony, and the tendency towards pes cavus or pes planus. The British Standard suggests that where there is a flat foot, the big toe should be dorsiflexed as far as possible, to see if this restores the medial longitudinal arch, and the result recorded along with indications of mobility or rigidity of the knee, foot and ankle joints. Peculiarities in the heel shape along with plantar surface contours, tender areas and any abnormalities in the sole of the foot should also be noted.

The hosiery which has been removed for this examination needs to be replaced before measurements are taken.

All notes need to be recorded at least in duplicate or in triplicate on a suitable measurement chart. Most footwear manufacturers will supply suitable drafting charts free of charge. They are in duplicate books with adequate room to include outlines of both feet on one page. The charts also include boxes in which to record specific information. The charts include instructions and, if completed fully and accurately, should ensure that the footwear manufactured meets the patient's needs. All measurements indicated on the chart are necessary if the finished product is to fit adequately. One copy of the chart needs to be sent to the manufacturer with the footwear order, but the other needs to be available for the measurer when the footwear is received for a trial fitting (Fig. 11.2).

Measuring and recording equipment

It is important that standard equipment is used so that the last maker knows which allowances are made. For example, it is important to take an outline of the shape of the foot using a standard sized pen, otherwise the finished footwear will not fit accurately. The British Standard suggests that the following equipment is used:

- A properly designed chart: usually available free of charge from footwear manufacturers.
- A ball point pen, 7 mm (0.28 inches) in diameter (pens with tapering bodies are unsuitable).
- A metric measuring tape between 6 mm (0.23 inches) and 10 mm (0.4 inches) wide.
- A metric length gauge (size stick).
- Plaster of Paris bandages or similar impression material and cast-taking equipment.

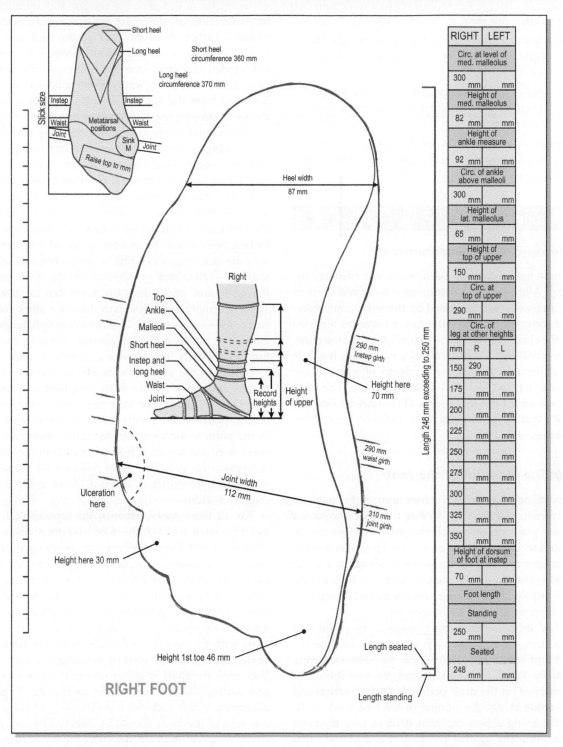

Figure 11.2 Drafting chart showing completed measurements for a shoe for the right foot. Note the position of markings for the tape measure and girth measurements at the instep, waist and joint circumference points.

- A malleable strip.
- A suitable metric height gauge to measure the height of toes and other prominences on the foot.
- A set of blocks for measuring and checking elevations used to accommodate limb length discrepancy.

Further aids which may be helpful are proprietary foot measurement gauges, appropriate photographs and X-rays.

Measurements

Allowances on measurements

Actual measurements need to be recorded on the chart. Allowances on measurements for manufacturing purposes will be added by the last manufacturer and recorded on the chart. Any allowances required by the clinician need to be clearly stated on the chart. These will include allowances for orthoses. It is best to write onto the chart the depth of any orthotic which is to be included in the footwear. The girth allowance for the footwear will then need to include twice that depth (see Ch. 7 for detail on prescribing orthoses).

Outline diagram of the foot

An outline diagram of the foot needs to be made on the measuring chart. To do this, the ideal is to have a raised platform on which the patient's chair can be placed so they can sit in an elevated position, and the measurer can also be comfortably seated at a lower level while taking the measurements. If no platform is available, the measurer will need to sit or kneel on the floor to take the measurements.

The measurement chart needs to be positioned on a firm, flat surface in a position near the patient's seat and onto which the feet can be positioned comfortably. When making the draft, the foot should be positioned on the draft pad with the leg vertical and the ankle at 90°. An outline of the foot needs to be made, using a pen of 7 mm (0.28 inches) diameter held vertically against the foot. It is important that the foot outline is continuous and unbroken at the back of the heel. The best way of ensuring this is for a right-handed measurer to start the outline on the

left-hand side of the chart, approximately 50 mm (about 2 inches) from the back of the heel, and to draw clockwise around the foot. Conversely, for a left-handed measurer, start the outline on the right-hand side of the chart, approximately 50 mm (about 2 inches) from the back of the heel and draw anti-clockwise around the outline of the foot.

This outline needs to be taken with any padding or dressings which are worn regularly in place, and the patient should be wearing the hosiery they intend to wear in the shoes. If the draft is taken barefoot, note that fact on the draft and inform the last maker of this fact. It is also necessary to record on the chart the length of each foot in millimetres or inches, both when the patient is seated and when they are standing. Once this is completed and with the foot maintained in position on the draft pad, the girth and width measurements can be taken. These are more extensive than those for stock footwear. Measurements at the metatarso-phalangeal joints and instep are taken as with stock footwear but, additionally, the waist measurement, immediately behind the metatarsal heads, is also taken. It is then necessary to take both long heel and short heel measurements. The long heel extends from the central point on the plantar-retro-calcaneal junction to the point at which the instep girth measurement was taken, and the short heel extends from the same retro-calcaneal junction to the point on the dorsum of the foot immediately in front of the ankle joint (Figs 11.3–11.5).

For all these measurements, the tape should be tightly drawn around the foot and then released slightly so that the tissues are not compressed. It is then also necessary to indicate the presence of any anomalies which may affect the ankle. For example, oedema may be indicated by including a broken line indicator comprised of two semi-circular outlines drawn around the oedematous area onto the chart with the pen at a 45° angle. Similarly, narrow ankles should be indicated by drawing two concave lines onto the chart at either side of the ankle area, and adding 'XX' to denote the narrowing. Valgus deformity, which includes a unilateral narrowing to one side of the heel, should be denoted by using a single concave mark on the chart on the narrowed side (Fig. 11.6).

Where boots are to be prescribed, additional measurements are needed, including the circumference

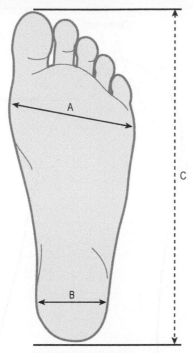

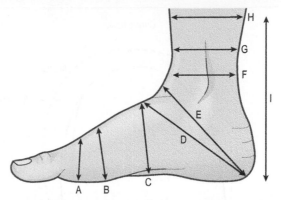

Figure 11.4 Foot girth measurements should be taken at the following points: A, joint circumference (first to fifth metatarso-phalangeal joints); B, waist circumference (from a point just behind the heads of the first to fifth metatarsals; C, instep circumference (at a point which corresponds to the first metatarsal – medial cuneiform joint); D, long heel measurement; E, short heel measurement. Additional measurements for boots: F, malleolar circumference; G, ankle circumference just above the malleoli; H, at a point 130 mm above the ground level (I on the chart). For boots with higher quarters, additional measurements should be taken at 25 mm intervals up the leg until the boot height is reached.

Figure 11.3 Foot length and width measurements: A, width at metatarso-phalangeal joints; B, width at heel; C, length of foot from heel to longest toe.

horizontally around the malleoli at the level of the medial malleolus, the circumference around the ankle just above the malleoli and the circumference at the top of the upper. It is also useful to record the circumference of the leg at regular intervals throughout the height of the boot quarter. The required height of the finished boot should also be indicated. Once girth measurements are completed, width and height measurements need to be recorded. The width of the foot at the metatarso-phalangeal joint needs to be noted, as does the width across the heel at the position of the malleoli. The height of any prominences over the toes or at any other position on the foot should be included on the chart and a note of any special features which the shoe maker will need to take into account. The malleable strip may be used in the case of any anomalous condition, to record the shape of the retro-calcaneal profile extending up along the back of the leg. This shape may then be traced onto a free part of the measurement chart, with labelling indicating what it is and which is the proximal and which the distal end of the curve (Fig. 11.7).

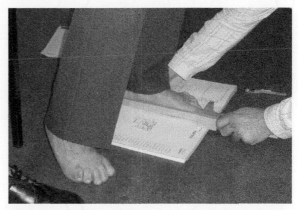

Figure 11.5 Taking foot length measurements when drafting for bespoke footwear.

The footwear manufacturer will also need to consider whether any orthoses are required, and if so, details of the allowance required needs to be included in the manufacturing instructions being sent. Details of any elevations required must also be included. These measurements must include the height of the heel elevation directly inferior to the

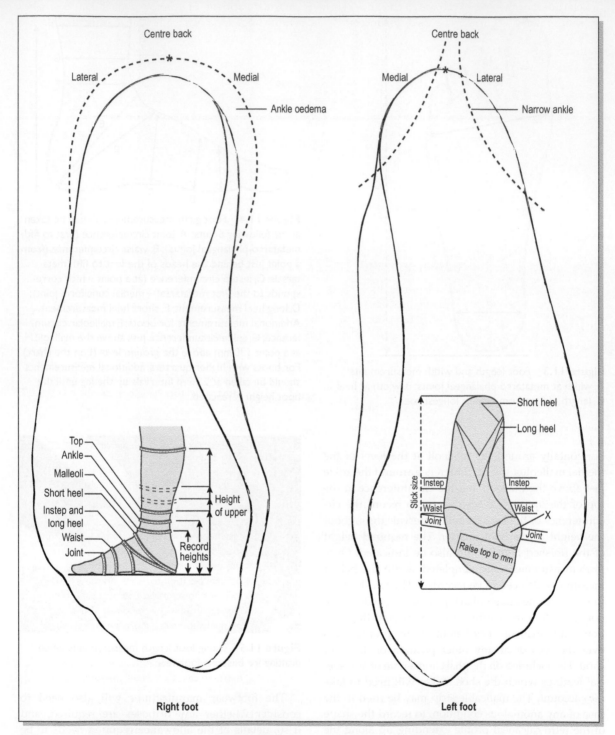

Figure 11.6 Note the indications for ankle oedema on the right foot and for a narrow ankle on the left foot on these incomplete drafts. Where the oedema is not evenly distributed around the ankle, measure from the centre back of the heel to both medial and lateral sides separately, and indicate the distribution on the chart. Recording this information helps the pattern designer to shape the quarters correctly.

Figure 11.7 Drafting where the foot is unable to make full contact with the draft pad. Note that the heel outline has been estimated on the chart. A plaster of Paris impression will need to be sent to the manufacturer with this chart.

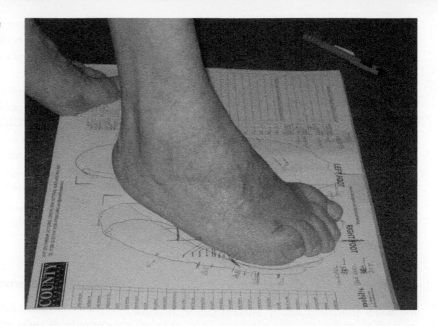

lateral malleolus, and the height of raise required at the metatarso-phalangeal joints and at the toes (see Ch. 9). In describing the raise required, it should be stipulated whether the raise is to be included as an external raise to the footwear, as an internal raise within the shoe or a combination of both.

Circumferential measurements

Circumferential measurements need to be noted in small units of measurement and the millimetre is suggested as the best unit. If using imperial measurements, be sure to state this on the chart. When taking the measurements, the tape should be pulled tight enough to compress the tissues a little and then released sufficiently to allow the normal elasticity of the tissues to bring the tape back to the correct measurement tension. Read the measurement off the tape measure when the tape is held at the correct tension.

When taking the circumferential measurements, the position of the foot on the chart must remain unchanged. The foot must remain in the position in which the outline was taken, as this allows the position of the tape measure also to be recorded on the chart, making it easier for the last manufacturer to accurately capture the data.

Circumferential measurements need to be taken at the following points:

- Joint circumference: this is an oblique measurement running from the first to the fifth metatarso-phalangeal joints.
- Waist circumference: the waist of the foot is the smallest girth measurement of the forefoot and is the circumference measured immediately behind the heads of the first to the fifth metatarsals.
- Instep circumference: this is measured at the centre point of the medial longitudinal arch with the tape measure passing over the point of articulation between the first metatarsal and the medial cuneiform.
- Long heel circumference: starting from the same point on the dorsum of the foot as for the instep measurement, the tape measure is taken around the back of the furthermost point of the heel where it touches the ground retro-calcaneally.
- Short heel circumference: this is measured from the same furthermost point of the heel (as in the long heel measurement) to the point on the dorsum of the foot on the anterior surface of the ankle joint which gives the smallest measurement.

Additional circumferential measurements for boots

Where boots are prescribed, additional measurements need to be taken. These include:

- Malleoli circumference: this measurement is taken horizontally around the bony prominence at the level of the medial malleolus. The height of the measurement position above the base of the heel needs to be noted on the chart.

- Ankle circumference: this is the circumference just above the malleoli. The height of the measurement position above the base of the heel needs to be noted on the chart.

- Top: this is the circumference at the top of the upper.

The height of the upper above the base of the heel for boots (normally about 140 mm (5.5 inches) for men and 130 mm (5 inches) for ladies) needs to be noted. If the height of the upper exceeds 150 mm (6 inches), circumferential measurements should be taken around the leg at every 25 mm (1 inch) interval to the top of the upper.

Foot length measurements

The overall length of each foot should be measured using a metric (or suitable imperial) length gauge (size stick). Two overall length measurements need to be taken and recorded for each foot, one in the standard seated measurement position and one in the normal standing position. These should both be taken while the foot is still in position on the chart, with the length measured from the medial side of the foot and the position in which the measurement was taken (i.e. the placement of the size stick) marked on the chart.

Height measurements

- Abnormal prominences on the dorsum (e.g. hammer toes, claw toes or swellings) need to be measured with a height gauge and their position correctly marked on the outline diagram of the foot. In the case of pes cavus, the height of the highest point of the dorsum also needs to be measured with a gauge and be recorded on the chart.

- The position of any abnormalities on the plantar surface (e.g. bony prominences, ulcers, etc.) need to be indicated on the outline diagram of the foot.

- When measuring for shoes, any abnormalities of the hind foot (e.g. inverted and everted feet) need to be indicated by taking measurements of the height of the distal extremity of both the medial and lateral malleoli, so that any abnormal shape of the upper at these positions can be included in the last.

- Where measurements cannot be taken accurately, plaster of Paris impressions should be taken.

Other requirements

Where the retro-calcaneal profile is abnormal, for example in cases of Haglund's deformity or other heel bumps, the shape of the back of the heel needs to be recorded.

When the back of the heel is abnormally shaped, there will be difficulty with fitting unless the upper is correctly cut. If necessary, a malleable strip of material can be used to denote the presence of abnormalities at the back of the leg. The malleable strip will need to be placed at the back of the leg and bent to the shape of the heel and leg. This shape should then be copied onto the measurement chart.

In difficult cases, again a plaster of Paris impression of the foot should be taken.

Measuring for limb length discrepancy

Before prescribing any footwear, it is advisable to consider any other factors which may influence choice of style of shoe, shoe upper materials and the type and style of soling which would best suit the patient's needs and lifestyle. It is also essential to note the type of hosiery normally worn and to note any other relevant information including allergies to materials which might normally be included in the footwear manufacturing process. If a limb length discrepancy is suspected, it should be measured before proceeding any further. With the patient supine, using a flexible tape, measure the length in millimetres from the ziphoid process of the sternum to the medial malleolus of each leg (the ziphoid process is

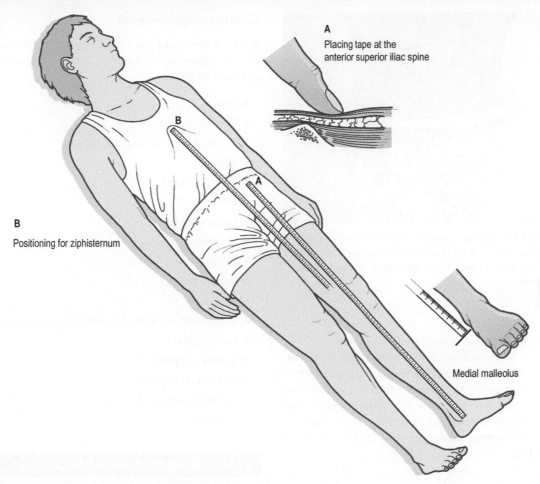

A

Placing tape at the
anterior superior iliac spine

B

Positioning for ziphisternum

A

Medial malleolus

Figure 11.8 Measuring for limb length discrepancy.

preferred to the umbilicus as the point of reference as it is more likely to be central). Next, take a measurement in millimetres from each anterior superior iliac crest to the medial malleolus of the same leg. Compare these measurements and evaluate the extent of any limb length discrepancy (Fig. 11.8) (see also Ch. 13).

Using blocks of non-compressible material which equate in height to the measured discrepancy, place the blocks to elevate the foot of the shorter limb, and extend the raise forward under the foot using the formula detailed in Chapter 9:

- Heel raise = 1 unit
- Raise at metatarso-phalangeal joints = 0.5 unit
- Raise at toe = 0.25 or 0 unit.

Ask the patient to stand with the shorter limb on this elevation and offer support if the patient is unsteady. Ask the patient whether it feels comfortable with the shorter limb elevated to this height. Pay particular attention to any spinal discomfort that may be experienced.

The aim of the raise is to allow the limbs to function symmetrically. To check this, use a pelvic level This instrument is comprised of a curved bar with moveable arms. The bar includes a spirit level placed on its top surface. The curved bar is held in front of the abdomen so that each of the arms of the instrument can rest on the relevant anterior superior iliac spine. Once in position, check the spirit level reading and adjust the height of the blocks under the shortened limb. Where patients have accommodated

167

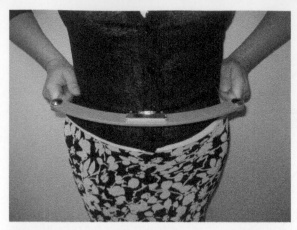

Figure 11.9 Using the pelvic level. The arms of this instrument are held on the anterior superior iliac crests, while the level is read off the spirit level on the front of the device.

a limb length discrepancy over many years, it may be better to allow them to function with a slight discrepancy rather than giving them a full raise. Over the coming years, as biomechanical accommodation changes, the full height of the required raise may be gradually prescribed. Having determined the height of raise required, note it on the patient record (Fig. 11.9).

Additional essential information to be recorded on the measurement chart

The following information should also be recorded on the chart:

Constructional requirements

- Whether boots or shoes are required.
- The colour of the footwear.
- Type of footwear, the style of upper, type of upper material, the type of lining required, inlay material, bottom material, substance of bottom material, height of heel, method of construction (i.e. welted or cemented), method of fastening, toe shape, puffs and stiffeners.

Clinical requirements

Relevant details of the positioning and dimensions of the following clinical requirements should be recorded on the chart:

- Socket
- T-strap
- D-ring for toe-raising appliances
- Stiffener
- Extended heel
- Flared heel
- Metatarsal bar
- Wedge
- Rocker sole
- Rocker bar
- Sole plate
- Shoe insert orthosis, e.g. Ankle-foot orthosis
- Loose inlay
- Valgus support
- Metatarsal support
- Felt or sponge pad
- Elevation.

Prescribing footwear elevations

- Details of elevation requirements should be given. The two important measurements for an elevation (raise) are those under the heel and under the metatarso-phalangeal joints. A toe measurement can be given, but this will usually be determined by the toe spring required. Where possible, give measurements of a previously satisfactory elevation and include them on the chart.

- Heel measurements should be taken from the centre of the base directly under the lateral malleolus, and not from the extreme back of the heel.

- Joint measurements need to be taken from a point directly under the metatarsal heads.

- For a short leg with a normal foot and ankle joint, the patient may require, typically, an elevation of 50 mm (2 inches) at the heel, 25 mm

Figure 11.10 Bespoke footwear: casting a patient with ankle equinus. Note the heel elevations in place and the horizontal and vertical cast markings which allow the last maker to correctly orientate the impression. Another vertical line will be drawn at the back of the cast to ensure that the cast can be correctly orientated in the three body planes.

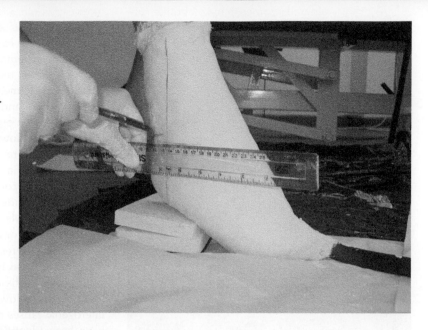

(1 inch) at the joint and as little as 10 mm (four-tenths of an inch) at the toe.

- In cases of a fixed equinus, a plaster cast is essential. This cast needs to extend far enough up the leg to clearly reflect the angle of the foot to the leg.

- In cases where the leg lengths are equal, but a fixed equinus results in the forefoot extending beyond the foot of the normal leg, it will be necessary to raise the normal side in order to level the pelvis.

- In general, elevations may be inside the footwear, outside the footwear or a combination of both.

Taking casts

In certain cases where bespoke footwear is needed (but not all), it is advisable not only to take a draft of the feet but also to take an impression of the feet in plaster of Paris or similar impression material. Where plaster of Paris foot impressions are required, it is first wise to wrap the patient's leg in cling film or similar material so that the skin is protected from the impression material. It is then useful to tape a plastic protector strip to the front of the patient's leg so that removal of the cast using either a cast saw

or scissors may be done without causing any damage to the patient's leg. The preparatory work is now complete. Position the patient with the foot plantargrade, but with an appropriate block representing the required heel height of the finished footwear in place under the patient's heel while the impression is setting (Fig. 11.10).

The cast should then be marked with a vertical line through the lateral malleolus and a true horizontal line also marked on the cast below the vertical line. Another line should be drawn on the back of the cast indicating the vertical. From this, the last maker will see whether there are any inversion, eversion, valgus or varus deformities to be taken into account. This will help in determining the positioning of the sole of the shoe. These lines correspond to the cardinal body planes and should capture deformity in the sagittal, transverse and frontal planes. Once dry and able to hold its shape, the front of the plaster of Paris cast should be marked with a series of horizontal lines crossing the plastic leg protector positioned before the cast material was applied. The cast should be removed from the leg using cast scissors or a cast saw along the protective line of the plastic strip, and afterwards the cast should be re-joined using more of the casting material, ensuring that the horizontal lines previously drawn meet across the front of the impression (Fig. 11.11).

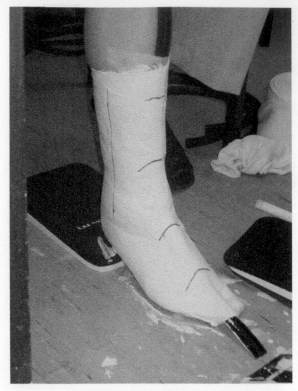

Figure 11.11 Taking a plaster of Paris impression for bespoke shoe manufacture. Note the protective plastic strip in place and the horizontal lines marked across the front of the cast to allow for correct re-joining of the impression once it has been cut off the leg.

To cast or not to cast?

When a foot has relatively normal angulations, casts may not be necessary and drafts alone may be adequate for the last maker to manufacture a bespoke last. The draft provides a two-dimensional foot shape, and the measurements of width and girth at specified points on the foot provide adequate detail where there are no severe deformities of joint position. However, there are cases where taking a cast impression of the foot is absolutely essential to obtaining footwear which fits adequately and drafts alone would be insufficient. Casts are absolutely essential in cases of equinus deformity, valgus deformation of the midfoot, inversion or eversion deformities, Charcot changes or in any case where the foot displays an abnormality of shape. If in any doubt, it is wise to take a cast of the foot.

Fixed equinus deformities are such conditions where casting is essential. Mild equinus deformities may occur in females who wear high-heeled shoes and experience tissue shortening of the posterior muscle compartment of the leg. However, this is usually not severe and not a permanent deformity and may be reversed over time by using a gentle stretching regime and lowering the heel height of footwear gradually. Severe equinus deformities, however, usually occur as a result of a neurological condition which may be congenital or acquired. Congenital causes may include conditions such as talipes equino varus, Charcot-Marie-Tooth disease, Duchenne muscular dystrophy or cerebral palsy. The condition may be acquired as a result of infections such as poliomyelitis. It may also be seen as a result of cerebrovascular accident, disseminated sclerosis and following fractures of the lower aspects of the tibia and fibula. Iaterogenic causes may also be considered, and cases have been identified following surgical fixation of the ankle joint, following casting where the foot has been held in plantarflexion for a period of time, and as a consequence of forefoot amputations where the insertions of foot extensors have been lost and the flexor group lack an antagonistic pull.

Severe equinus deformity seen today is often in the elderly whose congenital foot problems were untreatable during infancy and youth, and in immigrants from countries where medical care to treat the condition was unavailable in the early years. Congenital problems in economically secure nations today are usually successfully treated during infancy, and any residual condition may be minor.

While any condition which restricts ankle joint dorsiflexion to less than 10° of dorsiflexion from the subtalar neutral position may be defined as equinus, some patients are seen with severe deformity where the ankle is fixed with the foot in plantarflexion and heel–ground contact is impossible. Obtaining footwear for people with a fixed equinus condition can be challenging, and where these problems are present, bespoke orthopaedic footwear may be the only option. Such footwear can provide an extremely successful outcome but the prescription and fitting requires skill and expertise. The footwear prescriber is faced with the need to use a systematic approach to measurement and impression taking.

The first stage in the process must be to evaluate limb length in both anatomical and functional aspects.

It is possible, if the equinus is congenital or acquired in early life, that both limbs will have developed to different lengths to the malleolar point, but to similar lengths to the metatarso-phalangeal joints when the feet are load-bearing. If the problem was acquired in later life, it is more likely that the limbs will be of equal length to malleolar level but the equinus deformity may make the affected foot functionally longer, requiring the individual to modify gait to accommodate the dysfunction. It must be considered that bilateral symmetry is essential for fully effective gait. Where asymmetry is present, compensation will be required which may in turn cause joint misalignment and damage. A pragmatic approach to limb length evaluation is best. Examine limb lengths from the ziphoid process and from the anterior-superior iliac crests to the medial malleoli. Examine the spine for compensatory curves and assess the level of the pelvis. Once a discrepancy has been identified, use blocks under the heel of the shorter limb to assess the effect of the height of the raise on pelvic level, and on other compensatory features previously identified such as spinal curvature. It is then wise to ask the patient about the level of comfort which the raise offers and to adjust accordingly. In cases of fixed equinus, it will be necessary to balance the two limbs extremely carefully to ensure that the functional length of the limb with fixed equinus is the same length to heel–ground contact as the other unaffected limb with the raise in place.

The difficulty in taking measurements where there is ankle equinus is that the foot cannot be placed flat onto a draft pad. Nevertheless, it is important to place the parts of the foot which normally contact the ground onto the draft pad and to draw around those and then to use a dotted line dropped vertically from the raised areas of the foot (the heel), identifying their relationship with the remainder of the foot. Width and girth measurements should be taken as normal and noted onto the chart (metatarso-phalangeal joint, waist, and instep girth, and width at the metatarso-phalangeal joints and heel). The apparent length of the foot will also be less than the actual length, as the foot will be held in an arched configuration. However, the true length of the foot can be measured using a tape measure carefully held against the plantar surface of the foot from the heel to the longest digit. This measurement and the position from which the measurement was taken should then be transferred to the draft. Long and short heel measurements, ankle and

malleolar circumference measurements and leg circumference measurements at stated heights will also need to be taken when boots are required.

It is absolutely essential to take a plaster of Paris impression of the equinus foot as this will capture all three dimensions of the foot (length, width and girth), and will also capture the relationships between the various segments of the foot. This is required to allow the last maker to replicate the foot shape in the last. When taking the impression, the positioning of the foot is paramount. The leg must be positioned in the frontal plane, and immediately following the application of the plaster of Paris bandage, before it begins to set, the required elevation needs to be placed under the appropriate heel and the foot positioned with the forefoot in contact with the ground and the heel in full contact with the elevation blocks. A vertical line must then be drawn from the lateral malleolus proximally along the leg, and then a line at the base of this vertical which marks the true horizontal position. Another vertical line should be drawn at the back of the cast to ensure that the frontal plane position is accurate. This will enable the shoe maker to ensure that the last is made in the correct position with heel elevation identifiable from the cast and, most significantly, the tread line accurately located. It is also useful to photograph the patient's feet and to send a copy of the photograph with orders to the footwear manufacturer (Figs 11.7, 11.10).

Send the cast to the manufacturer with the foot drafts and measurements. When sending casts, always ensure that they are allowed to dry thoroughly before packing, as this will minimize any possible distortion. Inserting packing material inside the casts will also help in ensuring that it reaches the manufacturer in good condition, and a cushioning agent such as bubble wrap is also helpful in ensuring safe transportation.

The trial fitting

Bespoke footwear will be made to a trial fitting stage. Here, the upper of the shoe will have been completed but it will be attached to a temporary inner sole, will have no outer sole in place and will have a temporary heel loosely held in position (Fig. 11.12).

On receipt of the footwear, check against the order and the retained copy of the chart with the detailed

Figure 11.12 Footwear at fitting stage. Note that there is no outer sole in place and note the attachment of a temporary cork heel.

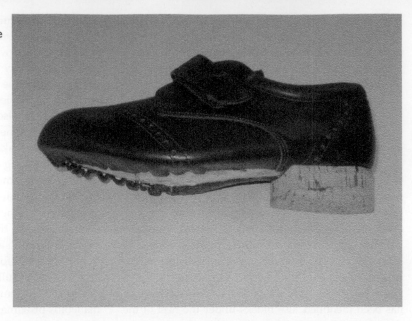

outline and measurements of the patient's feet. Ensure that the shoe style, material and colour are correct, the fastening is as requested and that the measurements match those on the draft. Also check that any raises required are planned to be added to the correct side. The footwear will be received at fitting stage without the raises in place. The British Standard states that raises should be available at this stage, but this is rarely practicable for shoe manufacturers.

The footwear needs to be tried on the patient's feet with any orthoses or cradles intended to be worn with it put in place. The patient should also be wearing appropriate hosiery; that which will normally be worn with these shoes or boots. The footwear should be fastened firmly using either the laces, straps or Velcro® fastening attached to the shoes. The patient should be asked to stand, with help if necessary, and to walk, again with help, for a few steps to evaluate the fit during gait. The footwear will be slightly unstable because of the temporary heel attachment and the lack of outer soling, so care is essential to ensure that the patient does not trip or fall during the trial fitting. Assess the fit using the criteria detailed in Chapter 13 and, when satisfied, return to the manufacturer for adjustment or finishing with full instructions on what is required. Any adjustments required to be made to the upper should be marked on the upper leather using a special effaceable pen, and full details should be recorded in the

patient's notes and on the trial fitting form which will come with the footwear from the manufacturer. It is essential to keep a copy of every instruction to the manufacturer, particularly to ensure that, in the case of repeat orders, all modifications are included.

It is also worth checking on the outer sole requirements to ensure that the original prescription is still valid. It is possible to have the prescription changed at this stage, provided it does not alter the toe spring/heel height relationship.

Fitting footwear at this stage will be difficult for patients with high unilateral raises. In such cases, the shoe for the shorter length limb can be assessed only during weight-on if a large, firm block of material which matches the height of the raise can be provided for the patient to stand on. Trying this footwear during gait is difficult unless the patient already has an existing shoe with a raise for the shorter limb. If so, the new shoe at fitting stage for the longer limb can be tried. The new shoe for the shorter limb can only be tried in the weight-on position, but usually this is sufficient to ensure adequacy of fit, particularly as, in cases where high raises are required, foot motion will be controlled by using a rocker sole.

Detailed notes of any alterations required, giving exact measurement wherever possible, should be recorded on a triplicate trial fitting form designed for this purpose. One copy of this form needs to be available for the measurer at subsequent fittings.

It is extremely important that detailed notes of alterations made at trial fittings are recorded in the patient's records by the manufacturer. If this is not done, and trial fitting information is not correctly recorded, there is a great danger that repeat orders for the patient will repeat the original mistakes.

Critical evaluation of British Standard measurement charts

It is essential to draw a very clear and accurate British Standard chart for bespoke items. If the foot outline is not accurate (if the line is broken or irregular, or the measurements taken are not quoted accurately in millimetres but are rounded up to the nearest centimetre), the footwear is unlikely to fit. The skill required to take a draft can be developed by practising and should take the competent practitioner only 15–20 minutes to complete.

Once the chart is completed, it is useful to be able to evaluate it. Critical evaluation will identify missing measures, wobbly lines and confusing instructions. It is essential to identify them and correct them while the patient is still in the clinic, because the consequence could be footwear which does not fit, and this could be quite expensive in terms of time, patient satisfaction and in financial terms.

Once the chart has been drafted, it is useful to perform an objective evaluation by asking the following questions:

- Has the correct equipment been used? There is a clear list of items in the British Standard to ensure reliability of measurement.
- What happens if a thicker or thinner pen than 7 mm has been used? A thick pen will add extra allowance onto the outline and this will be reflected in too large a shoe at the fitting stage. A thin pen has a similar but opposite effect in causing the finished result to be rather tight.
- Are all the required measurements listed? The drafting pads often include a useful checklist or boxes which need to be completed which act as an *aide-mémoire* so that no important measurement is missed. There is no need to measure above the ankle unless boots are being made, so when drafting for a shoe, a

few minutes may be saved in omitting these unnecessary measurements.

- What happens when measures are missed off the chart? By checking straight away before the patient leaves, the option of replacing the foot on the draft and adding any missing measures is available. Last makers have great skill in guessing the missing measures but would prefer to receive accurate detail. Their guess may lead to poorly fitting footwear.
- Does the last maker know if the tape has been correctly positioned? Learning the correct positions for the tape using bony landmarks as a guide is the best way to obtain good results. Marking the tape positions on the chart in addition to the measurements also helps the last maker, as he can take the measure in exactly the same position.
- Does it matter if the heel line is poorly drawn? A badly drawn heel line with wobbles or mismatched lines will affect the heel fitting and it is best to redraw the heel line and Tippex® out any misdrawn lines for clarity.
- Drawing a line from the medial side of the heel under the instep through to the first toe with the pen at 45° is suggested. What does it tell the last maker? This line helps the last maker to visualize the foot shape and the height of the arch area, as there are classic positions for foot shapes such as pes cavus and pes planus. It also helps clarify the heel width and joint width as the line should be drawn where the skin touches the ground.
- Should the position of the size stick be marked or only the reading noted? By placing lines at the top and bottom of the size stick, the last maker is then able to place his stick in exactly the same place for checking the sizes recorded. Remember there is no absolute standard in manufacture of size sticks so the last maker may need to remeasure using the one he is familiar with.
- What methods for marking unusual features can be used? Marking the feature with two bisecting lines at 90° to each other on the chart accurately marks its centre position. In addition, measure any heights or depths and write on the draft what they are and, where possible, take a

Polaroid® photo or electronic photo of the feet to send along with the chart.

- How necessary is this? Photos are not essential but prove to be an invaluable way of communicating unusual features.

- Does the last maker need a diagnosis of the foot condition? This is essential as the last maker needs to know details about the patient. A diagnosis of the condition will also help to get the prescription right: classic shapes such as pes cavus, a rheumatoid foot and a Charcot deformity immediately inform the last maker of the necessary alterations that will be required to the last.

- Has the prescription of the footwear been clearly listed with all the required fields completed? For boots, measure above the malleoli to the required top height. If the foot shape is grossly abnormal or the heel position is severely in varus or valgus, then casts to support the chart are essential.

- If an elevation is required, are all the details of the heights, inside or outside, and the type of elevation required stated? If a cradle is required, then so is a cast labelled with horizontal and vertical lines and the patient's name.

- Where oedema is significant, especially around the ankle, is the heel profile or heel width defined? Use the size stick to grip the sides of the heel and measure the space created carefully. Drawing the contact point of the heel to the floor adds a very useful dimension to a swollen heel area.

- Has the first joint width been clearly marked on the outline? Joint width in addition to joint circumference is necessary as it enables the last maker to allow the correct width under the first joint. This can be deducted from the measurement of the joint circumference. Similarly, if the heel is very wide or very narrow, the heel width measure can be very useful.

- Is the heel-to-ball length easily seen on the chart for the last maker? An extra line indicating the position of the first metatarso-phalangeal joint is useful for the last maker to check heel-to-ball length.

Effects on the footwear

If the draft is badly drawn or incorrectly completed, the resulting fit may also be problematic. The last maker assumes that a standard 7 mm pen has been used to mark the foot outline. Using a different pen size will change the measurements and will result in a larger or wider fit being produced.

A snug heel fit is essential, and if the whole last is too wide, then heel slip will be inevitable. This is difficult to correct without a major last alteration. This adds cost.

Failing to place the tape measure in exactly the correct position, particularly for the instep, will affect the placement of the footwear top line and facings when the pattern is made: this can cause them to be too close to the ankle, catching it as the foot dorsiflexes, or to be too low, allowing a loose heel fit and slippage.

Check every detail required by the British Standard and ensure that each has been met. The manufacturer can only work on the information given.

At the trial fitting stage, should there be significant problems with the fit, then recheck the measurements by placing the foot back onto the draft outline and re-measure. Look for any differences, as these may be the reason why the footwear is either too tight or too loose. If the foot measurements are still the same as the original, check the positions of the tape measure on the chart. If the tape is wrongly placed, the footwear made from the measurements may not fit.

Are the measures clearly written and is the unit of measurement clearly identified on the chart as millimetres or inches?

It is occasionally worthwhile to redraw the chart and to compare the original with the new one and identify and evaluate any differences that might appear.

Other information required by the manufacturer

The features of the outer sole required must also be identified and specified at the measurement stage. In addition, the style of shoe or boot, the colour and type of upper and lining material, the extent and positioning of stiffeners, the fastenings required, and additions such as callipers and calliper entry sockets and T-straps must also be included in instructions. The footwear will be made without the outer sole in place and this will give an opportunity for fitting to the patient. If the fit is less than perfect, adjustments may be made by indicating those required to the factory. The soling unit may then be added. The choice of soling unit and of finish may be slightly less extensive than in the case of stock and certain modular shoes. As soles also need to be bespoke, mass-produced injection moulded sole units are usually unsuitable for bespoke footwear. However, the available materials should ensure that the therapeutic needs of the footwear are met.

One additional specific feature which may be included in bespoke footwear relates to the inclusion of various modifications in the actual inner sole of the footwear. In particular, sinks for prominent metatarsal heads (most commonly the first), valgus supports or metatarsal domes or bars may be added at the manufacturing stage. This means that the inner sole will reflect the contours of the plantar surface of the foot rather than being a flat pitched surface.

The positioning of the modifications required need to be indicated on the measurement chart and confirmed with either a plaster of Paris impression of the foot or a phenolic foam impression of the plantar surface.

Summary

In summary, manufacturers hold a wide range of stock lasts which may fit a large number of patients requiring therapeutic footwear. It is possible to modify those lasts to accommodate minor foot deformities, but where the foot is outside this normal range, the guidance offered by the British Standard is extremely useful in transferring information from the clinician to the last maker and shoe maker, thus ensuring that the finished footwear meets the patient's needs. Communication is the key to successful last and shoe making. The British Standard provides an excellent guide and working tool indicating the system of measurement required for the successful manufacture of footwear that fits.

Fitting bespoke footwear

Clinical approach to fitting

All bespoke and modular footwear is available for a fitting part way through the manufacturing process. At this fitting stage, the upper is fully formed but is only loosely attached to an inner sole, and it is possible to have the upper modified in size and shape to meet any problems with fit when the footwear is tried on the patient's feet. This fitting stage is essential if the footwear is to fit well and provide effective therapy. A clear and systematic approach to testing the fit of the footwear is fundamental and will ensure that all parts of the shoe–foot relationship are examined.

While it is possible to modify the footwear at this stage, the fewer the number of alterations necessary, the better the outcome will be. In the ideal situation,

no changes will be necessary at fitting, but achieving a perfect fit at this stage will require accuracy of initial measurements, well-drafted charts, good casts and all other relevant details logged. The manufacturer's high level of skill in interpreting these data and in preparing lasts and patterns of appropriate dimensions is also essential for good-fitting footwear.

Ultimately the goal of fitting is to achieve footwear of adequate width and length, with a snug heel fit, comfortable top line, properly aligned fastenings and correct depth for the instep, toes or any deformity, using the fitting principles already described in Chapter 5. The most successful approach to checking fit relies on an initial assessment of the overall fit when the footwear is first placed on the foot. Where a fitting seems to have several problems which need to be corrected, the best approach is to make the changes so that the correct heel fit is obtained first. Other areas may then be adjusted later. If there are several other areas where fit seems poor, they are best addressed one at a time. This will mean that more than one fitting appointment is necessary but this is the only way to ensure adequate fit of the completed footwear. When one part of a shoe is altered, that alteration may have a consequential effect on other parts of the shoe. For example, reducing the instep circumference will alter the way the facings lay, and if too many changes are made at one time, the end result may be quite unexpected – a shoe which is unwearable.

Identifying fitting problems and finding a solution are vital to the successful outcome of the footwear being provided. There are a number of common fitting issues that can be identified and these are easily solved by identification of the factors that may be the cause. Table 12.1 at the end of this chapter will help you to identify the most likely solutions to the most common problems. The table works through the main fitting areas, starting at the heel counter and progressing to the toe box.

The purpose of trial (or rough) fittings

The trial fitting is designed to assess and record accurate information about the fit of the shoe that can be clearly understood by the manufacturer. It should enable all the modifications necessary to correct the fitting to be carried out. A comprehensive understanding of the technical terminology and a sound communication pathway with the manufacturer are both essential components of a successful clinician–manufacturer partnership. Prescribing and manufacturing bespoke footwear is complex and detailed, and there may be times when a written note describing the modifications needed does not clarify what is required, whereas a discussion with the technical manager may lead to better understanding and a solution may be found that the clinician was unfamiliar with.

In addition, photographs of the footwear on the patient's foot can also help the manufacturer to understand the nature of the fitting problem. Working this way gives the clinician the opportunity to learn about the technical aspects of footwear manufacture and thus learn about the best approach to prescribing footwear that will fit. Learning more about the complexity of footwear manufacture combined with regular visits to the factory to see the processes being performed, and observing, discussing and participating in the making of an item are invaluable experiences which can inform future clinical practice. This builds valuable expertise in footwear measurement and prescription and reduces the likelihood of problems at the fitting stage, saving time for the clinician and patient and also saving money.

A systematic approach to fitting will include the following:

- **Visual examination:** looking at all the relevant areas for good or poor fit on weight-bearing and when walking.
- **Feel:** the ease with which the shoe goes onto the foot tells much about how well it fits. Feel to check for tight spots or excessive leather.
- **Ask:** the patient for comments on comfort, fit, appearance, painful areas, support, inlays, etc.
- **Mark:** the points at which adjustment needs to be made on the shoe using an effaceable leather marking pen. Make the pen marks clear. For example, circle over a tight spot on the dorsum of a hammer toe: draw exactly the position on the shoe where it may need to be taken in, for example behind the first metatarso-phalangeal joint in a case of hallux valgus.
- **Write:** in addition to the marks on the shoe, write a fitting note detailing exactly what needs to be done to the shoe. On this note, include all measurements in millimetres. Marks alone are insufficient information.
- **Photograph:** a visual image is invaluable where the description is complex. Take photographs using an instant Polaroid® camera or electronic camera and send them to the factory with the shoes to be modified. The factory technicians are only too pleased to be able to visualize what is wrong via a picture.

What to look for in a trial/rough fit

Using the principles of fitting, systematically check the footwear for all the areas of fit, noting anything that needs altering. First, check that the shoes received match the order for this particular patient. Remove all packaging from inside the footwear. Start with the patient seated and remove the inlay from the footwear.

Inlays

Use the inlay as the first point of evaluating fit, to check the length and width of the footwear. Place the foot onto the inlay carefully, allowing a small gap at the back for the heel curve. It is then easy to check the heel width, instep and waist width and length,

Figure 12.1 Mismatched feet: right hallux valgus.

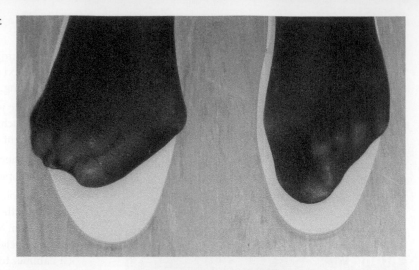

heel-to-ball position, joint width and overall length. Any obvious problems that show up on the inlay should help to determine clearly where there may be problems with the footwear on the foot (Fig. 12.1).

For example, where the large toe joint is too far forward on the inlay and there is a gap behind the joint, it suggests that the heel-to-ball length of the shoe is unlikely to be suitable. If this is the case, there will be creases behind the joint area where excess leather has twisted behind the joint. It is likely that the heel-to-ball is short and the instep length is too long, suggesting the wrong last has been selected. At this point, it would be better not to attempt altering the footwear but to return it, fully describing the fitting fault. A new last will need to be used to correct the proportions of the fit. There is no point in spending time altering a shoe that is fundamentally incorrect as it will never be right in the end.

Placing the shoe onto the foot

Just how easily the shoe slides onto the foot often tells the fitter if it is too snug or much too large, even before the patient fastens it or stands up in it. With experience, the fitter develops a sense of feeling for the right amount of space required as the shoe first goes on. It is also very important and useful to ask patients to put the shoes on themselves, to assess how well they can manage to don the shoes and fasten them up securely. If they do not have help at home, the ease of fastening becomes critical to the design of the footwear.

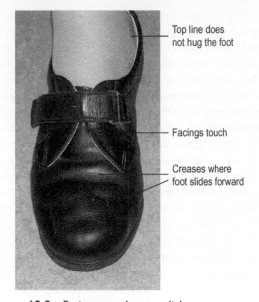

Top line does not hug the foot

Facings touch

Creases where foot slides forward

Figure 12.2 Facings too close: medial counter exposed.

Fastenings

The next step is to fasten the footwear onto the foot securely but not too tightly. Check the alignment of the facings on the foot and evaluate the ease of fastening.

Depending on the style, the typical space between facings on a lace shoe is approximately 1 cm. For lace styles or Velcro®, check for the following:

- Facings: touching; overlapping; too far apart (Fig. 12.2)
- Eyelets: lined up correctly; or are they twisted

Figure 12.3 Top line cutting into the Achilles tendon.

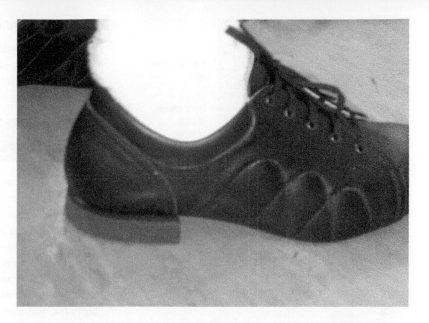

- Velcro® straps: too short; too long; correct angle and lay properly over instep
- Stay stitching at base of facings: does this allow ease of entry into the shoe? Does it need to be placed differently?

Heel fit

The heel fit is the most important area to get correct first. The way the foot is held at the heel determines the position of the foot distal to it. Once the heel fit is correct, an evaluation of the way the foot relates to the proportions of the last can be made.

Once the shoe is fastened, check the heel counter and look for a snug, comfortable fit. Check that the counter does not catch the Achilles tendon and cause pressure. Ensure that the counter is not causing pressure under the malleoli. Note that compression in this position can be very painful.

Any gaping at the side or back, or exposure of the top line, suggests that the heel fit is not good. Evaluate whether the counter flow round the foot reflects the profile of the heel, as it should do (Figs 12.3 and 12.4).

Throat/entry

The ease with which the foot slides into the shoe gives the first indication of how well the shoe

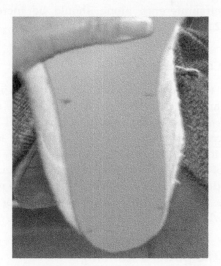

Figure 12.4 Inlay demonstrates a narrow heel seat.

fits. If the foot does not enter the shoe easily, remove the inlay. This often solves the problem and suggests either that the inlay allowance is insufficient or that the circumference of the joint may have increased. To check this, go back to the chart and remeasure the joint. If one measure has changed then check the waist and instep as well. This will indicate whether the inlay allowance should be increased throughout the shoe or whether the

179

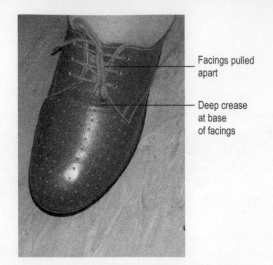

Facings pulled apart

Deep crease at base of facings

Figure 12.5 Tightness over the dorsum of the foot produces classic creasing at the base of the facings.

joint circumference alone should be increased (Fig. 12.5).

Vamp and toe area

Check that there is sufficient depth overall in the vamp and toe area. There should be adequate width across the first to fifth metatarso-phalangeal joints and across the toes. Check for adequacy of length at the toe end, the ball joint position and any overhang of the first metatarso-phalangeal joint and hallux abducto valgus prominence over the sole width. Ensure that there are no seams, stitching or tight spots which would irritate bony prominences.

With the patient standing

When the patient stands in the footwear, check the back of the heel for gaps, the counter height, the facings, the lay of the facings, heel-to-ball position, overall length, depth and joint width. Note any major creases.

On walking

Look for heel slip, bellows action, counter collapse and severe creasing on the vamp, and where an elevation (raise) is part of the prescription, check balance, comfort and toe-off action.

Ask patients for their views

Don't forget to ask patients for their views on general comfort, acceptability of style, overall fit, ease of donning and doffing, heel height, slippage, etc.

Writing fitting notes that make sense

It is important to use the correct terminology to describe exactly the part of the shoe to which the modification is required (i.e. vamp, inlay, facings). Only use medical terms that are known to be suitable: those involved in footwear manufacture are often unfamiliar with medical terms, therefore use alternative language when required. Familiarity with the chosen manufacturers is helpful, and time taken to visit them and to clarify the terminology they use is valuable.

The instructions to the manufacturer for the changes required following a fitting must be written in a neat and orderly way. This written instruction will go straight to the factory workbench and those working there need to understand it. They do not have time to read long and complicated explanations. They need facts.

It is essential to use correct terminology when describing the problem and the action that needs to be taken to remedy it. For example, a request to 'lower facings' can be interpreted in two ways: make the facing lower down on the vamp by moving distally; or make the facing open lower down the quarter, perhaps widening the stay stitch opening. Unless the alteration required is specifically described and confirmed by a clear pen mark on the upper, the interpretation could give an unexpected result.

To clarify this further, the following examples set out the terminology which should help to make alterations very clear to understand:

Inlays

- Mark on inlay any change of position of any pad included.
- State increase/decrease in pad thickness in millimetres if the pad included on the inlay is too thick.
- State changes in density of materials if those included are too hard or too soft.

- Write 'Reduce overall thickness by x mm' if the inlay is too bulky.
- Where there is insufficient depth for the inlay to fit, write 'Re-last adding full-length inlay allowance of x mm'.

Heel fit

Pressure on Achilles tendon

Where there is excessive pressure on the insertion of the Achilles tendon, write 'flatten out back curve shape to decrease pressure' (if this is the correct action). In this situation, it can be useful to take a cast, to photograph the problem area or alternatively to draw the back heel curve profile. This can be done by forming a flexible strip against the back of the heel and then tracing the outline of the flexible strip onto paper. Alternatively the heel seat may need to be increased in width (see Table 12.1 for more options).

Heel seat width

Where the heel seat width is too narrow, write 'Increase seat width between markings on inlay by x mm' (see Figs 12.3 and 12.4).

Ankle–foot orthoses or oedema

Where an ankle–foot orthosis (AFO) needs to be worn or there is oedema present, and the back heel curve needs to be straightened, write 'Straighten back curve to accommodate AFO (oedema)'.

Gap at back

Where there is a gap at the back of the heel, mark on the shoe top line exactly where the gap begins and ends and measure the depth of the gap in millimetres. Write 'Re-last counter to reduce gap at back' (Fig. 12.6).

Quarter height

- Where the counter is too high, write 'Reduce medial (or lateral) side height by x mm' (state whether this is on the inside or outside of the counter as these measurements will be different). To clarify, mark the side of the shoe with an effaceable leather pen.
- For more depth, write 'Increase depth of counter by x mm'. This will increase the depth all round the counter.

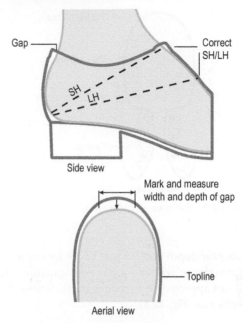

Figure 12.6 Gap at back of counter.

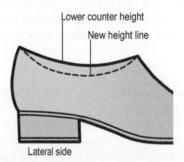

Figure 12.7 Reduce counter height.

- To increase the back height only, write 'Increase back height of counter by x mm'. Again, state if this is an inside or outside counter measurement.
- To reduce counter height under the malleoli, write 'Reduce counter height by x mm under (medial or lateral) ankle as marked on shoe' (Fig. 12.7).

Bellows action

- If caused by heel seat width being too narrow, write 'Increase heel seat width by x mm.'
- If caused by the inlay being made too bulky, write either 'Reduce bulk by x mm' or 'Increase

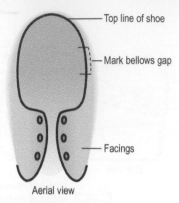

Top line of shoe

Mark bellows gap

Facings

Aerial view

Figure 12.8 Bellows gap: top view.

counter depth and/or seat width by x mm'. Consider which solution is best: sometimes it is not appropriate to reduce the thickness of orthotics (Fig. 12.8).

Slight heel slip

Where everything else is fine but the counter is still a fraction loose, consider using a reverse leather heel grip. Write 'Add reverse leather counter lining'.

Top line

Where this is loosely fitting, it needs reducing in overall circumference. Depending on the shape of the foot, this may only change one side of the top line, for example in a fixed valgus deformity, this may only change one side of the top. The instruction to the manufacturer must be clear. Write: 'Reduce top line circumference by x mm all round/medial side/ lateral side' as relevant.

Instep/waist

This could be either too narrow, too wide or the wrong depth:

- If it is too narrow, write 'Increase instep width of insole by x mm and/or increase waist circumference by x mm'. (Note: If the width is increased but not the circumference there will be no increase in the volume and the consequence may be overall tightness; however, if there is plenty of slack in the upper, then not increasing the circumference may solve the overall fit as, by default, the circumference will be reduced).

- If it is too wide, write 'Reduce instep width of insole by x mm and/or reduce waist circumference by x mm'.

Facings position

- Where the facings are too wide apart, write: 'Re-last to close in facings by x mm' (Fig. 12.9).
- Where the facings touch or overlap, write 'Re-last to 'set apart' facings by x mm'.

Entry

- To change the opening position for 'ease of entry', write 'Extend facings forward by x mm'. Note that this will also extend the stay stitch forward by the same measurement. Mark it on the shoe as well (Fig. 12.10).
- To change the position of the stay stitch only, write 'Set stay stitch apart to position marked' and mark it on the upper (Fig. 12.11).

Vamp/toe areas

Depth

- Where there is excess depth throughout the vamp and it is necessary to reduce the depth of the vamp overall, write 'Last down by x mm'.
- If it is necessary to reduce the circumference in a specific place on the vamp, write 'Reduce circumference (state from where to where, e.g. forepart up to instep or forepart up to joints) by x mm'.

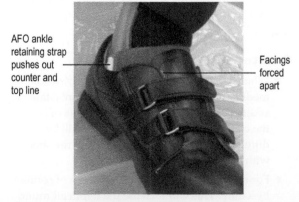

AFO ankle retaining strap pushes out counter and top line

Facings forced apart

Figure 12.9 Facings too far apart.

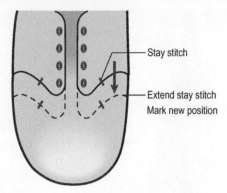

Figure 12.10   Extend stay stitch.

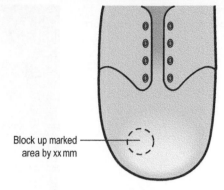

Figure 12.12   Block up specific area.

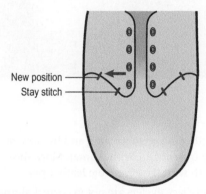

Figure 12.11   Set stay stitch apart.

- Where extra depth is required at the joint area only, write 'At base of facing add x mm to circumference'.
- Where extra depth is required all over the vamp, write 'Re-last forepart increasing depth by x mm'.
- Over a localized tight spot or prominence, write 'Block up over marked area by x mm'. This will then create a localized area of extra depth only which will not affect the overall fit if that is all that is needed (Fig. 12.12).

Width across joints

- Where the shoe is too narrow for the hallux abducto valgus joint, write 'Make sole board wider by x mm'. Mark the position of the alteration on the bottom of the shoe and on the removable inlay, indicating exactly where the extra is needed.
- Where the shoe is too wide for the hallux abducto valgus joint, write 'Make sole board

narrower by x mm'. Mark the position of the alteration on the bottom of the shoe and on the removable inlay, indicating exactly where the narrowing is needed.

Excess gap behind the great toe joint

Where there is excess material in the upper of the shoe behind the first metatarso-phalangeal joint, write 'Clip in behind joint by x mm'. Mark clearly on the upper where the material needs to be reduced.

Length of shoe

Heel-to-ball

Where the heel-to-ball fit is incorrect, write 'Adjust length to correct heel-to-ball fit'. Mark on the upper with an effaceable leather pen the position of the ball joint to show whether the heel-to-ball fitting is too long or too short.

Overall length

Where the overall length is inadequate, write 'Add or reduce half size (or 1 size = 4 mm) to toe end only'. This will add or take away from the toe box only and not affect the heel-to-ball length (provided that this has not been requested and that this part of the fitting is correct). Mark on the inlay the weight-bearing position of the toes so that the factory can clearly see how much excess or lack of space there is.

Where one foot is smaller than the other

Where one foot is smaller than the other and the longer shoe needs to be adjusted to contain the foot

Figure 12.13 Example of Velcro® straps that are too short.

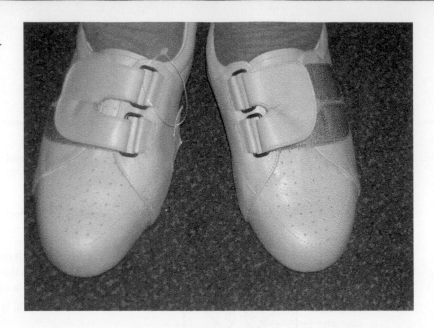

without altering the external appearance, write 'Add toe block to match length' (unless this was part of the original prescription, when the factory should do this automatically). Note there should be a 4 mm gap from the end of the toes to the block. The sole of the shoe may also need stiffening if there is a big difference in length. If so, write 'Add metal sole strip' (or carbon fibre insert – a lighter material). A rocker sole and compensating heel piece are often required to aid toe-off, where the flexion of the shoe has been removed.

Fastenings

- Where Velcro® straps are too short, write 'Please extend loop and hook by x mm'. This will extend both halves of the Velcro®. If the hook part only is to be extended, then state 'Extend hook only by x mm'. Mark the position of the strap where it passes through the D-ring or slot with an effaceable leather pen so that the maker can see where the strap returns on the foot (Fig. 12.13).

- Where Velcro® straps are too long, write 'Reduce length of strap by x mm' or request they add 'trim-back lines' (this will give you rows of stitching on the strap) so that the strap can be trimmed in length at the final fitting (if there are two or more straps, then state which ones need

lengthening or shortening and by how much, as they may not all be the same). Mark the excess length with the effaceable leather pen.

- Where lace eyelets are not in correct alignment, write 'Realignment of facings required' and mark the angle and the position of the facings onto the tongue of the shoe so the maker can see its position on the foot.

Summary

In writing the notes, certain other basic information needs to be included. It is essential to identify on which shoe the modifications requested are to be undertaken. When completing the notes, begin by stating which shoe the work is to be carried out on and then list all required modifications for that shoe clearly and unambiguously. Give exact measurements in millimetres for every alteration required. Mark the shoe upper to correspond with each modification. Enclose a Polaroid® photograph or take an electronic photograph, and either print a copy or send one electronically to the manufacturer. Complete the fitting form by indicating whether a further fitting is required or whether the shoe should be finished completely once the modifications have been completed.

Enclose one copy of the fitting form with the footwear for return to the factory and retain another with the patient's notes. Speak to the factory and to the person undertaking the footwear modifications if the work seems complex, or if there is uncertainty as to how to proceed or how to remedy a fitting issue.

Points to note: The factory will only carry out the modifications requested in the clinician's fitting note instructions. The factory needs all the information available from the fitting session. If the clinician has not requested a clear action or identified a fault, the modification *will not be made*.

Once the fitting note has been written (particularly in complex cases), it is helpful to read it to a colleague to ensure that it makes sense, and that the instructions are able to be interpreted correctly. If not, then it should be reworded to make it crystal clear.

Problem solving

It is inevitable that, at some time, a patient with very complex footwear needs will attend the clinic. Meeting such a patient's footwear needs satisfactorily will require expertise and experience. There is no substitute for experience, but this takes time to acquire. A deep knowledge and understanding of the construction techniques and of the technical aspects of footwear design and manufacture are required, but it is also useful to be able to draw on the knowledge of other colleagues, and both fellow clinicians and footwear manufacturers can provide invaluable assistance.

In complex cases, take time to gather a comprehensive history, noting all past footwear prescriptions and paying attention to the patient's subjective comments and experiences. If possible, examine footwear items previously made and worn. Much information can be gathered by looking at old footwear, even if it was not the perfect answer. It is especially useful to discover what did not work well and also what did. Much can be learned from a patient who has lived with a particular problem for a long time. Such patients may have solved niggling discomforts themselves. Some of their ideas can be translated into an inlay or made with much more suitable materials than those available to them. It may be that a seemingly complex problem can be resolved simply. Clinicians can occasionally be over ambitious

in their objectives, and at other times fall short of patient expectations. Personalities vary considerably and some patients are incredibly tolerant and grateful for any help, whereas others will not be particularly cooperative, even though the clinician may be doing everything possible to help them.

An example of the latter is a man in his fifties, who became hemiplegic through a car accident in his twenties. He spent much of his time in a wheelchair but could mobilize indoors with crutches. He could only use his right hand and wore an AFO on his left leg. The footwear clinic considered his footwear needs were fully addressed with low-opening Velcro® fastening boots. These were a fairly standard item, which accommodated the AFO easily and provided ankle support. Due to the accident, this man had difficulty in communicating and his well-meaning mother would always speak on his behalf. She was fiercely protective of her son but, in truth, became a barrier to the communication between the clinician and the patient. It was not clear why he seemed so upset about his boots so a decision was made to make an extra effort to connect with him and exclude the mother from the consultation. In order to achieve this, it was necessary to get down on the floor to make eye contact. His speech was slurred and difficult to understand and required careful listening. By gradually getting to understand him better, it became clear that he strongly disliked his boots because they made him look so 'crippled'. He also wanted to be able to dress himself and could not manage to reach the Velcro® straps and fasten them on both boots with one hand. It was quite surprising that he felt so strongly about the look of the boots considering he was in a wheelchair and had many other issues to cope with. It seems it was the last straw and he became very angry.

A mission was set to improve the footwear and to try and resolve both the appearance and practicality issues. After much discussion with colleagues and the manufacturer, boots were designed that had false laced facings which looked normal to the patient but, in fact, had a hidden Velcro® fastening under the facing which allowed the access to get them on. Crucially, the client could fasten the boots himself and he much preferred the way they looked (Figs 12.14 and 12.15).

This may seem an extreme example, but the overall clinical outcome is dependent on patient concordance and the will to wear the footwear prescribed.

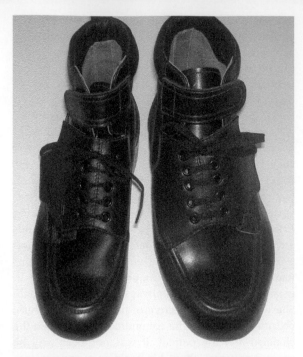

Fig 12.14 Velcro® boots disguised as lace ups.

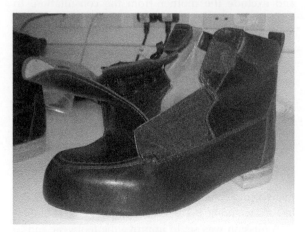

Fig 12.15 The same Velcro® boot as in Figure 12.14 showing low opening.

Failing to take the time and trouble to understand and communicate with the patient and, instead, relying on his mother was the wrong approach in this instance. It was a trap easily fallen into, as it seemed the preferable route initially. It seems that family members frequently speak on behalf of patients in the clinic and convey their own view rather than that of the patient. The opposite scenario may also be experienced where communication with the patient is very difficult. Calling a family member to attend the clinic session can be helpful, especially when the patient does not understand about the clinical approach to footwear. Unless the clinician and patient communicate well, the clinical outcome may be compromised. Because footwear prescribing is complex, features that seem possible to the patient may be impossible to prescribe.

Problem solving is much more than the technical aspects or design of the footwear. It is also about the whole process of connecting with patients and gaining their confidence and understanding.

Some golden rules

- Ensure that the heel counter is correctly fitted before making any other alterations. As the functions of various parts of the footwear are interlinked, changing one may have a consequential effect on another and too many changes at one fitting may cause many more problems than existed originally.

- Add new additions one at a time so that it is possible to examine the effect of that modification. For example, adding a sole modification such as a flare and also introducing orthoses at the same time may not work effectively. It will then take more time to identify which prescription was ineffective.

- While adding one addition at a time, make a note in the patient's file about the others that warrant consideration. This serves as an *aide-mémoire* but is also helpful if a different clinician sees that patient at subsequent appointments.

- Listen! Listen! Listen! to the patient and be sure of concordance before beginning to prescribe. If there are warning signs during the assessment that the patient is unlikely to be concordant, it may be better to defer the prescription and offer a recall at a later date when the patient has had an opportunity to give full consideration to the proposal.

- Explain the commitment expected from the patient: that they will be expected to attend all appointments. Discuss how the manufacturing process proceeds and how long it is likely to be before they go home with shoes. This could be between 48 hours or up to 12 weeks, depending on the type of item prescribed.

- Always check the facts and obtain current medical history from referring colleagues or the GP if necessary. Patients can misunderstand their own history. For example, patients may describe their leg length discrepancy in inches when, on measuring, it is found to be that same number in centimetres.

- Never tell patients the size of the shoe being issued as it almost always varies from the size they have bought previously. They may firmly believe that they need a specific size no matter what the actual dimensions of the size. It is simpler to inform them that orthopaedic sizing is different from retail sizing and the two should not be compared.

- In complex cases, involve colleagues at an early stage. Their experience may have involved a similar case and that expertise may save time, money and unnecessary mistakes.

- Do not change something that is working well, even if you think you know better (it is tempting to modify other people's prescriptions, but if the footwear works well, is comfortable and is effective then there is no point in making extra work for yourself and possibly creating problems that did not exist previously).

- Believe in your ability to prescribe successfully, enjoy the work and build empathy with patients. A successful footwear prescription can relieve pain, improve mobility and health, enable patients to better perform the activities which they enjoy and can dramatically improve their quality of life. After all, it is not 'just a pair of shoes'.

Table 12.1 Fitting solutions

Area of shoe	Difficulty identified	Visual signs – could be any of these	Possible causes	Solutions
Heel seat	Too narrow	Flesh squeezed into heel counter, shows signs of creasing, or dragging of skin.	Incorrect draft: heel outline may have been poorly drawn.	Provide an accurate draft of the heel outline.
			No heel width shown on draft.	Measure the heel width and send to the makers for alterations to be made.
		Feels very tight. Heel may not be able to sit properly on the seat.	Foot has become oedematous since measuring or dressed in bulky bandages since measuring.	For stock items, choose a wider heel fitting; look for a maker who offers choice of heel widths.
		Counter may bulge at the sides and become distorted by forcing the heel down into the counter.		Use the inlay against sole of foot to check how much increase in width is required and also evaluate whether the increase is needed as far as the instep area as well. Mark the inlay clearly and note the changes.
Heel seat	Offset by form of last	As the shoe is eased onto the foot, the heel is positioned to the outside of the counter. The heel has to be forced into the shoe.	The last may be straight lasted or the forepart wider on either the medial or the lateral side. If this does not match the foot shape then a conflict of pressure will result. Varus or valgus heel position, club foot or major rear foot deformity cause heel position to differ from standard last.	Examine the shape of the foot and the shoe form, to see if they correspond. If stock footwear is indicated from foot measurements, check whether straight-lasted shoes are available for improved heel shape – test them for suitability. Bespoke may be necessary, where the foot shape appears unusual. Full accurate drafts and casts will need to be taken.
Heel counter	Cutting into Achilles tendon	Flesh bulges over the topline.	Heel-to-ball ratio is too short, forcing the foot into the counter.	Check the heel-to-ball length and overall length, to be sure these are correct. If heel-to-ball is short, then ask for a re-last to correct this, showing the ball position. For stock, change to another last where heel to ball fitting is longer.
		Discomfort felt by wearer at the back of the shoe.	Overall length is too short.	If overall length is short, but heel-to-ball is correct, then *add length to the toe end only* – stating by how much in shoe sizes, e.g. half size.

		Symptom	Cause	Action
		Foot pushed forward by the counter top line, leaving a space in the counter below.	Curve or profile of counter is too short around top line.	For foot profile problems, take a Polaroid® or digital photo, draw the shape, or cast the foot and send to the maker for correction of the counter shape. Refit the shoe to check.
		Sides of counter 'bellow' below malleoli and the top line of the back is pulled into the tendon.	Heel seat width is too narrow, forcing top line to cut into Achilles.	Measure heel width and look for, or request, more heel width as a modular alteration.
			Depth at back of counter too deep.	Request reduction in counter depth or look for a brand that is lower. For stock shoes, consider if the foot is really suitable for 'ready made' or needs modular instead to achieve the correct fit.
Heel counter	Too high	Rubbing under either medial or lateral malleoli.	Height of malleoli not measured and stated on the draft. Unusually low malleolar heights.	Draw a line on the shoe counter with an effaceable leather pen, to show where it needs lowering. Give the measurement in mm, and request that the counter is lowered. This can be altered at fitting stage on bespoke or as an adaptation on stock items if there is no padded collar.
			Ankle fracture causing changes to bony prominences.	On bespoke items with a padded collar, request re-last of heel counter to lower height and state measurement required. Stock: check other makes to find one that is lower, rather than altering the shoe, especially if it has a padded collar. On a finished item, add 3 mm cork heel lift under inlay to lift heel higher in the counter to relieve any pressure. Ensure malleolar heights are recorded on future orders.
		Catching the Achilles tendon.	Presence of 'heel bumps' or bursae over Achilles tendon.	Soften the counter with chemical softener, and use ring and ball stretcher to create a 'bump' in counter; encourage gradual 'wearing in' over a few days. Bespoke items can be ordered with a cavity in the counter stiffener to accommodate the bump.

(Continued)

189

Table 12.1 Continued

Area of shoe	Difficulty identified	Visual signs – could be any of these	Possible causes	Solutions
Heel counter	Too low	Does not grip the foot properly and foot comes out of the shoe too easily. Feels unsafe in wearing.	Counter depth sits too low on the foot.	On unfinished footwear, request counter depth to be increased and give measurements.
			Inlays may be too thick under heel, and lifting foot out.	Stock items: choose different maker.
			Inside heel raise is too high for the counter.	Reduce inside heel raise height, and add balance to external heel height, or change to external shoe raise only.
			Excessive oedema affects how the heel sits down in the counter.	Request modular or bespoke only. Straighten the back curve to accommodate oedema and increase width of heel seat.
Heel counter	Pinches soft tissue	Top line cuts in to foot.	Drawstring type of fastening around top line pinches flesh.	Change style. This style should not be chosen for any vascular, oedematous or ulcerated cases.
			Long heel measurement is incorrect (too short).	Remeasure long and short heel; check for relationship. If within normal range for stock shoes, change last fitting.
			Proportions of long and short heel measurement should be between 1.5 and 2.5 cm difference, on average. If they are greater, or very close, then a bespoke last will be needed.	For bespoke, send in remeasured long and short heel lengths, and ask for remake of back quarters. Make sure that the long and short heel measurements are taken in the correct positions.
Heel-to-ball length	Too long	Footwear causes pain/discomfort; foot gets 'tired'. Creases too far back. Check for wear marks on sole behind flexion point.	Foot is flexing too far back in shoe; incorrect fitting.	If stock is being used, find shorter heel-to-ball last fitting. If bespoke, re-last on a last with a shorter heel-to-ball.
	Too short	Heavily creased vamp below facings. Toe puff may be creased as well. Toes often sore. 'Turned up' toe end. Heavy wear marks placed forward of flexion point.	Foot is flexing too far forward in shoe, incorrect fitting.	If stock is being used, find longer heel-to-ball last fitting. If bespoke, re-last on longer heel-to-ball fitting. (This problem is rarely found with bespoke footwear if drafts and measurements have been taken correctly.)

Area	Problem	Observation	Cause	Action
Ball joint	Limited range of motion (ROM)	Twisted or angled creases that seem unusual. Wear marks heavy to lateral side.	Check first metatarso-phalangeal joint: ROM may be fixed or severely limited.	Add rocker sole and compensating heel to aid toe-off.
Instep	Too deep	Facings overlap; excess leather around area. Creases along quarters.	Incorrect instep measurement (if oedema present, this can be variable).	Check measurements for changes from original draft. If these have changed then supply new measurements to maker and request accordingly. Refit.
		Foot slides down shoe causing gap at back of counter. Patient can sometimes feel toes at end and says shoes are too short. Deep creases appear at base of facings.	Incorrect long and short heel measurements – again, could be due to oedema.	For stock, try changing inlays, or add valgus filler. If the shoe fit is satisfactory elsewhere, a tongue pad may solve problem. For bespoke, request 'reduce instep circumference and set facings apart by x mm'.
Instep	Too shallow	Facings appear too far apart; tightness over dorsum of foot. Pressure on dorsum from fastenings.	Look for high-instep foot shape (e.g. pes cavus) or possible dorsal prominence.	Check draft and add instep height measurement and ensure the instep line is drawn in. Request 'increase over instep' (and give measurement in millimetres). Close in facings by x mm'. Refit.
		Velcro straps do not fasten over adequately. Lace facings have a wider space at top than the base.	Bulky valgus inlays. Too many inlays: stock shoes may have up to three layers.	Adjust inlays to try and correct the fit. Remake inlays if you consider the shoe to be satisfactory otherwise.
			Layered bandages are very variable and may cause extra bulk. Variable oedema.	Wait for dressings to be reduced or stockings to be supplied, and supply temporary healing shoe short term. Or ask for swelling cork to be added, which requires re-lasting with the addition.
		Deep crease at base of facings at level of stay stitch.	Instep measurements are incorrect. Also check position of tape measure. Was it too low?	Check measurements. Request increase in instep circumference giving measurement in mm. Look at alternative supplier for better fit.
			Instep strap styles can often be shallow.	Change style for a better fit, if style is unsuitable for foot shape.
Instep	Too narrow	Facings pulled apart at wrong angle. Very tight; may not get shoe onto foot.	Poor quality drafts, no instep line or the measurements were not recorded correctly.	Redraw draft and ask for re-last.

(Continued)

Table 12.1 Continued

Area of shoe	Difficulty identified	Visual signs – could be any of these	Possible causes	Solutions
		Quarters bulge on medial side.	Excess pronation may cause poor foot position in shoe.	Corrective inlays may help. Uppers will need re-lasting to accommodate these inlays. (A quick way to check before casting is to use prefabricated neutral orthotics within the existing fitting and observe any improvements to foot position and/or facings.)
		Incorrect style: does not suit foot shape or fasten properly.	Wrong style? Oxford facings can be very difficult to fit well, especially if instep is high. Instep bar or key-hole style can be shallow or narrow across instep.	Change style to Gibson or Derby instead. Reconsider style chosen, or redraft or cast to improve fitting.
Instep	Too wide	Facings feel loose; excess leather, particularly along medial side of quarter.	Fitting too wide. Entry probably too wide as well.	Change to narrower fitting, check foot on inlay for heel seat and instep fitting. Measure heel width: if it is narrow, it could also affect the instep.
		Facings butt or overlap. Foot not retained adequately into counter.	Incorrect long heel measurement, or reduction in measurement due to oedema or change of dressings, etc.	Check measurements. Reduce instep circumference and/or entry giving measurement in mm. Remove inlays and check fitting again. Trim back inlays if faulty, until they fit correctly. Adding a valgus filler or a moulded inlay may save replacing the shoe.
			Inlays too thin.	Increase inlays, but beware as this may compromise the fit elsewhere.
			Insole board may be too wide at instep.	Reduce width of insole board; draw line on underside of shoe to show where it should be reduced. Give measurements.
Entry	Too narrow	Foot can not pass down into toe box.	Joint width not shown on draft. Incorrect girth measurement.	Measure joint width, remeasure girth and request increase at entry giving measurement in mm.

	Symptom	Cause	Solution
	May not get shoe on.	Fitting incorrectly ordered or wrong fitting delivered.	Check the order. This may not be what was ordered.
	Pressure across toe joints.	Incorrect width measurement.	Reorder on wider fitting.
	Feels too tight	Inlays too thick	Remove inlays. This will give some indication of extra space required. Feel the sides of the sole board, under the first and fifth joints; check it is positioned under the joints properly. Request an increase in entry width across first to fifth metatarsal heads on the insole board. Give the amount of increase required in mm.
	Stretch creases visible across vamp at base of facings. Visible 'tight spots' especially over hallux abducto valgus.	Foot has changed since measured.	Solution as above.
Entry Too shallow	May not get shoe on.	Incorrect girth or joint measurement.	Request increase in circumference giving measurements in mm.
	Very restricted feel as foot enters shoe.	Foot may have altered due to oedema or dressing type being changed.	As above. Or issue temporary healing shoe, and wait for improvement.
	Width may be correct, but shoe feels too tight.	Inlays too thick	Try to reduce inlays. If padding required, request increased depth to accommodate this. Give measurements.
	Deep creases formed at base of tongue.	Indicates fitting depth is incorrect.	Increase depth by removing inlays. Request increase in depth, and give measurements in mm.
Entry Too deep	Foot slides forward to touch end of toe box.	Measurements may have changed.	Check draft again, and remeasure. Send new measurements and draft, and request relast to reduce excess depth.
		Incorrect inlays; may be too thin or not customized.	Try different inlays or order custom inlay. If required, give depth of materials to be used. Fit in shoe again before altering depth or fitting.

(Continued)

Table 12.1 Continued

Area of shoe	Difficulty identified	Visual signs – could be any of these	Possible causes	Solutions
			Insole board maybe too wide.	Check width of insole board and, if necessary, reduce width on the side of the extra width. Also request reduction in circumference by stating on the fitting note the number of mm required. To check the amount required, use 3 mm inlays until the fit seems better (note: one 3 mm inlay = 6 mm girth). Keep adding inlays until the fit is good. Remove them, add twice the depth of the insoles to the girth measurement and this will tell you how much to reduce girth.
		Excess leather across joints.	The last does not match the foot.	Check draft for changes, and request re-last to reduce entry.
		Deep creases on flexion. Deep creases at base of facings or bulge at base of facings.	Facings may be too wide apart. Excess leather in vamp.	Check position of facings to joint region, and check instep area. This is probably too wide as well. Reduce entry and instep and refit. If insole is correct width, and inlays are suitable, then reduce entry circumference. Check toe box depth as this may also need changing. If it is correct, then request 'no change to toe box depth'.
Vamp and toe box	Too wide	Feels big.	Change in measurements, or poor-quality draft supplied.	Check draft: remeasure if necessary.
		Excessive space around the toes.	Change in oedema or in hosiery or dressings.	If oedema is variable, then allowances are needed. Redraft and request 'add swelling corks' (removable 3 mm cork inlays that can be added or removed).
			Insole board is too wide.	Feel position of the forefoot in vamp. Draw with effaceable leather pen where the excess is situated. Request reduction of insole board in mm. Check depth as this may also need to be reduced.

Location	Type	Symptom	Cause	Solution
Vamp and toe box	Too deep	Deep fold creases on flexion.	Excess leather.	This is possibly depth not width. Feel the position of the foot in the vamp: if width is correct under first to fifth joints, then reduce circumference.
		Feels 'baggy'. Excess leather across dorsum. Deep creases on flexion.	Change in measurement; reduction of oedema.	Reduce whole forefoot area by 'lasting down' and refit. If joint width is correct, reduce distal to the joint circumference.
		Base of facings bulge up from vamp.	Instep/entry is also too deep.	
Vamp and toe box	Too narrow	Feels tight.	Toe box shape of shoe not compatible with foot shape.	Compare foot shape with shoe; request change in toe box shape, if necessary, to rounded or square. Use inlay to check for width.
		Forefoot squeezed.	Swelling may have occurred.	Refit once swelling has reduced, or monitor swelling until stabilized.
		Stretch creases.	Insole board too narrow.	Check insole board against foot and request increase in width if too narrow. Mark shoe with effaceable leather pen where more width is needed.
		Toe puff may press into toes. Toes bulge into upper on lateral border.	Too narrow in toe box, or toe box wrong shape for foot.	Request change of toe shape and re-last the upper. (Note: increasing the width will also increase the circumference.)
Vamp and toe box	Too shallow	May not get shoe on.	Incorrect measurement.	Check draft, remeasure and request increase in depth giving measurement in mm.
		Very tight.	Change in measurements.	Request increase in depth, giving measurement.
		Toes rub on vamp leather.	No toe box depth measurement given on draft.	Solution as above.
		One high toe may be pushing up on the upper.	Position of high toe not given on draft.	Mark tight area with effaceable leather pen, circle the area to be increased and request 'blocking up' of tight area, if rest of toe box depth is sufficient. Give measurement.

Treating patients with complex pathologies

Chapter contents

Many patients who have complex, multiple pathologies which affect their feet in some way will require footwear as part of their overall care plan. Historically, these patients formed a high percentage of the those attending for treatment at any orthotics clinic, but gradually the effects of many conditions have been minimized thanks to modern surgical techniques, technical innovations, immunization against diseases such as poliomyelitis and improved early-stage intervention for congenital conditions such as club foot and talipes equinovarus. Many children who have epiphyseal growth dysfunction, for example, who may have required a shoe raise in the early years are now offered corrective surgery before ossification is complete to correct the limb length discrepancy, thus eliminating the requirement for a shoe raise during adult life.

This inevitably has brought considerable changes to the type of footwear prescribed in today's orthotics and orthopaedic clinics. The consequence is that the number of highly skilled bespoke orthopaedic makers is in decline. Those with the skills are retiring and younger apprentices are not being trained to follow on. While modern technology has advanced and is able to cope with the majority of bespoke prescriptions, there are some complex ones that still require human expertise and a few traditionally skilled craftsmen remain.

Certain patients attending for footwear will have multiple pathology states. For example, some may have diabetes coupled with osteoarthrosis or rheumatoid disease, spina bifida and cardiac failure, renal impairment, lupus or post polio syndrome. Changing times and world travel have allowed many nationals to live, work and access health care in more modern countries and we are once again seeing patients with post polio syndrome and untreated congenital conditions. The challenge from such patients places high demand on the inexperienced footwear clinician and on the footwear manufacturer. The effects of these pathologies may be complex and it is essential that a comprehensive medical history is taken. This history will highlight the factors which are relevant to foot health, and by a process of clear thought and logical progression, the footwear prescription can be readily derived. The essential factors concern biomechanical function, circulatory status, neurological impairment and structural changes within the foot. Added to this, patients should be asked to identify the issues they have with footwear and also to identify their footwear needs. It may be that a patient needs simply to be provided with an item for indoor wear that is safe, supportive and well-fitting if they are house bound. Work-wear items may, however, be more complex. Once the purpose of the footwear is clear, decide on the prescription features that will be of most help to the patient, considering the level of risk of the pathologies in question; for example, if there is sensory neuropathy, a specification of softee leather, whole cut linings and rim toe puff will be indicated. If the patient has variable oedema, determine the smallest and the largest dimensions of the feet and identify whether adjustable footwear will meet both these dimensions or whether the volume change is so great that two pairs of shoes of different sizes are needed.

Once the features are clear, then decide on the style(s) which would best meet the patient's needs. Then begin to measure the patient's feet and decide whether they fit within the dimensions of stock orthopaedic footwear or whether the foot measurements are just outside that range, in which case modular footwear may be possible. If the foot shape is abnormal, drafts and casts using the British Standard system will be indicated (see Chs 11 and 12). This approach will help in identifying the qualities, shape and styling required in the shoe upper. The shoe outer sole will need to be prescribed, and this is best approached by using the information contained in Chapter 9. This also includes some useful charts which can help in identifying ways to approach the biomechanical anomalies identified.

Never assume the direction to take just from the medical history, but consult with the patient, family members and other colleagues to reach the best choice of action as, although the pathology is complex, the footwear need not necessarily be so.

This chapter includes an outline of some of the traditional ways of making cradles, raises and bespoke items. A clear understanding of how these are made may help to solve many a technical dilemma, even where materials available vary and bespoke skills are not readily available. The chapter will also consider the means of compensating for limb length discrepancy, the fixed equinus condition and use of cradles, and designing footwear for amputees. Many of the clinical guidelines given are, of course, a generalization, as each patient is individual and no two patients are the same, however the overall aims of any prescription are based on fundamental principles, and using these guidelines may prove a very useful tool in developing skills in prescribing for complex pathologies.

Limb length discrepancy

Limb length discrepancy (LLD) is one of the conditions most frequently referred to orthotic and footwear clinics. The majority of LLDs are already diagnosed, therefore the patient assessment strategy will include confirmation of the difference in the length of the two limbs.

However, as many patients referred for footwear have complex health pathologies, LLD may be overlooked because of other conditions or may be hidden by the patient. For example, those who need to use wheelchairs may be reluctant to move from the wheelchair during the consultation, and so the identification of LLD may be missed by the clinician. By becoming familiar with the clinical signs of LLD, using appropriate tests to evaluate the presence of related conditions such as fixed spinal deformities, hip dysplasia and resolved lower limb fractures which might lead to an anatomical limb shortening, and conditions such as unilateral hyperpronatory syndromes which might lead to functional LLD, the clinician will be able to identify the patients who would benefit from detailed limb length evaluation.

Aetiology

There are numerous causes of inequality of leg lengths and these may be classified as congenital or acquired.

Congenital conditions may include spina bifida, cerebral palsy, congenital dislocation of the hip, epiphyseal growth dysfunction, talipes equinovarus, hemiatrophy (lack of bone growth), hemihypertrophy (overgrowth) and hemimelias (longitudinal defects).

Acquired conditions will include the results of certain types of trauma, for example fractures, the results of infections such as poliomyelitis and Still's disease (juvenile rheumatoid arthritis), biomechanical conditions, including foot pronation, and surgical interventions, for example arthrodesis of the knee and hip arthroplasty.

It is also worth bearing in mind that existing limb length can reduce unilaterally. For example, in cases of osteoarthrosis of the hip where the patient is unable to use the two limbs equally, the limb on the side of the painful hip may shorten through asymmetrical loading. Similarly, in cases of post polio syndrome, the affected limb may shorten as the patient ages and is no longer able to load the two limbs equally in gait.

Blake & Ferguson (1992) suggest that LLD can be subdivided into two groups:

1. Anatomic or structural: where the bones are physically shortened from diseases like Perthe's disease or poliomyelitis, fractures or surgical intervention.

2. Functional or apparent: where the result of disease or injury causes each of the limbs to be used in a different way, but the bones which comprise those limbs may not actually be shorter. Examples include:

   • Joint deformity
   • Compensated posture
   • Scoliosis
   • Genu recurvatum
   • Extreme pronation.

The difference between an anatomic and functionally short leg is very concisely described by Valmassy (1995) (given with permission of the publisher):

1. An anatomic short leg tilts the pelvis down, producing a functional scoliosis with convexity to the short side. Balance is restored by lateral bending of the spine toward the longer leg. Axial rotation coupled with lateral bending twists the lowest intervertebral joint and its musculoskeletal ligamentous structures, resulting in inflammation and pain. This flexible scoliosis corrects in the sitting or lying position (Fig. 13.1).

2. A similar tilting of the pelvis with functional shortening of the leg can occur as a result of sacroiliac or iliosacral torsions. These are, respectively, dysfunction between the sacrum and the ilium or between the ilium and the sacrum. This problem requires correction of the sacroiliac dysfunction before levelling of the pelvis can take place.

3. Structural congenital scoliosis is not accompanied by limb length inequality or low

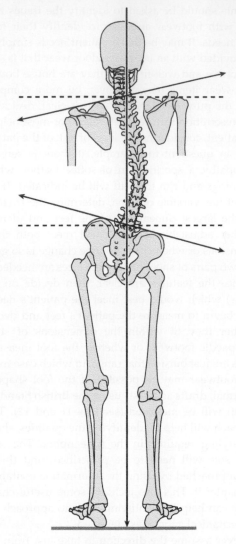

Pelvic tilt syndrome

Figure 13.1 Pelvic tilt syndrome. (Reproduced with permission of Valmassy 1995.)

back pain, and remains rigid or unchanged through changes of position.

The pelvic tilt syndrome is accompanied by other objective clinical findings. The short leg is characterized by the following:

• Usually on the right side
• Lateralization of the chronic low back pain
• Anterior rotation of the innominate bone (can lengthen by 6 mm)

- Reduced facet angle (produces degenerative joint changes)
- Inter-trochanteric bursitis
- Lateral knee joint degeneration
- Foot supination
- Pes cavus.

Compensation

As a result of acquiring short leg syndrome, the body will develop several ways of compensating to allow upright stance and reasonably balanced gait. If normal body symmetry is disturbed, particularly by LLD, then gait and posture are disrupted. If left untreated, this can lead to chronic problems.

Observation of any or all of the signs of this condition is an essential skill of the patient assessment and today's clinicians need to be thoroughly familiar with limb asymmetry.

The following signs may be present:

- The head remains level causing a 'C' curve in the cervical vertebrae.
- The elbow and hand positions may be uneven due to shoulder tilt.
- The foot will **supinate on the shorter side** and weight-bear on its lateral side.
- The foot may also function in the equinus position, preventing dorsiflexion.
- The foot will **pronate on the longer side** and weight-bear on its medial side
- The knee **hyperextends** on the short side.
- The knee **flexes** on the long side (Figs 13.2 and 13.3).
- The hip externally rotates on the short side.
- Circumduction occurs in the long limb.
- There will be ankle instability due to the supinatory position of the foot on the short side.
- Pelvic tilt will occur.

In order to determine which bones are shortened, details of the patient history gathered from written referral and information gained from the patient need to be considered first, but most important of all is clinical examination. Several diagnostic tests are helpful.

One example is Galleazzi's test: lay the patient supine and place the heels together with the knees flexed. Observe the knees from the side. If the femur

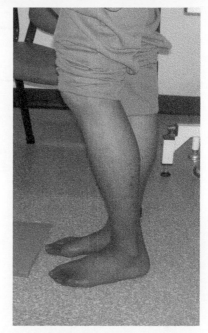

Figure 13.2   Example of LLD showing knee flexion on the long side.

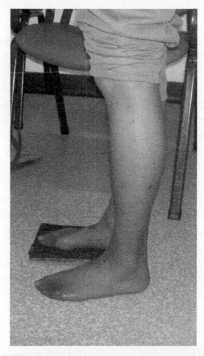

Figure 13.3   Example showing correction of LLD using a compensatory block.

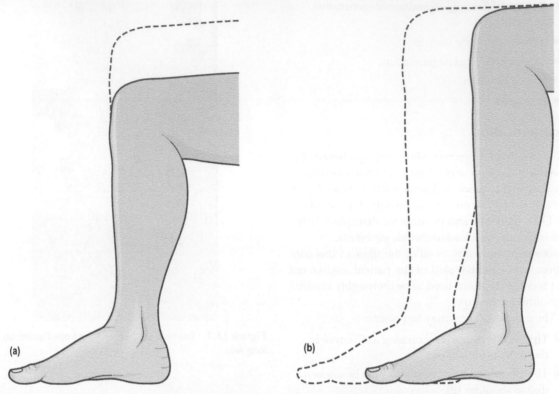

Figure 13.4 Galleazzi's test for limb shortening (a) below the knee and (b) above the knee.

is lower on the shorter side then the shortening is below the knee. If the tibia is further back, then the shortening is above the knee (Figs 13.4 and 13.5).

The significance of the discrepancy in LLD is a controversial topic and much of the literature on this subject reveals contradictory findings on the length of discrepancy that is likely to produce pathological symptoms (Lorimer et al 2004). Some authors believe that the body adapts well to the inequality and the deformity is best left untreated (Blustein & D'Amico 1985). Others believe that treatment for the deformity is essential to prevent further complications such as osteoarthritis (Blake & Ferguson 1992).

No catalogue of rules can possibly take account of all potential combinations and anatomical details, however there are certain universal clinical guidelines that can be applied (see p. 203).

Scoliosis

Scoliosis is a condition that involves complex lateral and rotational curvature and deformity of the spine.

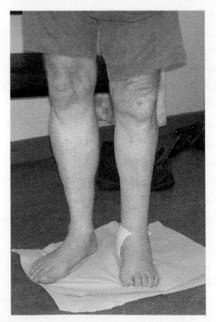

Figure 13.5 An example of shortening below the knee.

It may be congenital, idiopathic or a secondary symptom of another condition such as cerebral palsy, spina bifida or spinal muscular atrophy.

A normal spine, when viewed from behind, appears straight. A spine affected by scoliosis shows evidence of a lateral or sideways curvature and a rotation of the vertebrae, giving the appearance that the person is leaning to one side. The Scoliosis Research Society defines scoliosis as a curvature measuring 10° or greater on X-ray. Scoliosis is a type of spinal deformity and should not be confused with poor posture.

Blake & Ferguson (1992) describe three typical posture compensations in cases of scoliosis. The clinical features in each case are described below.

Type 1:

- The pelvis is tilted on the short side.

- The head and shoulders are tilted down on the long side causing cervical and lumbar scoliosis.

- The fingers are lower on the long side.

- The foot on the long side is more pronated and externally rotated.

- The hip and shoulder levels are uneven.

- There is a rib hump and/or prominent shoulder blade, caused by rotation of the ribcage in thoracic scoliosis.

Type 2:

- Similar to type 1, except only lumbar scoliosis is present and other compensations are less exaggerated.

Type 3:

- No spinal column compensation occurs.

- Head and shoulder tilt are to short side.

- The fingers are lower on the short side.

Fixed scoliosis

To differentiate between functional and fixed scoliosis, first check the spinal curves presenting in the standing position visually and by palpating the spine. Then seat the patient and observe the spine from the back view. If there are no changes in the curves, then it is 'fixed'. If the curves disappear, then it is not fixed but a compensatory scoliosis (Blake & Ferguson 1992).

Measurement of limb length discrepancy

Clinical and radiographic measurements

Clinical measurements of LLD remain unreliable in general, with no single method that can be used alone as an accurate method.

The most commonly used method of 'supine direct measurement' may be influenced by landmark palpation. This may prove difficult in obese patients. The measurement is taken from the anterior superior iliac spine to the medial malleolus of the same limb. Many authors now discount this method as being highly inaccurate.

Valmassy (1995) suggests that 30% of clinical measurements differ from radiographic measurements, the clinical findings indicating greater differences. To date, Valmassy considers the best radiographic technique (with accuracy to within 1.5 mm) to be an erect lumbosacral anteroposterior film, with the feet 6 inches apart and the beam perpendicular to the iliac crest, visualizing the femoral heads. The leg length difference is measured by dropping a perpendicular to a horizontal line joining the most superior points of the femoral heads. The sacral base plane inclination is measured by dropping a perpendicular through the top centre of the femoral heads and intersecting it with a line joining the most posterior part of the promontory of the sacrum and comparing the right and left sides. X-ray films should not be done until pelvic mechanics are corrected.

Computerized axial tomography (CAT) scanning is also suggested as a current gold standard method, but is a very expensive use of this equipment which cannot necessarily be justified unless the scan is required for more than just LLD measurement.

Measurement of LLD remains controversial, and is generally a case of X-ray methods versus the tape measure.

Compensation in the spine, foot and limbs influences the vertical position, and the LLD changes as the body adapts itself as best it can without external support. In real time, checking the LLD at least two different ways, and then giving the client one trial shoe raise or internal lift works well in practice. This approach allows for any natural compensation which is asymptomatic to be accommodated, thus reducing the visible raise.

Should measurements be taken with the patient prone, supine or upright? Should a tape measure be used or are advanced diagnostic techniques preferred? The location of bony prominences can be difficult, but X-rays carry exposure risks, are costly, create a time delay for the patient and are possibly an inappropriate use of this diagnostic tool. A pragmatic alternative needs to be considered, and using a tape measure but checking the measurements by using a variety of bony landmarks is a sensible clinical choice.

Clinical methods

Supine (direct method)

- Lay the patient supine (on the back), completely flat on the examination couch.
- Palpate the anterior superior iliac spine (ASIS) or the ziphoid process of the sternum.
- When measuring from the ASIS, hold the tape measure between the thumb and forefinger and trace the inguinal ligament upwards until the thumb catches in the notch below the ASIS. When measuring from the ziphoid process, hold the tape measure in the same way, placing one end of it on the central point of the process.
- With either method, hold the other end of the tape measure in the other hand and trace the tip of the thumb along the medial side of the calcaneus to the notch below the medial malleolus.
- Record the length.
- Measure both legs in this way and note any difference in length.
- Repeating this three times in succession allows for slight variations in the lengths recorded, and using the average of the three measurements is sensible (see also Ch. 9 and Ch. 11).
- However, as it is not totally accurate, the measurement should be backed up by measurements taken with the patient upright – the vertical method.

Vertical (indirect method)

- Stand the patient barefoot (if crutches or a stick are essential to stand straight, it is helpful to have a staff member to help support the patient).
- Ask the patient to look straight ahead, not down at the feet.

- Observe shoulder height, arm length and the spine for scoliosis curves. Check for fixed scoliosis. Examine the knee positions for flexion and extension, and also the gluteal and knee skin creases and foot positions for supination and pronation.
- Palpate the ASIS on both sides: press your hands down firmly on each side and observe which side is lower. If you have a pelvic level instrument, this can be used instead of observation alone, but caution is needed here because uneven pressure on the level as it is positioned firmly on the ASIS could give a false reading. The level requires great accuracy in positioning and requires that pressure is exerted evenly. Practice is required to ensure that it reads accurately.
- Place raise blocks (a firm material of wood or high-density ethylene vinyl acetate (EVA), in graduated heights) one at a time under the short limb until the pelvis is level, checking as above.
- Check the knees for locking and stability and ensure that there is even weight distribution through both limbs.
- Ask the patient whether it feels comfortable once the limbs are levelled. Is the patient comfortable or is there spinal discomfort?
- Measure the height of the blocks used as this will be the prescription height for the elevation or raise.
- If a tapered raise is to be used, then change the blocks under the foot to replicate the tapering (lower under the metatarso-phalangeal joints and toes) and evaluate for comfort and stability.

Point to note: Some bony prominences can be difficult to locate accurately. In some instances, alternative measurement points have been identified. When the patient is supine, measurements may be taken from the greater trochanter to the lateral malleolus. In cases where the malleolus is not palpable, measurement can be taken to the plantar surface of the heel with the foot fully dorsiflexed. When taking measurements with the patient upright, the symmetry of the shoulders, hands, anterior superior iliac spines, iliac spines, iliac crests, posterior superior iliac spines, gluteal folds, popliteal creases, patellae and tibial tubercules may be assessed or measured (Lorimer et al 2004) (Fig. 13.6).

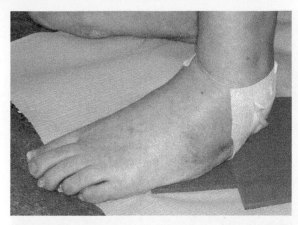

Figure 13.6 Example of a mild equinus being assessed with raise blocks to establish the required height.

Who should take measurements?

Measurements of limb length may be taken by any health professional who refers the patient for a shoe raise, or even patients themselves. However, British Standard 5943 states that the surgeon/consultant should make the initial measurement and it is preferable to receive a referral that has quantified the LLD and gives detail of the lengths of each limb.

Once the patient has been referred to the footwear clinic, the clinic may then remeasure to clarify and confirm the discrepancy. It is not unusual to differ in opinion on measurement, and measurements taken by different practitioners at different times have been known to vary. The amount of variance is usually minimal and may be about 5 mm.

It is not unusual for patients to tell the footwear prescriber of the length differences they have, but very often they have misunderstood or confused centimetres and inches and the measurements they offer can be wildly inaccurate.

Clinical guidelines for managing limb length discrepancy

The clinical aims of managing LLD are to enable the patient to:

- Mobilize safely
- Achieve a level pelvis
- Improve or maintain existing limb and foot function
- Bear weight fully and equally on both legs
- Achieve locking of both knees
- Find footwear, including any necessary raise, which is cosmetically acceptable.

Where a good range of motion (ROM) is present in the ankle joint, a tapered raise is usually prescribed. In this case, the raise will be of full height under the heel and will include half the measured heel height at the joint and half again at the toe (e.g. heel elevation 6 cm, joint elevation 3 cm, toe elevation 1.5 cm). This produces a comfortable raise, reducing unnecessary bulk and weight. In some instances, adding a back rocker (or heel striker) to the heel can increase the ankle ROM and improve gait further. Limb length discrepancies of 3–4 cm (1.2–1.6 inches) are treated most frequently by modifying the client's own footwear (Münzenberg 1985) (Fig. 13.7).

Where the ankle ROM is severely limited, a full-length raise is generally more comfortable but a good toe-off is still essential. The raise should be the same at the heel and joint and only reduced at the toe (e.g. heel elevation 4 cm, joint elevation 4 cm, toe elevation 2 cm). Limb length discrepancies of 5–8 cm (1.65–3.2 inches) require a prescription shoe as the raise must be built into the structure of the midsole. Retail items are not sufficiently robust to take a medium-to-high raise safely.

In instances where the patient has very limited ankle ROM, but also knee and/or hip limitations, and possibly relies on a walking aid such as a frame for support, then a total full-length raise may be necessary (e.g. heel elevation 4 cm, joint elevation 4 cm, toe elevation 4 cm) to provide complete stability, as very little toe off is possible during gait (Figs 13.8 and 13.9). At these heights, a prescription shoe may be the safer option, although this option may not always be as acceptable to patients as adapting their own shoes. A block heel shape is essential for stability at this height and the heels of many retail shoes will not be sufficiently stable.

With any raise, the foot needs to be secure and not slip on any internal support. To control this, Münzenberg (1985) offers the following advice:

- The heel area should be deeply padded (Fig. 13.10).

Figure 13.7 Example of a tapered raise: heel elevation, 3 cm; joint elevation, 2 cm; toe elevation, 1 cm. This external raise is inserted into a micro rubber sole. It is not covered with the shoe upper material and appears as part of the shoe sole unit.

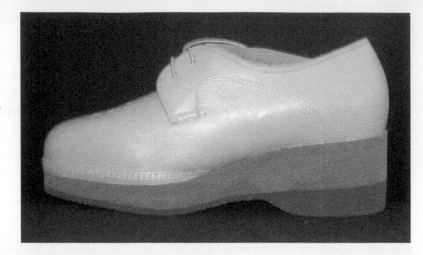

Figure 13.8 Example of a full-length raise with toe-off. The raise is outside and made of leather covered cork.

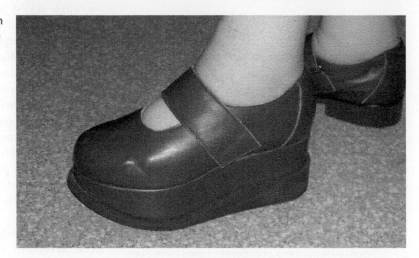

Figure 13.9 Example of a full-length raise of 1 cm with no toe-off. The external raise inserted within the existing sole unit allows the surface of the sole unit to retain its profile and surface characteristics.

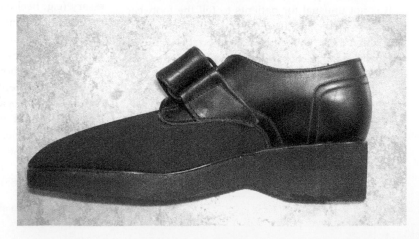

Figure 13.10 Example of an equinus cradle with a padded deep heel seat. (Reproduced with permission of Jane Saunders & Manning.)

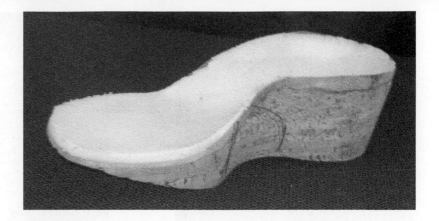

- A toe grip bar within the shoe is often helpful (not a metatarsal pad as this may be uncomfortable).
- The dorsum of the foot should be firmly gripped by the upper of the footwear. Therefore, a fully functional fastening is essential.

The greater the compensation required, the more the shoe sole and heel should be flared laterally (for every 1 cm height = 1 mm lateral flare) (Münzenberg 1985). This recommendation is based on the fact that during transfer from heel to toe, lateral forces develop which could bend the shoe over and the lateral flare counteracts this. However, this again can be unacceptable to the client as it adds bulk and weight and becomes very clumsy in appearance. By eliminating the lateral flare, the overall cosmetic effect is more acceptable but is functionally less stable (Fig. 13.11).

The higher the degree of ankle equinus, the shorter the anterior lever arm (Münzenberg 1985). The compensatory raise needs to be equivalent to the height that the heel is elevated off the ground when the forefoot is loaded. In prescribing bespoke footwear for patients with high degrees of equinus, it is essential to take a plaster of Paris cast to capture the equinus position and achieve the correct pitch from heel to joint in the finished footwear. If possible, the cast should be taken weight-bearing. Before the cast is removed, it is vital to mark horizontal and vertical reference lines on it relating it to the ground, to allow the last maker to evaluate the cast and position it correctly, so that the finished footwear will relate to the ground surface accurately. Without these lines, it

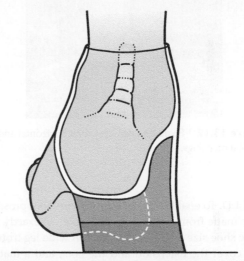

Figure 13.11 Lateral flare to counterbalance equinus with a varus heel. (Reproduced with permission of Münzenberg 1985.)

is impossible to position the foot in its plantargrade position. The resulting footwear will be of incorrect heel fit and the pitch of the footwear and of the cradle will be inaccurate (Fig. 13.12).

The short anterior lever may be supplemented by adding a partial foot prosthesis to balance the front part of the shoe. In severe equinus, this prosthesis/filler needs a flexible midsection to improve the toe-off action. The patient will need to be familiar with using such a filler, as its use will involve considerable changes to the gait pattern.

The O'Connor boot illustrated in Figs 13.13–13.15 accommodates both the equinus foot position and

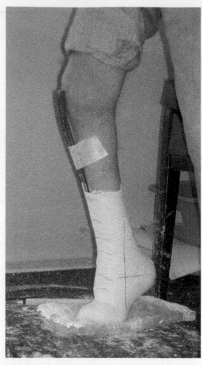

Figure 13.12 Fixed equinus cast with horizontal and vertical markings.

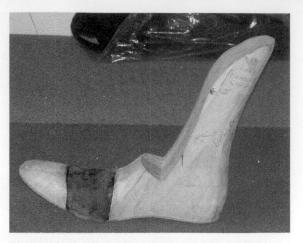

Figure 13.13 Example of a prosthetic foot with flexible midsection, to become part of an O'Connor boot. (Reproduced with permission of TayCare Medical Ltd.)

the LLD. To enable normal toe-off, a full foot prosthesis is made from leather covered wood, to exactly the same shoe size as the normal foot. A wide leg trouser will cover the extension and the boot, and a matching pair of retail shoes is purchased by the patient to wear on the unaffected limb and over the prosthesis in the normal way.

In cases where the LLD is longstanding and where the patient has worn no accommodating raise to level the limbs, initial management of the LLD should not necessarily attempt to provide full height compensation immediately. In cases such as this, the patient will have adopted compensatory strategies in gait and these may have resulted in compensatory tissue shortening and the development of antalgic gait patterns which cannot easily be reversed. The addition of a full height compensatory raise may cause discomfort in both the foot and the low back. Each patient should be assessed on an individual basis, and in such cases, it may be advisable to prescribe a lower raise and reassess as appropriate until the most satisfactory solution is reached.

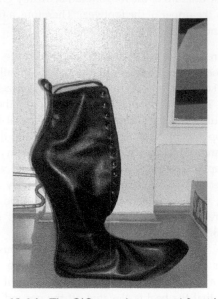

Figure 13.14 The O'Connor boot at mid fit with the prosthetic foot inside. (Reproduced with permission of TayCare Medical Ltd.)

In the majority of cases, *the aim is to achieve full locking of both knees* during gait and *equitable weight-bearing* through both legs. Patients may need to be encouraged to break the habit of always flexing the longer limb at the knee and may need to re-educate their weight-bearing strategy to ensure that they stand with their weight distributed through both

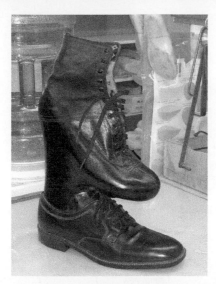

Figure 13.15 Example of a double O'Connor boot with a retail shoe fitted to the prosthesis. (Reproduced with permission of TayCare Medical Ltd.)

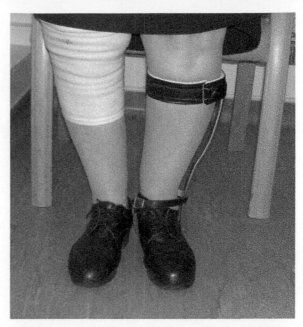

Figure 13.16 Example of a patient with Paget's disease fitted with a left internal raise and outside stabilizing below-knee calliper. Knee flexion is limited.

legs equally. Physiotherapy input may be helpful to assist in developing the muscular strength and appropriate gait pattern. It is also useful to ask patients to stand and walk towards a full-length mirror so that they can view their stance and gait and identify the modifications that need to be made (Fig. 13.16).

Where a patient with LLD also has genu valgum or limited ROM of the knee, the LLD should not be fully raised as this could compromise gait rather than improve it. A raise of 1–1.5 cm less than the measured height is recommended to help with toe clearance in such cases (Münzenberg 1985). A tapered raise may be adequate but the heel height may still need to be reduced. If the height required is under 2 cm, then the client may be better without a raise, or alternatively a simple three-quarter length heel lift within the shoe may be adequate (Fig. 13.17).

'Functional foot orthoses should be prescribed with built-in heel lifts when the foot and limb pathology warrant such intervention' (Lorimer et al 2004). If internal heel lifts are prescribed they should be strictly for a short term only (max 6 months), and provided the patient follows the regime recommended, the expected outcome is that the heel lifts should not be needed permanently. Regular reviews and possible modification of the orthoses is essential.

Points to note:

- Raises higher than 1 cm ideally should be tapered through to the toes in order to prevent excessive pelvic tilt and ensure good balance (Blake & Ferguson 1992). This tapering also protects against further shortening of the Achilles tendon and the possibility of causing a fixed equinus foot position. Such raises are best included in the outer sole of the shoe. However, many patients are reluctant to have a visible raise and, consequently, an internal raise is often prescribed which, because of the limited internal accommodation within a shoe, may fail to deliver the necessary compensation.

- Advising a patient to place 'some kind of padding' under the heel to raise it is very poor practice (but often said and frequently seen) and should be discouraged. When this scenario presents in a clinic, the padding (pieces of foam, felt, cut-up insoles, layers of cardboard, etc.) should be removed. The LLD should be measured clinically and the patient prescribed a proper internal heel lift made from cork, high-density ethylene vinyl acetate or other suitable durable material.

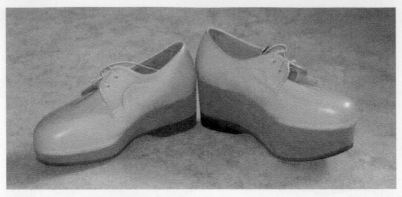

Figure 13.17 Example of footwear for left-sided equinus with equal limb length. The right side has a compensating raise. (Note: colour match is poor and unacceptable to the patient.)

- Internal heel lifts need to be correctly designed to provide the raise at the correct position under the heel. The full height of the raise needs to be extended sufficiently distal under the heel to be in line with the malleoli before it begins to be tapered down.
- In cases where LLD is less than 6 mm, heel lifts may be inserted into the heel of the shoe with the full height of the raise supporting the calcaneus and a bevelled distal edge positioned further forward (be aware that many ready-made items are too short and do not fully support the calcaneus). Where the LLD is between 6–10 mm, raises are better provided as three-quarter length inlays, tapered off proximal to the metatarsal phalangeal joints.
- It is important to note that the maximum raise which can be included in most retail footwear is 1 cm. A higher internal raise may be acceptable in deep footwear, such as trainers with a high top collar, ankle boots or any design that has more depth in the heel/ankle area accompanied by good foot entry access and a functional fastening (Figs 13.18–13.21).

Measurement for footwear elevations

The British Standard 5943 (1980) makes the following statements in relation to measuring a LLD (for elevations):

- Details of the elevation shall be given by the surgeon, but it may be necessary for the

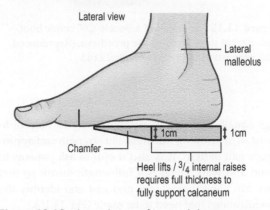

Figure 13.18 Lateral view of internal three-quarter shoe raise, demonstrating the height required under the calcaneum before tapering starts.

measurer to give particulars of the height after consultation with the surgeon.

- The two important measures are the heel and joint.
- A toe measurement may be given but this will usually be determined by the toe spring required.
- Heel measurements should be taken from the position below the malleoli, not the centre back.
- Joint measurements should be taken from a point directly under the metatarsal heads.
- In cases of fixed equinus, a plaster cast is essential. This cast should extend far enough up the leg to give clearly the angle of the foot to the leg.

Figure 13.19 Example of a modified stock shoe with internal tapered raise. (Reproduced with permission of Klaveness.)

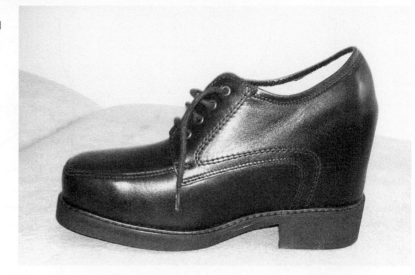

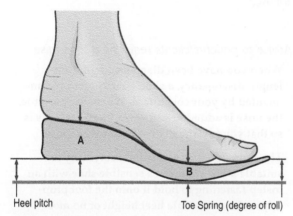

Heel pitch   Toe Spring (degree of roll)

Figure 13.20 Typical internal shoe raise; unilateral. (Reproduced with permission of BS 5943 1980.)

- In cases where the leg lengths are equal but a fixed equinus results in the forefoot extending beyond the foot of the normal leg, it will be necessary to raise the normal side in order to level the pelvis.
- In general the elevations may be inside the footwear, outside or a combination of both.

Points to note:

- In functional mechanical terms, the anterior lever arm of the foot becomes shorter as the degree of equinus increases, so in severe cases, it may be necessary to address this function more drastically, by adding a forefoot prosthesis (Münzenberg 1985).

- All LLD patients are effectively in equinus to some degree until they are levelled, so it is essential to assess the ROM not only in the foot and ankle, but also in the knees and hips to ensure that any raise will cause an improvement to gait, and not be a hindrance to it.

- There are some authors who advocate that if a LLD of 2 cm or less is asymptomatic it will not require treatment (Blustein & D'Amico 1985; Münzenberg 1985). However, Subotnick (1981) and Blake & Ferguson (1992) suggest that clinical benefits have been proven in patients prescribed raises where their LLD is between 1 and 2 cm.

- In all LLD cases, it is recommended therefore to measure and prescribe a raise on one pair of shoes only, advise the patient to wear the raised item for 6–8 weeks and then review to evaluate its clinical effectiveness. Clinical judgement in many of these cases errs on the side of prescribing a lower raise than the LLD, especially where it is long established and has been untreated. A gradual adjustment to the raise should take place over several months.

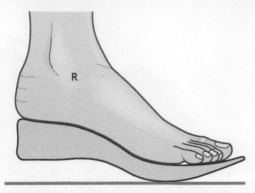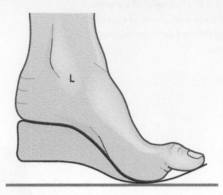

Figure 13.21 Typical internal raise with fixed equinus and no LLD requiring compensating raise. (Reproduced with permission of BS 5943 1980.)

In the majority of cases, these low shoe raises or internal heel lifts are very helpful and patients benefit, finding relief of chronic symptoms, particularly of low back pain.

Footwear requirements

- A LLD up to 5 cm can be treated by modifying a retail shoe (see notes below on retail shoe purchase), unless complex foot pathology exists, in addition to the LLD, that requires a prescribed shoe.
- Raises between 5 cm and 8 cm require a therapeutic shoe or modified stock shoe. The raise needs to be part of the shoe construction if it is to be stable and safe in wear. It also needs to be attached to an inner sole which is much firmer and stronger than those found in retail footwear.
- Raises above 8 cm may require an in-shoe prosthesis, and a bespoke therapeutic shoe/boot or an O'Connor boot.

Retail footwear

Footwear suitable for added raises

When patients are advised to obtain footwear to which a unilateral raise can be added, they have very little knowledge of what will be suitable. In addition to offering verbal advice about the necessary features, it is very helpful to be able to provide patients with a printed leaflet which covers this topic.

The following guidelines describe the type of information that patients need to understand and follow.

Advice to patients/clients requiring a shoe raise

When you have been diagnosed with limb length discrepancy, a shoe raise is often recommended by your consultant. Whenever possible, the raise is added to your own footwear. This is so that your existing shoes can still be worn.

The shoes must be of a suitable style. By suitable style, we mean a sensible shoe with an instep fastening to hold it onto the foot properly and a reasonable heel height of no more than 2 inches (5 cm) that is not too tapered or too narrow.

The fastening is required to keep the shoe securely on the foot. The added raise will inevitably add extra weight to the shoe so a slip-on style is very likely to fall off the foot at the heel. The shape of the heel is important because the higher it is raised, the narrower it becomes, in a tapered shape, and this will be unstable to wear (Fig. 13.22).

The fastening can be:
Laces
Velcro®
Strap and buckle
High elastic gusset.

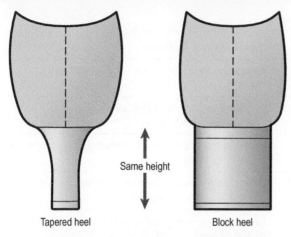

Same height

Tapered heel   Block heel

Figure 13.22 Same heel height but different shapes demonstrating increase in ground contact.

The style can be:

Simple tie-up shoe
Trainers
Bootees (ankle height)
Most boots, except safety workwear (see Ch. 6)
'T' bar
Mary Jane
Moccasins with a high vamp

Sandals with very secure instep fastenings (i.e. adjustable straps, lacing and preferably with a proper heel counter in the back)

Indoor slippers; these can be raised as long as they are fastened on with Velcro® or a strap and have a firm rubber type sole unit rather than a soft spongy sole.

The sole can be:

Rubber
Leather
Commando
Ethylene vinyl acetate
Injection moulded
Synthetic soling like polyurethane.
The sole *must not* be:

Stitched through to the inside, as the sole needs to be split to have the raise inserted into it and the stitched soles will fall apart when split.

Have inserted 'air bubbles' or 'lights'
Multi striped (some trainers are like this)

Very thick injection moulded soles: these are difficult to split as they are very often a honey-comb construction inside and cannot have extra layers added.

Cautionary note: rather than raising the shoe on the shorter leg, some people may want to consider lowering the sole and heel of the shoe worn on the longer leg. It is generally inadvisable to do this. For example, the technician cannot lower a platform shoe because of the way the shoe is con-structed. By attempting to lower the heel of any shoe, the effect is to increase the toe spring and unbalance the roll through of the shoe. Conversely, a heel raise without an equally high rocker bar will reduce the toe spring, causing foot slap.

Therapeutic footwear is not routinely prescribed just for a shoe raise to be added. There are strict criteria for prescribing special footwear, and unless you have other complicating conditions that require special shoes to be made, you must continue to buy your own shoes in the normal way.

These guidelines are to help you to buy the best possible type of shoe for adaptation. The clinic will always offer additional advice if required and will check the suitability of any new shoes that you have bought before they are adapted.

The clinical staff will check every pair of shoes brought in for the addition of a raise. They will advise you on the suitability of the style and the quality of the fit. They will reject footwear if it is unsuitable, badly fitting or too worn.

Point to note: The above guidelines refer primarily to adults, but they are suitable for children as well (see Ch. 6).

Clinically, the ultimate goal in paediatric cases, where the LLD is in the mild-to-moderate category, will be to minimize the risk of a permanent equinus foot position and encourage full ankle ROM. To this end (depending entirely on the diagnosis), prescribing a lower raise than measured and encouraging muscle stretching exercises with regular follow-on reviews is a sound clinical plan. The raise prescribed may be half of the measured height in many instances.

Table 13.1 Comparison of external and internal raise options

External raise options	Internal raise options
Inserted into the existing sole (by splitting the sole open and re-gluing) (Fig. 13.7).	Added to an inlay (e.g. heel lift) (Fig. 13.18).
Uncovered (material exposed) (Fig. 13.7).	An inside levelling cork (e.g. equinus) (Fig. 13.20, 13.21, 13.24, 13.30, 13.31).
Tapered (reducing in height towards the toe end) (Fig. 13.7).	Moulded contact inlay incorporating an elevation (raise) (Fig. 13.30).
Made from cork, high-density plastazote, micro-soling material, ethylene vinyl acetate (Fig. 13.7).	Split in height with an outside raise to lessen the obvious appearance (Fig. 13.19).
Leather covered to match the shoe (Fig. 13.8).	Limited in use with retail footwear to height of back quarters.
Full length (no taper at toe) (Fig. 13.9).	Cosmetically more acceptable (Figs. 13.19, 13.24).
Stuck-on to the existing sole (Fig. 13.9).	Part of a prosthetic foot (Fig. 13.36).
A bridge shape (cut out through the centre) (Fig. 13.23).	
Heel raise only (not recommended as toe spring is lost) (Ch. 9).	

Many children with LLD are offered surgical lengthening before they are fully grown to correct any residual discrepancy, thus removing the need for a shoe raise for the rest of their adult lives.

Prescribing shoe raises

There are many combinations of shoe raise that can be prescribed, depending on the construction of the footwear, the height required, weight and build of the wearer, occupation, etc. Table 13.1 summarizes the options available.

When ordering a shoe raise

It is very important to state accurately the type of raise required, for example inserted, full length or tapered, whether internal or external (especially on semi-bespoke or bespoke footwear). The manufacturer will need full information on the height required, and heights throughout the raise should always be stipulated in the following order: heel, joints, toe (H = x mm, Jt = x mm, T = x mm).

Bear in mind that the shoe for the longer limb will have a degree of raise in its existing sole and heel. The shorter limb needs a raise additional to these heights. It is essential to state only the height of the elevation

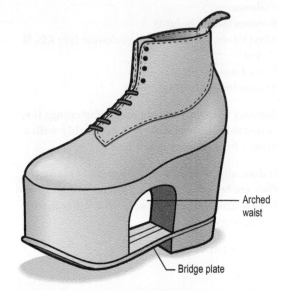

Arched waist

Bridge plate

Figure 13.23 Bridge plate and arch waist on a very high external raise. (Reproduced with permission of MHM 50 1980, part B, pp 32–35.)

to be added to the shoe of the shorter limb and not the total height of the finished raised heel. Technicians are trained to add what is requested to the height of a shoe and not to subtract the one height from another. Finally, ensure that the shoe is clearly labelled with

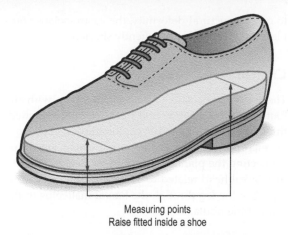

Measuring points
Raise fitted inside a shoe

Figure 13.24 Example of a typical full-length internal raise. (Reproduced with permission of MHM 50, part B, pp 32–35.)

the patient's name, the raise heights required and where it has come from (i.e. clinic or hospital name). It then stands a very good chance of not being lost and the factory will also know where to send the invoice for the work if the shoe becomes detached from the paper order which will accompany it.

On receipt of the raised item

A few basic suggestions may seem obvious, but time may be wasted unnecessarily if errors are unnoticed before the patient arrives to be fitted with the raised shoe:

- Check that the heights added to the footwear are accurate at the heel, joint and toe and that they match the order submitted.
- Check that the raise has been added to the correct shoe (left or right).
- Check that the raised footwear sits flat on the floor and is stable.
- Check that the overall cosmetic finish is acceptable (i.e. colour matching, appearance).

A shoe raise should never be issued to the patient without trying the adapted item and examining the effect which wearing the raise has on the patient's gait. Ensure that the patient is standing level when the raise is worn (if that is your aim) and advise the patient that wearing the raise will seem strange at first.

Points to note: Patients need reassurance that the raised footwear is cosmetically acceptable and that

their gait will improve as they adjust to walking with limbs of equal length.

The patient should also be reminded that, as the raised sole is both stiffer and thicker, they cannot rely on feeling through the sole for edges of kerbs, stairs, etc. Patients should be advised to walk slowly initially and should use their eyes to look down for such things. Patients should wear the raise for short times initially and should gradually increase wear times over a 4-week period. Their progress should be reviewed a few weeks later.

Equinus conditions

Ankle equinus may be defined as 'any condition either structural or functional that restricts ankle joint dorsiflexion to less than 10 degrees with the subtalar joint (STJ) in neutral position and the mid tarsal joint (MTJ) fully pronated' (Figs 13.25 and 13.26).

Antony (undated) qualifies this further by stating 'during the mid stance period just prior to heel lift, 9–10 degrees of ankle dorsiflexion is required for normal progression to occur without compensation

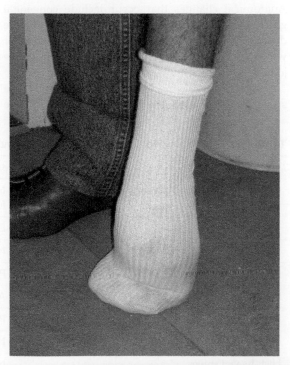

Figure 13.25 Example of a severe equinus on the left side.

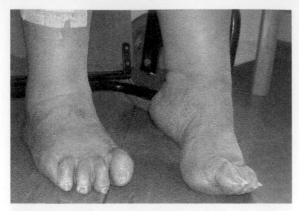

Figure 13.26 Example of a mild equinus.

at another level'. This requirement occurs at a time when the subtalar joint has reached neutral and is slightly supinated, the knee has reached full functional extension, the hip is 10° hyperextended and the tibialis anterior is not active.

Aetiology

Anatomical changes that occur include congenital gastro-soleus shortening and talar trochlear surface deformity (i.e. flattening of the top of the talus, or widening of the top surface causing locking of the joint early in dorsiflexion) (Table 13.2).

Point to note: If the foot is functioning with the subtalar and midtarsal complexes fully pronated due to other structural deformity, the gastro-soleus complex will relax and subsequently shorten.

Clinical test

The condition is said to be present when, with the foot in neutral position and the knee fully extended, the foot has less than 10° of dorsiflexion. The lines of reference for taking this measurement are a line connecting the plantar surface of the heel to the fifth metatarsal head related to a line bisecting the lateral aspect of the leg through the lateral malleolus to the head of the fibula.

Differential diagnosis

In order to make a differential diagnosis of limited ankle joint dorsiflexion:

- Test ankle joint dorsiflexion with the knee flexed and again with the knee extended.
- Where insufficient dorsiflexion of the ankle joint occurs when the knee is extended, but dorsiflexion is sufficient when the knee is flexed, the likely cause is gastrocnemius equinus.
- Where insufficient dorsiflexion of the ankle joint occurs in both flexion and extension of the knee, the likely cause is either an osseous anomaly or inadequacy of the soleus muscle.

To differentially diagnose between soleal and osseous equinus, feel the end of the range of motion in

Table 13.2 Comparison of functional aetiology in equinus conditions

Contracture state of gastro-soleus complex caused by:	
Clonic spasm (e.g. upper motor neurone lesion)	Needs supporting and stretching programme to prevent further tightening
Tonic spasm	Delivers pain in varying degrees
Vasospasm	Muscles need better arterial flow (e.g. intermittent claudication)
Fibrosis	Post injury complication
Prolonged bed rest	Avoidable if heel protection is used
Post below-knee casting leaving ankle in plantarflexion	Post injury complication
Athletic hypertonicity	Muscles may shorten with excess exercise such as running
High-heeled shoes	Never walking without high heels can lead to muscle shortening in years to come

the ankle. An abrupt block may indicate an osseous problem, whereas a spongy end range of motion would suggest the equinus condition is related to soleal inadequacy.

Compensation

Apart from the ankle joint, the only joint within the foot that has significant sagittal plane motion is the midtarsal joint through its oblique axis. Some dorsiflexion is available by subtalar joint pronation, but this is inadequate to compensate the whole equinus deformity. However, pronation of the subtalar joint will result in additional motion at the midtarsal joint, which may be used to compensate for the deformity.

In equinus conditions, the longitudinal arch of the foot is generally more pronounced than normal, and there is often either a valgus or varus heel deformity present.

In terms of functional mechanics, severe equinus is characterized by the fact that the weight-bearing surface of the foot is reduced to the area under the metatarsal heads. Consequently, rollover is only possible via the ball of the foot.

Measuring the equinus

When prescribing footwear for this condition, the extent of the equinus is determined by standing the patient erect and assessing the level position of the pelvis (measurement of limb length discrepancy, p. 201). The limb presenting with the equinus condition may be longer than the unaffected limb and thus a raise may be required under the unaffected limb. Measurement of the equinus can be achieved by using compensating blocks under the opposite limb to achieve a level pelvis. The height of the blocks required can then be measured and the height of the equinus can be determined. It is important to achieve the correct perpendicular (sagittal) position. The sagittal line must start from the hip joint, pass just in front of the knee joint axis during standing and continue to behind the metatarsal heads. Once levelled, the clinician is able to assess for the first time exactly what compensation and level of raise are required. It is particularly useful to allow patients to view themselves with the blocks in place in a full-length mirror. They may be surprised at the height of the required raise, or alternatively they may appreciate the improvement in their posture and the relief of back

pain. If the patient indicates that they would find such a raise unacceptable, there is little point in proceeding further. Patients may well need time to adjust and return to the clinic in the future if the condition causes a high level of discomfort.

If the patient is fully committed to the process, the prescription can begin. The BS 5943 requires a full plaster of Paris cast to be taken for equinus conditions. The cast is generally taken with the foot and lower leg suspended above the floor to capture the foot's fixed position. The knee joint should be flexed to 90°. The cast is marked with both horizontal and vertical lines bisecting the lateral malleolus, using a long ruler and cast marker. This is essential for the last maker to relate the leg position to the horizontal plane when the cast is sent to the manufacturer (Figs 13.27 and 13.28).

Clinical guidelines for the management of equinus

The clinical aims of managing the equinus condition are to enable the patient to:

- Mobilize safely
- Achieve a level pelvis
- Improve or maintain existing foot function

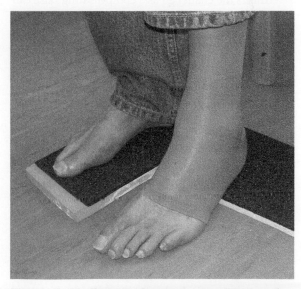

Figure 13.27 Example of measuring an equinus on the left side, using compensating blocks for the right leg.

215

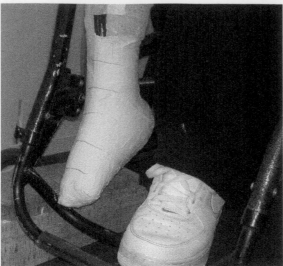

Figure 13.28 Example of casting a fixed equinus, maintaining full flexion at the knee of 90° with the foot suspended off the ground.

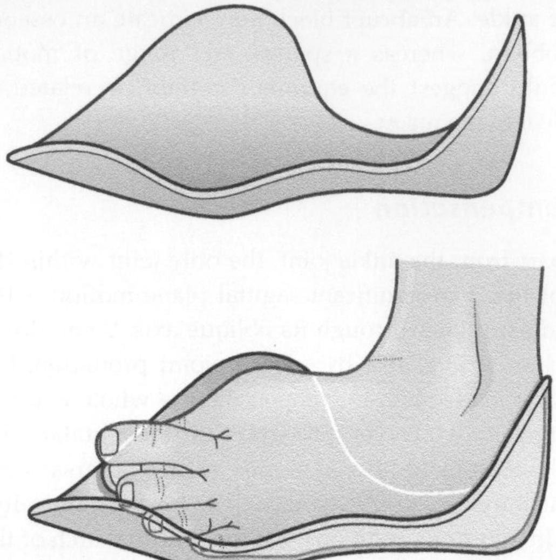

Figure 13.29 Typical levelling cradle cork. (Reproduced with permission of MHM 50.)

- Redistribute load-bearing on the affected side
- Be able to fully weight-bear on both legs/feet (a compensating raise may be required where there is no actual LLD in addition to the equinus)
- Achieve locking of both knees
- Wear footwear that is cosmetically acceptable (this is the challenge as a compensating raise can be hard to accept, especially as it is on the non-affected side).

The prime objective must be to distribute load-bearing as far as possible over the entire sole of the foot. This is often achieved by making an internal levelling cork cradle to the cast supplied and a suitable shoe or boot to accommodate this. In most instances, a full plaster of Paris cast is required, but a phenolic foam impression can sometimes be adequate to capture the plantar contours and heel pitch, if this low. The double-depth phenolic impression box may be helpful, but, as it cannot capture the rear heel profile, it becomes a poor substitute for plaster of Paris (Figs 13.29 and 13.30).

The levelling cradle allows the horizontal plane to be achieved between the foot and the ground, despite any degree of deformity.

Any relative limb shortness of the contralateral leg should ideally be corrected with a compensating raise, always provided that this is not cumbersome or cosmetically unacceptable. Where a compensating raise is not acceptable, the true height of the equinus raise may not be achievable, but this will leave the patient with a flexed knee position, which is less than ideal. Sometimes compensation of the unaffected limb becomes too clumsy and is not tolerated well, and, consequently, the management of the equinus with therapeutic footwear reaches its limits. In such cases, surgical intervention may be the only acceptable outcome.

Where some degree of motion is available, it should not be restricted provided that it is not painful. The shoe supplied may require full rocker action to allow this movement rather than be limited by the stiffness of an internal levelling cradle. The heel height should be the lowest possible, accounting for the plantarflexion available.

In cases where there is extensor impairment of the knee joint, often due to tissue shortening following many years of coping with LLD, the equinus cannot be fully compensated as this would require normal knee extension during gait (Münzenberg 1985).

Footwear requirements

The following examples often present in the clinic.

Figure 13.30 Example of an internal levelling cradle 'cork'. This example was constructed from high-density Nora®.

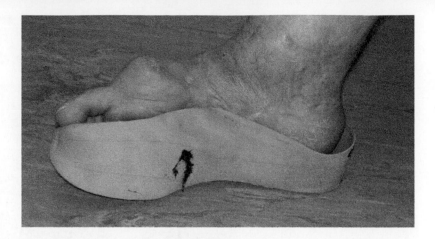

Mild fixed equinus (<2 cm) without limb length discrepancy

- Simple internal three-quarter length shoe raise of up to 1 cm with any additional height added to the external heel with a balanced rocker sole just proximal to the flexion point at the metatarso-phalangeal joints.
- Internal raise should be tapered to 0.5 cm at the metatarso-phalangeal joints.
- Compensating raise to non-affected limb is minimal, but it is needed to allow good toe clearance to affected side.
- Retail footwear may be suitable for these patients.

Mild fixed equinus with limb length discrepancy

- Establish the LLD as described above.
- Measure the required height (<2 cm probably does not need casting).
- Wearing the footwear to be modified, stand the client on blocks under the affected side and recheck for level pelvis, posture and compliance (see Fig. 13.27).
- Prescribe the raise: either all external or split.

Point to note: Remember if the height is split between an internal and external raise, it will double the cost, but in most cases, this is the most acceptable option and can usually be applied to retail footwear.

Mild to moderate fixed equinus (2–5 cm) without limb length discrepancy

- Compensating raise to unaffected limb is essential to achieve a level pelvis and toe clearance (see Fig. 13.17).
- The equinus foot may need the lever arm extending by adding a toe block to match foot length.
- Secure fastening style (preferably laces) and block heel shape for stability.
- May not be possible to accommodate in retail footwear in all cases (depending on height) (see Fig. 13.19).
- Where client's own shoes are used, ensure they are reasonably new, firm in the counter, have a secure fastening style and fit well.
- Wearing the footwear to be modified, stand the client on blocks to both sides and recheck for level pelvis, posture and concordance.
- Prescribe lightweight materials to reduce overall shoe weight.

Moderate to severe fixed equinus (5–7 cm) without limb length discrepancy

- Compensating raise to unaffected limb is essential to achieve a level pelvis and toe clearance.

Figure 13.31 Example of a levelling cradle in construction. (Reproduced with permission of TayCare Medical Ltd.)

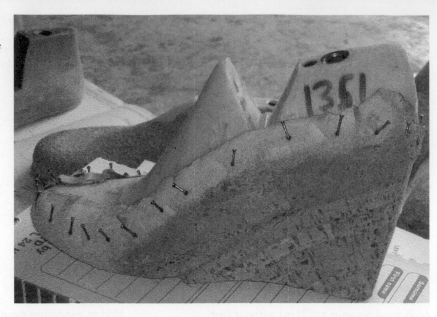

- As the effective mechanical foot length (lever arm) is shortened, it is often necessary to make a partial foot prosthesis with an extended shank up to the flexion point of the shoe.
- Adding a rocker sole will help compensate for reduced ankle joint movement. If the footwear creases badly as a result of the rocker, then the whole sole should be stiffened to prevent the shoe from bending upwards. This can be done by adding a carbon fibre sole plate and resoling the shoe.
- The cradle should pad and support the heel firmly to reduce the risk of slippage. Also ensure that the counter depth is adequate to hold the heel securely.
- Where necessary, a toe grip bar or ankle retaining strap may help to reduce movement inside the shoe or boot, however ensuring the footwear fits very well across the instep is the best way to keep the foot from sliding forwards (Münzenberg 1985).

Extremely severe equinus (>7 cm) without limb length discrepancy

- If surgery is completely out of the question, bespoke footwear will be necessary, ideally ankle-high boots.

- Casts and British Standard chart should be taken.
- Follow points made for 5–7 cm height, above.

In summary, laced ankle boots are the preferred choice of footwear for moderate to severe equinus, along with high counter stiffener and internal levelling cork cradle, rocker sole and extended shank or stiffened sole, and possibly a compensating raise to the other foot (Fig. 13.31).

Extremely severe equinus (>7 cm) with limb length discrepancy

In these extreme cases, where the foot is in severe equinus, the ball of the foot may not be in contact with the ground when the pelvis is levelled and the knees can lock. In addition to the above points, note the following:

- The prosthetic in-shoe levelling cradle also needs to incorporate a full-length internal raise, pitched under the metatarsal area as captured by the plaster of Paris cast.
- The toe filler should extend sufficiently to balance the lever arm propulsion if not to match shoe size evenly.
- The toe filler needs some flexibility, and can be made from a flexible material

(i.e. medium-density Nora® or ethylene vinyl acetate) (sometimes referred to as a Downey prosthesis).

- A deeper toe pitch to create a good rocker action is vital, and may take several attempts to perfect this so that the client is able to walk as well as possible.

Limb length discrepancy above 12 cm

The O'Connor boot was designed for the extreme LLD and incorporates a cradle for the equinus foot to be supported at the angle most comfortable. A false foot prosthesis is built below the cradle with the intervening height matching the individual measurements. The prosthetic foot is most often made to fit a matching pair of good retail shoes with the bespoke section made to hold and support the short leg and foot. This is often hidden by either wearing a long skirt or wide leg trousers so that only the retail shoes are seen. However the gait when wearing the O'Connor boot is slow and laboured, due to the height and not inconsequential weight (see Figs 13.13–13.15).

Compensation for amputation surgery

Providing footwear for the foot after amputation

Münzenberg (1985) states that 'Loss of the great toe or part of the foot in the metatarsal or tarsal region results in shortening of the anterior lever arm, in a similar way to a severe equinus'. However, in addition to creating a lever arm of normal length to improve the gait pattern, care must be taken of the stump and an assessment of its capacity to bear weight or stress is vital. Also, the location of scars and previous ulcer sites or skin grafts, for example, make the management of these patients highly complicated.

The prime clinical guidelines for management can be generalized *but* each case must be given individual assessment in order to provide the most appropriate footwear, taking into account medical conditions, risk factors, cosmetic preferences, occupation, age, mobility and concordance.

Clinical guidelines for the management of the foot after amputation surgery

The clinical aims of managing the foot after amputation surgery are to enable the patient to:

- Mobilize safely
- Achieve a level pelvis
- Improve or maintain existing foot function, especially on the non-affected side
- Redistribute load-bearing on the affected side
- Be able to fully weight-bear on both legs/feet
- Achieve locking of both knees
- Wear footwear that is cosmetically acceptable.

The prime objective must be to allow weight-bearing and mobilization on the amputated stump, reduce pain and protect the foot to a degree that improves quality of life and reduces further damage.

Patients with metatarsal and tarsal stumps seek a shoe or boot that is designed to protect and accommodate the stump in such a way that it is undetectable to others. Semi-bespoke or modular footwear is now readily available and is often appropriate and more cosmetically acceptable to the patient, particularly where one foot is normal. It is also quicker to supply, thus possibly saving the foot from further trauma, than waiting for the slower bespoke option of the past (Figs 13.32 and 13.33).

In principle, the anterior lever arm can be substituted by a stiffened full-length sole (Münzenberg 1985). A high metatarsal bar or rocker sole may also help to achieve proper roll over. It is vital that the foot prosthesis matches the original foot length. The shorter the stump, the longer the force transmission plate required, extending from the foot prosthesis to the lower leg. A partial foot prosthesis with a flexible joint, as described for equinus, is often required and can be requested for modular footwear.

All movement between the stump and the prosthesis must be eliminated. This can be very difficult with tarsal stumps particularly, but can be helped by:

- Good support under the heel area from a moulded cradle.
- Holding the stump back in the counter (possibly using a retaining strap if not at risk of causing further tissue damage). A very close-fitting

counter helps and a style that encloses the foot securely is preferable.

- Keeping padding anterior to the stump end rather than underneath it.

A cast is essential and extreme care must be exercised in taking impressions to protect the stump from any damage during the procedure. Fully trained cast technicians may be required to do this work.

Loss of a great toe or lesser toes can be compensated for by prescribing an orthotic or moulded inlay with toe fillers. This can be fitted into a correctly fitting retail shoe which has a functional fastening, providing the risk of recurrent ulceration is low.

Where all the toes have been lost, then a semi-bespoke or bespoke shoe should ideally be prescribed following the British Standard charting system. The clinician must only accept footwear which fits perfectly. No compromises can be allowed. A great deal of skill and dedication are needed to prescribe and fit this type of high-risk footwear.

Footwear requirements

Features that can help in the construction include the following:

- Extended medial and/or lateral counter stiffeners, but only use if truly necessary.
- High stiffeners: may be required but try to avoid pressure over scarred areas. Either a unilateral medial or lateral high stiffener will probably be sufficient, but do not use these if ankle instability is evident.
- Cushioned toe block.

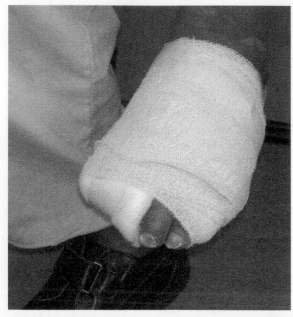

Figure 13.32 Example of diabetic patient with great toe amputation healed and still being dressed for protection.

Figure 13.33 Same diabetic patient as in Figure 13.32 fitted with modular depth footwear that accommodates the foot and dressings effectively.

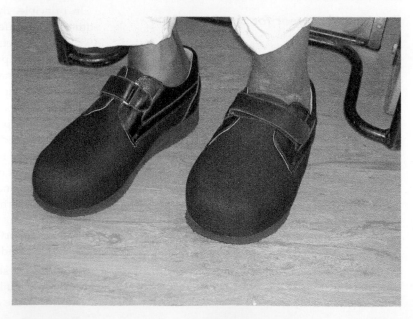

- Moulded inlay which is not bulky around the heel area: this can affect the counter fit and cause heel slippage.

- Rocker sole with compensatory heel: but check LLD as well so as not to unbalance the client inadvertently.

- A very soft non-slip lining: gives comfort to the vulnerable foot. In some instances, the leather lining can be reversed to grip better, especially in the counter area, as long as there are no skin lesions.

- A functional fastening with an adequate opening: laces are preferable as these are more effective than Velcro® at holding the foot back.

- Footwear that allows full ankle movement: a midtarsal amputee may still retain full ankle movement so the footwear needs to enable this to continue. The footwear most suitable would include quarters which finish just above the ankle, to enable close fit and retention of the foot in the counter.

The prosthesis needs a flexible midsection to help toe-off and this may be preferable to a high rocker sole (Figs 13.34 and 13.35).

An ankle retaining strap may be helpful, but be very cautious. Good soft padding to protect the skin

helps, but sometimes the bulk and direct pressure can be more of a hindrance.

The shorter the stump, the higher the top line of the footwear needs to be to ensure secure retention of the stump in the counter and to distribute pressure over a larger area. High-top boots are essential in these cases. In cases of peroneal nerve paralysis,

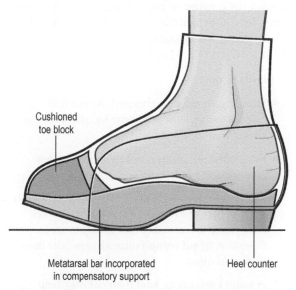

Figure 13.34 Features of a simple shoe construction for an amputee. (Reproduced with permission of Münzenberg 1985.)

Figure 13.35 Example of a Downey prosthesis with a flexible mid section. (Reproduced with permission of Jane Saunders & Manning.)

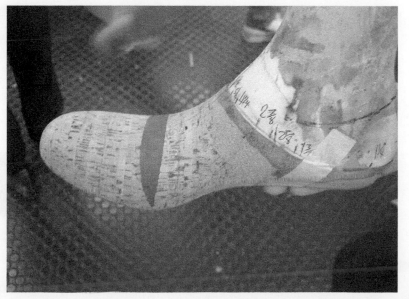

a boot quarter height of 18 cm is recommended as a minimum.

In some instances where an ankle–foot orthosis is combined with the prosthesis for full limb support, a shoe can be worn rather than a boot, as the footwear is accommodating rather than fully supporting the ankle (Figs 13.36 and 13.37).

Extra padding can be added to the tongue and around the counter to protect the stump from pressure. This is in addition to a cushioned prosthesis ideally using a mouldable material to eliminate any surface defects (Fig. 13.38).

Points to note:

- Shoe length must be checked. A common error is to make the footwear too short for the amputated foot.

- Ensure the remaining toes or stump are not compressed against the end of the shoe or filler.

- Check that the height above the ankle is not too high. Where the stump is at metatarsal level, a lace shoe is less bulky and heavy to wear, therefore, to aid compliance, always bear these factors in mind.

- A softer cushioning heel material may help reduce shock impact and this may be better

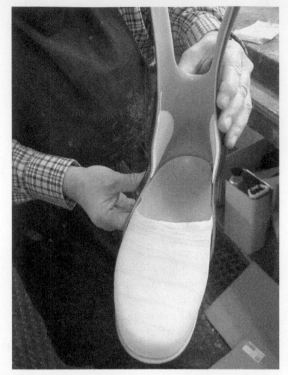

Figure 13.36 Example of Nora® partial foot prosthesis placed onto an AFO. (Reproduced with permission of Jane Saunders & Manning.)

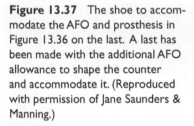

Figure 13.37 The shoe to accommodate the AFO and prosthesis in Figure 13.36 on the last. A last has been made with the additional AFO allowance to shape the counter and accommodate it. (Reproduced with permission of Jane Saunders & Manning.)

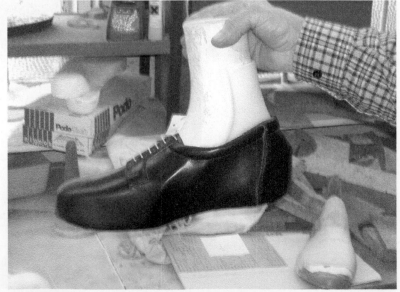

Figure 13.38 Example of an amputee cradle cork base with soft Nora® lining. (Reproduced with permission of Jane Saunders & Manning.)

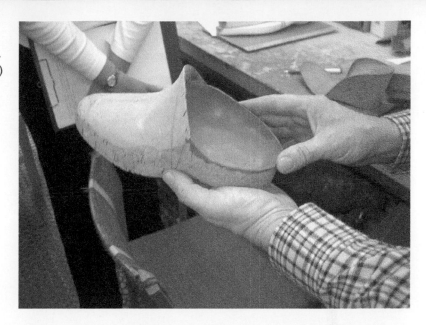

added to the external heel than under the calcaneum. There are buffer materials that can be used and manufacturers should be able to advise on availability.

Points to consider in evaluating footwear include:

- Has the footwear reduced any existing ankle motion more than is helpful?
- Is the heel height consistent with the toe spring or has the rocker affected this?

And finally the all important question:

- Has the client ended up with wearable, functional, comfortable footwear? If not, why not?

References

Blake RL, Ferguson H 1992 Limb length discrepancy. JAPMA 82(1):33–38.

Blustein SM, D'Amico JC 1985 Limb length discrepancy: identification, clinical significance and management. JAPMA 75(4):200–206.

Lorimer D, French G, O'Donnell M, Burrow JG 2004 Neale's disorders of the foot. Edinburgh, Churchill Livingstone, 123–125.

Münzenberg KJ 1985 The orthopaedic shoe: indications and prescription (translated by Beattie O). Weinheim, VCH Verlagsgesellschaft.

Subotnick SL 1981 Limb length discrepancies of the lower extremity (the short leg syndrome). J Orth Sports Phys Ther 3(1):11–15.

Valmassy RL 1995 Clinical biomechanics of the lower extremities. Edinburgh, Churchill Livingstone.

Internet articles/Web sites

La Trobe University Faculty of Health Sciences Department of Podiatry. Ankle equinus: *www.latrobe.edu.au/podiatry/Ankleequinus.html*

Bird AR, Payne CB 1999 Foot function and low back pain. The Foot 9:175–180.

BUPA UK Scoliosis, treatment of adult & congenital spinal curvature: http://hcd2.bupa.co.uk/fact_sheets/scoliosis.html

Leg length discrepancy: *www.orthoteers.co.uk/Nrujp-ij3331m/orthopeadlld.htm*

Scoliosis: *www.methodisthealth.com/Ortho/scolio.htm*

TIS The Hip and Pelvis Chs 7 & 9 (2002): *www.therapyedu.com/orhto/chapter*

The hip surgery: *4t.com/20.6htm*

Wikipedia.com free online encyclopaedia

For further reading on a specific topic search on Elsevier Health book site

Case studies

Chapter contents

In this chapter, a series of case studies is presented. They range from relatively simple cases to the most complex and are intended as a guide to problem solving when prescribing and fitting orthopaedic footwear.

Case study 1 (stock orthopaedic footwear)

Patient X is a 74-year-old gentleman with a history of type 2 diabetes which is insulin treated. This was diagnosed in 1980; it was first treated by diet alone, then with the use of oral hypoglycaemic agents, with transfer to insulin therapy some 3 years ago. HbA1$_c$ levels are now at 6.1 which represents good control.

He is a retired civil servant who had a sedentary job and his activities include normal day-to-day shopping, swimming and occasional gentle walks.

Patient X, however, has peripheral neuropathic changes affecting both feet. There is no response to testing with 10 g Semmes–Weinstein monofilament and no response to neurothesiometry values at the threshold value of 25 V when applied to the medial and lateral malleoli of both feet and to other distal bony prominences. There is also evidence of motor neuropathy with clawing of the lesser toes, mild triggering of the hallux and some autonomic neuropathy indicated by disturbances in sweat production and extremely dry skin. He has a history of plantar ulceration underlying the first metatarso-phalangeal joint of the right foot. This has healed following weight redistribution strategies, including the use of an Aircast® walker with bespoke orthotic insert, regular debridement and dressing with inadine. Additionally, there is evidence of peripheral ischemia with an ankle brachial pressure index (ABPI) of 0.75 on the left limb and 0.80 on the right. The feet are cold to the touch but there is no evidence of tissue atrophy or of intermittent claudication (Fig. 14.1).

The patient presents with the classical neuro-ischaemic foot with callous evident over the plantar surface of both first metatarso-phalangeal joints. The hallux has begun to adopt a triggered form and the

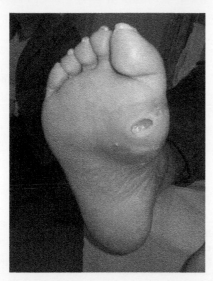

Figure 14.1 Patient with diabetes: first metatarso-phalangeal joint ulcer.

dorsal surface of the proximal interphalangeal joints of the second and third toes on both feet show signs of irritation from footwear.

Patient X was referred for special footwear as his own footwear was identified as being inadequate and was seen as a likely contributor to the development of greater digital problems. Plantar pressure redistribution was particularly required to minimize the likelihood of ulcer recurrence in the high-pressure areas of the plantar surface of the first metatarso-phalangeal joints. Orthoses to achieve pressure redistribution could not be accommodated within his existing footwear. The implications of special footwear were discussed with the patient. He was apprehensive at first. He did not wish to wear 'hospital' shoes which he described as heavy with deep toes, but he did not wish to suffer recurrence of his ulcer which had limited his activity. It was confirmed that it was his decision as to whether he wished to proceed, and it was also suggested that he might wish to take time to think about the need for special shoes and return to the clinic at a later date if he wished to proceed. It was suggested that foot measurements should be taken so that his footwear needs could be evaluated. He might then look at a selection of shoe styles which would be considered suitable for him. Foot measurements were recorded as shown in Table 14.1.

The shoe required specific qualities including a vamp and lining free of seams to prevent any

irritation to the forefoot, a rim toe puff to reduce the risk of pressure on the dorsum of the toes, adequate heel counters, padded top line and minimal seaming in the quarters. The upper and lining should be made of leather while the sole unit should be of ethylene vinyl acetate (EVA). Bearing in mind the above criteria and the measurements taken, it was decided to suggest shoes from manufacturer A. The patient was pleased with the selection and appreciated that the footwear looked similar to that which he would normally have chosen from a retail outlet. Phenolic foam box impressions were taken of each foot with the foot in a neutral position, and an allowance made on the shoe girth measurement of 20 mm to accommodate an orthotic of 1 cm in depth.

A size 9 deep brogue-type style in black leather was chosen with the snug-fit heel facility to ensure a good fit at the rear part of the shoe. The last measurements for this footwear are shown in Table 14.2. With the additional requirement for the orthoses of 20 mm girth throughout, these dimensions would meet the patient's needs.

The shoe has a standard heel height of 1 inch, which was adequate in view of the ankle joint motion available. The orthoses required were made in advance of receipt of the shoe as inner sole templates from this manufacturer were available. On receipt of the footwear, the orthoses were matched with the inner dimensions of each shoe. Total-contact orthoses were made with an EVA base of shore 50 and depressions for each first metatarso-phalangeal joint which were filled with poron. The orthoses were top covered with cross-linked polyethylene foam to provide a degree of cushioning throughout and to insulate the foot, keeping it warm and minimizing risk of circulatory damage.

The manufacturer's inner soles were removed from each shoe and checked against each foot to ensure adequate heel-to-ball fit, width at the metatarso-phalangeal joints, ball-to-toe measurement and overall length (Fig. 14.2).

The shoe inner soles were not replaced in the shoe, but the total-contact orthoses manufactured for the patient were placed within the shoe and the shoes donned. The adequacy of the shoe fastening and the top line fit was first assessed. This should be snug with no areas which gape. The width over the instep and across the metatarso-phalangeal joints was also checked. Then the toe box depth was evaluated

Table 14.1 Case study 1: foot measurements

	Stick size		Joint width (mm)	Joint circumference (mm)	Instep circumference (mm)
	Semi-weight-bearing	Weight-bearing			
Left	8.5	9	102	275	250
Right	8.5	9	103	270	250

Table 14.2 Case study 1: last measurements

Size	Joint width (mm)	Joint circumference (mm)	Instep circumference (mm)	Toe depth (mm)
9 deep	103	283–295	252–270	47

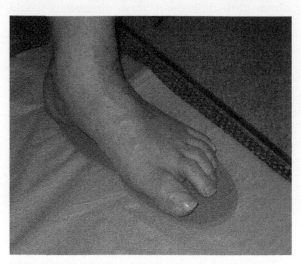

Figure 14.2 Matching foot dimensions to the shoe inner sole template.

to ensure that the vamp did not cause any compression over the clawed toes and triggered hallux. The patient was then asked to walk and the footwear was assessed for position of the toes on weight-bearing and ambulation, for heel slip, for stability at heel contact and for flexion at the appropriate point – the tread line. All were adequate.

The patient was satisfied with both the appearance and fit of his shoes. He was given advice on wear of his shoes (Appendix 1) and asked to return to the clinic in 4 weeks for evaluation. On return, all was satisfactory. The shoes had been worn for increasing lengths of time and cumulated in wear for several entire days. A second pair of shoes from the same company and made on the same last plus duplicate orthoses were ordered and issued some 4 weeks later. The patient is comfortable. The inflammatory response on his toes is reduced.

Case study 2 (modular orthopaedic footwear)

Mrs B is a 45-year-old lady who was diagnosed with rheumatoid arthritis about 8 years ago. Her initial symptoms included stiffness on walking, especially noticeable when first getting up from bed each morning, the feeling of walking on stones under both her feet and difficulty in dressing herself because her shoulders were painful.

After some months of complaining of worsening symptoms, her GP referred her for hospital tests and the results indicated that she was rheumatoid factor positive. Mrs B needs to work to support her family. She is a single parent of two children both in their teens. She works as a shop assistant and needs to spend much time standing. She complains of discomfort on the plantar surface of her feet, but, significantly, finds it difficult to find footwear to fit her changing foot shape.

On examination, Mrs B was found to have hallux valgus with plantar callous affecting the plantar metatarso-phalangeal joint area, hammered, overlying second toes and clawed lesser toes, and feet which were warm to the touch. There was also evidence of the early stages of rear foot changes, with the hind foot indicating that it was beginning to function in a pronated position. It was thought that she might benefit from footwear deep enough to accommodate the lesser toe deformities, wide enough to accommodate the medial foot changes associated with hallux valgus and adequate for the accommodation of orthoses necessary to cushion the metatarsal heads and control the rear foot motion. The footwear would be best with wedged through soles and heel for rear foot and midfoot stability, but should provide forefoot cushioning (Figs 14.3 and 14.4).

The foot measurements were recorded as shown in Table 14.3.

The sizing of Mrs B's forefoot is within the normal range for stock orthopaedic footwear, but note that her instep girth was the maximum measurement allowed within the footwear (see measurements in Table 14.4). Mrs B wanted shoes with an external decoration, and from the shape of her foot, it was determined that either a shoe from manufacturing company B or manufacturing company C would suit her best. The stock footwear available from these suppliers is generally similar in overall style, and before showing catalogues to patients, it is best to identify the manufacturer whose shoes would most closely match the patient's foot shape. The shoes from company C were chosen as they were leather lined and fairly durable. The rim toe puff is fairly firm and the soling material is also durable. The quality of the leather uppers is also excellent and wears well.

In this instance, a stock shoe was inadequate to accommodate the patient's foot when wearing the required orthoses, and modular footwear was ordered. An additional 15 mm instep girth was requested to be added to the last, to accommodate both the foot girth at the instep plus the accommodation for the orthotic. The additional accommodation also required for the hallux valgus deformity was requested and bunion pockets of 6 mm were prescribed for both shoes. This size of shoe contained 40 mm of toe depth which would accommodate her hammered and clawed toes plus the necessary orthoses to treat the plantar callous. There was no stock shoe available to try on Mrs B, but clinician familiarity with sizing from various suppliers and the calibration of the size stick used was known to accord with this manufacturer's measurement notation. While clinicians were confident of the sizing, nevertheless the shoes would be very carefully fitted and checked against Mrs B's feet on receipt.

Orthoses of 5 mm depth from heel to ball and then tapered to 2 mm under the toes were also prescribed for use within the footwear. An additional 10 mm girth for accommodation of the orthoses within each shoe was also added to the prescription measurements. While Mrs B wanted shoes with an external decoration, it was important that the shoe linings were seam free. The shoes needed to be free of any internal seams in the vamp to prevent any irritation or damage from footwear to the forefoot, especially in the region of the deformed toes and the medial prominence of the first metatarso-phalangeal joint resulting from the hallux valgus deformity. The shoes also needed a heel height of about 2.5 cms. Mrs B found the shoe styles in the brochure acceptable – similar to those she would have purchased from a retail outlet. Impressions were taken of Mrs B's feet using phenolic foam so that orthoses could be made to fit within the shoes. The orthoses were designed

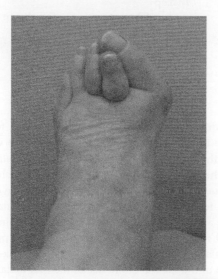

Figure 14.3 Hallux valgus with overlying second toe.

Figure 14.4 Footwear with wedged through sole and heel unit.

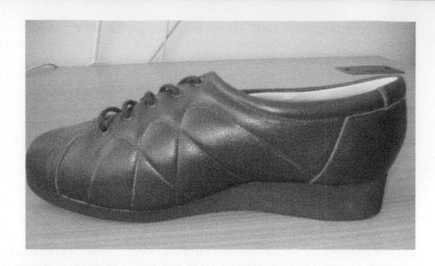

Table 14.3 Case study 2: foot measurements

	Stick size		MP joint width (mm)	MP joint girth (mm)	Midtarsal joint girth (mm)
	Semi-weight-bearing	Weight-bearing			
Left	5	5.5	95	265	260
Right	5	5.5	95	260	260

MP, metatarso-phalangeal

Table 14.4 Case study 2: stock shoe last measurements

Size	Joint width	Joint circumference (mm)	Instep circumference (mm)	Toe depth (mm)
5.5 wide and deep	95 mm	257–276	240–260	40

to help cushion the plantar metatarsal area but should contain a firm rear foot control. They were prescribed to be made of 3 mm thermoplastic sub-ortholen, a semi-rigid material, extended to provide a cushioning forefoot of 5 mm poron, reducing in depth anteriorly under the toe area.

The shoes were received within 4 weeks of the initial order. Mrs B found the footwear quite acceptable. The inner soles, reflecting the length and width of the footwear, were removed from both shoes and placed underneath Mrs B's feet. The heel-to-ball measure on both was checked against the feet to ensure that the shoe flexion line (tread line) would be in the appropriate position on the feet (aligning with the metatarso-phalangeal joints). The width of the inner soles was also checked against the width of the feet, particularly at the metatarso-phalangeal joints, and the toe shape was measured against the digital formula of Mrs B's feet. The bunion pockets were also checked for adequate width and accommodation of the medial eminence of the first metatarsal. These dimensions matched well.

The shoes were fitted with the orthoses which had been made from the impressions taken of Mrs B's feet on first consultation. The footwear containing the orthoses was then fitted to her feet. The heel fit was first checked to ensure that, with the shoe fastened, the heel sat back and was contained by the heel counter. The long heel fit seemed adequate. The facings were checked to ensure that they were in apposition with the laces fastened. The top line was checked to ensure that there was no gaping and that it did not irritate the malleoli or the retro-calcaneal area. Next Mrs B was asked to stand, and the girth was checked by careful palpation of the foot and toes within the shoe, paying particular attention to the hallux valgus deformity. This was made easier by the rim toe puff and the resulting soft upper over the dorsum of the toes. Mrs B was then asked to walk so that the shoe could be checked for heel slippage. The footwear seemed satisfactory and Mrs B was given printed wear and care instructions in addition to verbal instructions on the wear and care of her shoes.

Mrs B attended 5 weeks following the issue of her footwear to assess wear and identify any problems which might have arisen. She had followed the wear instructions given. There was no reported rubbing or redness from the footwear. On examination of her feet, there were no signs of trauma from the footwear. The orthoses were also examined for wear patterns and both width and length measurements of the footwear appeared to match those of the feet. The shoes were also examined for wear marks. The top line was checked for signs of any undue wear, the lining of the shoe was checked for any wear or irregularities and finally the outer sole and heel were examined for wear marks. These were normal, with wear demonstrated on the posterior–lateral aspect of the heel top piece and across the middle part of the tread line of the sole. The degree of wear accorded with the length of time that the shoes had been worn. However, there was one point for consideration. There was a slight slip of the heel in the shoe on walking. This was addressed by the insertion of a heel grip into the shoe. A piece of leather was adhered to the inside of the heel of the quarter with the suede side next to the foot (Fig. 14.5). Following this addition, the fit of the shoes and the wear observed appeared satisfactory.

When prescribing therapeutic footwear, each patient is considered an individual and any foot pathology, pain and preferences are considered. Lifestyle factors, mobility and other medical conditions

Figure 14.5 Footwear with heel grip inserted.

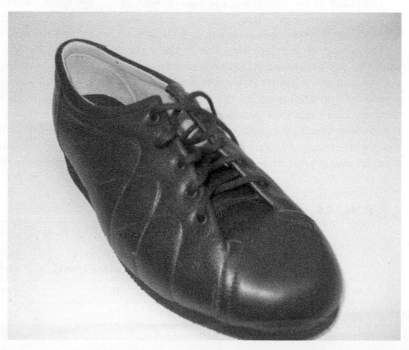

are all considered. The aim is to provide footwear that patients are happy and able to wear, that will enable them to walk better, reduce discomfort and prevent further complications and thereby improve lifestyle.

Case study 3 (modular orthopaedic footwear)

Mrs Gt is a 59-year-old lady with type 2 diabetes. She is a housewife who lives in the countryside and does not have access to a car. She therefore relies greatly on public transport and frequently walks considerable distances. The amount of exercise she gets is good for her health generally, but despite this her HbA1$_c$ levels are 9%. Due to the relatively poor control of her diabetes, she has retinopathy with resultant reduced visual acuity and a sensory neuropathy affecting both feet proximal to her ankles, accompanied by microvascular disease. Proprioception is also impaired and she tends to experience repeated ankle sprains. Her own footwear had caused ulceration on the dorsum of both fifth toes. She also presented with diffuse plantar callous over the metatarsophalangeal joints, with thicker areas of callous under the first and fifth metatarsals on both feet.

The shape of her feet was quite 'square' with little differentiation in the length of each of her toes. Measurements were taken as shown in Table 14.5.

The sizing of her feet was within the normal range for stock footwear. It was necessary to address the issue of the repeated ankle sprains. Ideally this would be best addressed by the use of boots with reinforced heel counters and heel floats (flares), but this patient found boots unacceptable. The shape of the toe box required to accommodate the square toe formula also needed to be taken into account. It was

also necessary to consider the fact that her footwear would be subject to considerable wear due to the amount of walking she does.

The footwear available from suppliers is generally similar in overall style, and before showing catalogues to patients, it is usually best to identify the manufacturer whose shoes would most closely match the patient's foot shape. In this case, it was considered that company D's footwear would be the best option as the toe box shape is rounded and less tapered than those of other manufacturers. This manufacturer's footwear also contains rim toe puffs rather than those extended more proximally back over the toes. It was felt that this would be the best option as there would be less danger of irritation of the dorsum of the toes with a soft upper without stiffening over the toe dorsum. We had a sample of this manufacturer's footwear in the clinic (6.5 wide), but when tried on the patient, it was too large. Unfortunately there is no standard between the measurements used by footwear manufacturers and clinicians frequently need to rely on experience to guide them to the actual size required from a particular manufacturer. It can be useful to maintain a stock of footwear from each manufacturer in a range of sizes so that the size suggested by the measurements taken can be tried on the patient before ordering. This, however, requires storage space – a commodity which is in short supply.

The sizing from company D has usually been found to be very generous and, so, when ordering the footwear for Mrs Gt, the size was reduced to a size 6 deep. In addition, orthoses of 7mm depth were prescribed. The accommodation for the orthoses would then require an additional 14mm girth within both shoes. The size 6 with extra depth from company D would meet her foot needs and already included sufficient accommodation to house the orthotic The last measurements are shown in Table 14.6.

Table 14.5 Case study 3: foot measurements

| | Stick size | | | | |
	Semi-weight-bearing	Weight-bearing	MP joint width (mm)	MP joint girth (mm)	Midtarsal joint girth (mm)
Left	6.5	7	96	235	240
Right	6.5	6.5	97	240	240

MP, metatarso-phalangeal

Table 14.6 Case study 3: stock shoe last measurements

Size	Joint width (mm)	Joint circumference (mm)	Instep circumference (mm)	Toe depth (mm)
6 deep	97	251–269	236–254	41

The shoes needed to be free of any internal seams in the vamp and have a low heel height of about 2.5 cms. Bilateral float outs (flares) on the heels of both shoes were prescribed to try to minimize the ankle sprains, and the manufacturer was also requested to manufacture the shoe outer soles and heels of a durable material. There was the option of having a commando-type sole unit, but Mrs Gt was concerned about the appearance of her footwear and wanted a sole unit which looked normal. She found the styling of the company D trainer-style shoes acceptable and wanted to have laced shoes rather than Velcro® fastening. However, the sole modification needed meant that this was a modular shoe prescription rather than a stock footwear prescription. This would involve extra cost, but the therapeutic needs of the patient are paramount.

Impressions were taken of Mrs Gt's feet using phenolic foam so that orthoses could be made to fit within the shoes which would help reduce the plantar pressures which were contributing to the development of callous.

On receipt of the footwear, the shoes were shown to Mrs Gt and she was pleasantly surprised by their appearance. The inner soles reflecting the length and width of the footwear were removed from both shoes and placed underneath Mrs Gt's feet. The heel-to-ball measure on both was checked against the feet to ensure that the shoe flexion line (tread line) would be in the appropriate position on the feet (according with the metatarso-phalangeal joints). The width of the inner soles was also checked against the width of the feet, particularly at the metatarso-phalangeal joints, and the toe shape was measured against the digital formula of Mrs Gt's feet. These dimensions seemed to match adequately (Fig. 14.6).

The shoes were then fitted with the orthoses which had been made from the impressions taken of Mrs Gt's feet on first consultation. They were then fitted to Mrs Gt's feet. The heel fit was first checked to ensure that, with the shoe fastened, the heel sat back and was contained by the heel counter. The long heel fit seemed adequate. The facings were checked to ensure that they were in apposition with the laces fastened. The top line was checked to ensure that there was no gaping and that it did not irritate the malleoli or the retro-calcaneal area. Next Mrs Gt was asked to stand and the girth was checked by careful palpation of the foot and toes within the shoe. This was made easier by the rim toe puff and the resulting soft upper over the dorsum of the toes. Mrs Gt was then asked to walk so that we might check the shoe for slippage.

The heel flare was discussed. It was suggested that Mrs Gt might find the benefit from this broadened heel base and that it might reduce the incidence of her ankle sprains. She was given an instruction sheet and also given verbal instructions on the wear and care of her shoes.

Mrs Gt attended 4 weeks following the issue of her footwear to assess wear and identify any problems which might have arisen. She had followed the wear instructions given. There had been no incidence of rubbing or redness from the footwear. The heel float outs were not problematic. She had become used to them within a short period of time and early indicators were that her ankle problems were reducing.

She had examined her feet as asked, with help from her husband (because of reduced visual acuity) and this foot examination is now part of her daily foot-care regime. She was asked to remove her footwear and we first examined her feet for any sign of trauma from the footwear. None was apparent. We next removed the orthoses from her footwear to look at wear patterns on those. This is a really useful way of identifying whether the width and length measurements of the footwear match those of the feet. All was fine. We next examined the shoes for wear marks. The top line was checked for signs of any undue wear, or bleeding or exudate from lesions, the lining of the shoe was checked for any wear or irregularities and,

Figure 14.6 Orthopaedic footwear in trainer-style with bilateral heel floats (flares).

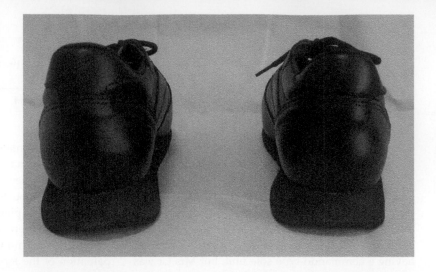

finally, the outer sole and heel for wear marks. These were normal, with wear demonstrated on the posterior–lateral aspect of the heel top piece and across the tread line of the sole. The degree of wear accorded with the length of time that the shoes had been worn. This is found to be a particularly useful exercise, as sometimes patients may mislead us about the number of occasions and the length of wear time their shoes have been used over the first assessment period.

We were satisfied with the fit of the shoes. Had there been any redness or rubbing over the dorsum of the toes then we would have stretched the offending area using a ring and ball stretcher and either steam or leather stretching solution. Any more serious problems would result in a re-prescription of the footwear.

Had the shoe begun to slip slightly at the heel, we would have considered using a reverse leather heel grip adhered into the shoe. Had there been any problems on the dorsal surface of the midtarsal area, we would have considered using a tongue pad for cushioning.

The decision to use lateral heel float outs seems to have been effective; had this not been the case, then alternative strategies would have been considered.

Generally a good first fit ensures that problems at this stage are minimal, but on rare occasions, issues which cannot be remedied are identified. In such cases, we would replace the footwear with shoes of the correct length and fitting.

Mrs Gt will now be offered a second pair of shoes made to the same prescription. Patients with diabetes-related foot complications are footwear patients for life, and all patients are given rapid access to clinics if ever they are concerned about their foot health or about their footwear. They can telephone and are given an appointment at the next clinic during the same week. All being well, Mrs Gt will be seen 6 months following the issue of her second pair of shoes and then annually.

Unless her diabetes is controlled, it is likely that Mrs Gt's foot health will deteriorate. She has been advised about caring for her feet and about ensuring that her blood glucose levels reach and are maintained at an acceptable level. One of the concerning factors is that, with the tendency to ankle inversion, she may injure her feet and may develop Charcot neuroarthropathy. This should be minimized with the heel float outs added to her shoes, but there may be times when she fails to wear them – at social functions, for example. There may also be danger if she wears slippers at home. Additional to this is the fact that, in the presence of motor neuropathy, foot shape changes over time and this requires careful re-evaluation of foot health and foot dimensions at each visit.

As with all patients, Mrs Gt must understand the need for her footwear. These shoes are not 'just shoes'; they are an essential therapy if her foot health is to be improved and maintained at an acceptable level.

Case study 4 (bespoke orthopaedic footwear)

Mr L is a retired engineer, born in 1938, who developed diabetes mellitus in 1983. The complications of the condition have affected his feet and he presents with a considerable sensory neuropathy affecting both feet and legs to the midcalf region. Mr L developed ulceration on the first metatarso-phalangeal joint of his left foot in 1996. This failed to respond to treatment; it became infected and resulted in a forefoot amputation. Some 2 years later, Mr L developed ulceration on the apex of the right second toe and the distal phalanx of this toe was also amputated.

In 2000, Mr L developed ulceration on the plantar surface of the right hallux and this toe also was subject to amputation. There were problems with healing of the site on the left foot, but this healed following regular debridement, treatment with appropriate wound dressings and the use of Pullman® trauma boots which contained total contact orthoses. The total contact orthoses were made with a rocker function by using a carbon graphite footplate shaped to give toe spring underneath them. This was necessary to prevent the forepart of the boot doubling up, to prevent Mr L tripping during gait, to use a boot which had the correct dimensions in the rear part, correct dimensions in the heel-to-ball length for the foot prior to amputation, and to facilitate a normal gait pattern. A block was made for the forepart of his left foot. Using this combined approach, the amputation site healed within 4 weeks. It was then necessary to measure for permanent footwear and it was suggested to Mr L that boots would probably provide the most successful outcome for his foot condition. The forefoot on the left foot in particular is so short that it would be difficult to ensure that shoes had an adequate area over which to grip the foot. Nevertheless, Mr L wished only to wear shoes. In such cases, where the patient is adamant that the ideal prescription choice is not acceptable, it is advisable to try to accommodate their wishes.

Foot measurements were as shown in Table 14.7.

In instances where the forefoot has been amputated, it is essential that the long and short heel measurements are accurate and provide a good fit around the heel and top line of the shoe.

Mr L's foot measurements indicated that bespoke footwear was required. These were prescribed and

drafts taken following the British Standard measurement system. The manufacturers were asked to match the shoe length to Mr L's former foot size (size 8) and to make a toe block for the amputated forefoot. Rigid rocker soles were also requested. phenolic foam impressions were taken and total contact insoles were ordered. The shoes were tried at fitting stage with the orthoses and block in place. They were found to be adequate and were returned to the manufacturer for finishing.

Mr L was fitted with his footwear, was given wear instructions and was asked to return to the clinic in 4 weeks. At this appointment, it was found that his left foot was slipping slightly in the shoe and a thin heel grip was added. Apart from this adjustment, all was well. Mr L had gradually increased wear time on a daily basis as suggested, and had worn the shoes all day for several days in succession towards the latter part of the 4-week period. The amputation site had remained healed and there was no evidence of any trauma from footwear. A second pair of shoes was ordered from the same prescription but with information also supplied about the necessary adjustment to obviate the need for the heel grip. These shoes were satisfactory.

Two years later this patient returned for a third pair of shoes. The prescription remained unchanged. But during the time between the receipt of his second pair and attending for measurement of his third, his eyesight deteriorated and he underwent cataract surgery. The patient failed to attend his subsequent appointment for shoe fitting. He attended the clinic again 12 weeks later. During these weeks, he had undergone further amputation of the remainder of the second toe and the fifth toe on his right foot. He had also developed ulceration under his right fifth metatarso-phalangeal joint, which was almost healed. These problems had arisen as Mr L was doing work in his local church. He had been working up a step ladder for several days and the angulation of his foot on the rungs of the ladder had caused him to alter the normal position of his foot within the shoe and had resulted in compression injuries. The ulceration had developed but Mr L had not sought help. He also then went on holiday to Devon. He was admitted to hospital in Devon when the ulcers became infected and they advised amputation of the remainder of the second toe and of the fifth toe. Unfortunately, on his return home, the area had not healed and there

Table 14.7 Case study 4: foot measurements

	Length seated (mm)	Length standing (mm)	MP joint width (mm)	MP joint girth (mm)	Waist girth (mm)	Instep girth (mm)	Long heel (mm)	Short heel (mm)	Heel width (mm)	Malleolar circumference (mm)
Left	186		–	–	–	275	360	335	65	255
Right	250	250	101	275	275	260	360	330	65	250

MP, metatarso-phalangeal

Figure 14.7 The patient in case study 4.

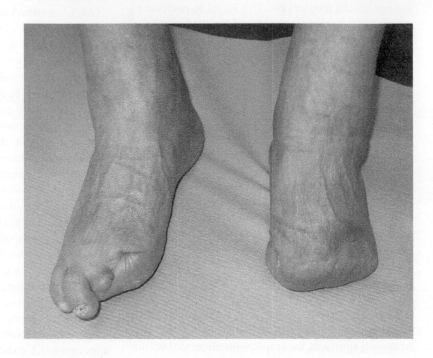

appeared to be complications. On further investigation, a sequestrum of bone was identified. This was surgically removed and the area healed. The ulceration under the fifth metatarso-phalangeal joint later healed following rest (Figs 14.7 and 14.8).

Further measurements were taken for new footwear. Again the patient wanted shoes rather than boots and his wishes were acceded to. The manufacturers were given the style of shoe requested, were asked to include cradles containing a toe block for the forepart of the left shoe and to use rigid rocker soles. Where patients have profound sensory neuropathy, it is difficult to assess fit of footwear and particular care must be taken to ensure that the finished shoe will not cause compression on any part of

the foot. Ill-fitting footwear has been cited by many clinicians as a major factor in the causal chain which leads to ulceration and to amputation.

Mr L's shoes were received from the manufacturers for fitting without an insole template and so templates were cut from firm card so that we might assess the position of various anatomical features of the foot against the template. The heel-to-ball measurement of the right foot was adequate and an estimate of the same measurement on the amputated left forefoot also appeared satisfactory. Width measurements also seemed accurate, as did length for both feet. The positioning of the block was evaluated on the insole template with the block placed at the forepart. The shoes were tried on Mr L's feet with the orthoses in

Figure 14.8 Phenolic foam foot impressions of the patient in case study 4.

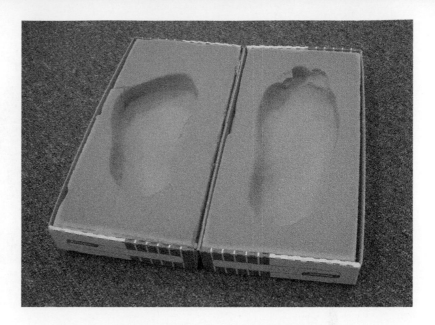

place. The top line fit was adequate, which was especially important in this case if the feet were to be held back within the shoe and the shoes were to stay on the feet. The long heel fit was good, the facings met correctly across the instep, but the fit at the base of the tongue was a little tight and an additional 5 mm girth was requested at this point on both shoes. The shoes adjusted as requested were returned from the manufacturer and fitting appeared to be good. Mr L attended for fitting and, again, Mr L's heel was comfortably held back in the counter with the orthoses in place. The fitting across the instep seemed satisfactory, the facings were in the correct position and, on palpation, there appeared to be no area on the vamp which might compress the foot or the remaining toes.

The shoes were returned for finishing with the addition of rigid rocker sole units. Mr L attended for final fitting and issue. The previous fitting evaluation was repeated and all was well. Mr L was given wear instructions for his footwear and a telephone contact number in case of any problems. He was instructed to wear the shoes for no more than 30 minutes and to examine his feet carefully after that time to identify any areas of redness or rubbing. He was asked particularly to look at the forepart of his left foot and to ensure that the toe block had caused no damage to his foot. If all was satisfactory, he was advised to increase wear by an additional 1 hour each day but to telephone

immediately and to cease wearing the shoes if any problems developed. He was reviewed 4 weeks following issue, when Mr L reported that he had worn the shoes as agreed. The shoe wear signs were positive – the orthoses reflected the adequacy of width and length in both feet, the shoes were not slipping during wear, there were no signs of any trauma affecting the feet and the sole and heel wear marks were as anticipated with normal wear at the posterior–lateral part of the heel top piece and under the metatarsal head area of the sole of the right shoe (Figs 14.9–14.11).

With careful management, it is hoped that Mr L will suffer no further trauma to his feet. He has experienced some sobering events and will now be more circumspect in agreeing to undertake DIY jobs for anyone at all, especially if they involve standing on ladders.

Case study 5 (bespoke orthopaedic footwear)

Mr R is an 82-year-old gentleman with an interesting podiatric history. In his late teens, he suffered a motorcycle accident and had a compound fracture of the lower section of his left tibia and fibula. The open wound became infected and Mr R was prepared for lower limb amputation. However, with administration of distaquin and surgery to pin the tibia and fibula, the

Figure 14.9 Shoes with toe block: case study 4.

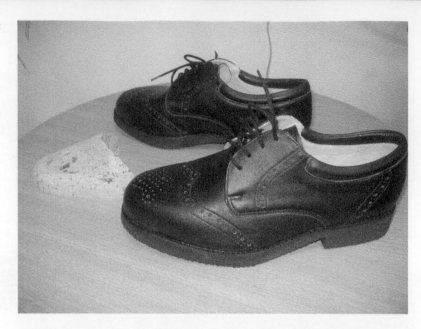

Figure 14.10 Shoes containing orthoses and toe block: case study 4.

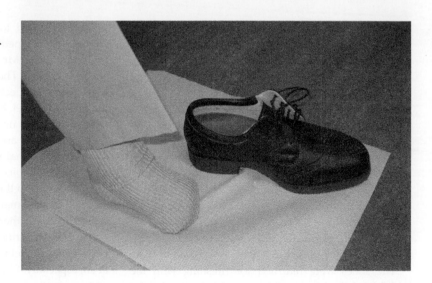

infection resolved and amputation was avoided, but the foot was inverted on his leg, and in order to walk effectively, Mr R was given surgical footwear and callipers. In 1972, further surgery was undertaken in an attempt to bring the foot to a plantargrade position, and his ankle was fixed at 90°. Following a considerable time in a plaster of Paris cast, Mr R began to mobilize and no longer needed surgical boots or callipers. The limb now has a prominent lateral malleolus, the

foot tending to inversion with the lateral border of the heel making ground contact to the exclusion of the medial aspect. An area of the heel is subject to periods of repeated ulceration which heals and then re-ulcerates. There is underlying osteomyelitis which is treated symptomatically with various antibiotics. The exciting factor in the re-ulceration saga is considered to be high pressure on an area which is denuded of the normal plantar heel tissue which

Figure 14.11 Patient in case study 4 wearing the shoes prescribed.

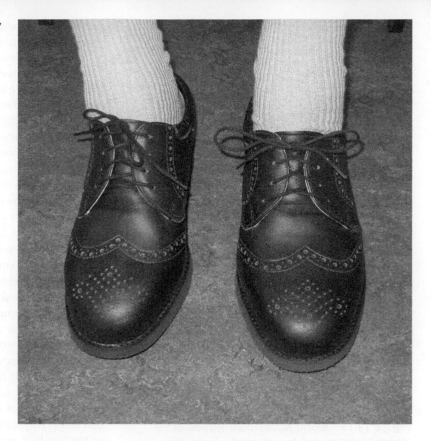

would 'pad' the area and thus absorb the ground reaction force present on heel contact.

The ulceration has been treated using a range of approaches. Environmental wound dressings and Allevyn heel cups have proved successful when coupled with trauma boots containing astrene lateral heel cushioning for shock absorption accompanied by total contact insoles made of 70 shore EVA covered with a cross-linked polyethylene foam. The ulceration improved and Mr R attended for measurements for bespoke footwear. It was noticed that Mr R was walking with one shoulder at a lower level than the other: the spinal inclination was evaluated and it became evident that we should look for a limb length discrepancy. The left limb was found to be 10 mm shorter than the right. On using elevation blocks of 10 mm (Figs 14.12 and 14.13) under the

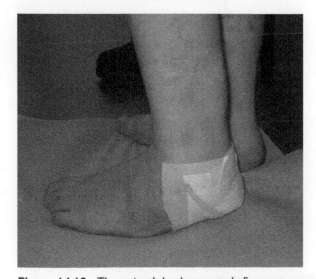

Figure 14.12 The patient's heel: case study 5.

an increased plantar surface contact area, with an extended heel cup for the left and a 10 mm heel raise for the left. Because of a slightly compromised circulatory status, polyethylene foam was chosen to insulate the feet and a base of 70 shore EVA. The orthoses were similar to those included in the trauma boots.

At fitting stage, the boots were found to fit adequately and were returned for finishing without adjustment. A more detailed evaluation of the footwear at fitting stage is included below. The orthoses were made with the underside of each reflecting the dimensions of the inner sole of the appropriate boot, the upper surface reflecting the contours of each foot with a high cup for the left heel. This is designed to ensure that the surface contact area of the feet is increased, thus equalizing the force to which unit areas are subjected in load-bearing. This should, therefore, reduce the pressure taken by the damaged left heel and produce an environment which encourages healing. The heel raise included on the underside of the left orthotic will also address the limb length discrepancy to provide greater symmetry of limbs, so reducing stress throughout the kinetic chain. The footwear will have a major role in ensuring that each foot is allowed to function at an optimal level. The ankle fixation, the altered architecture of the left heel and the overall dimensions of both feet have been addressed.

While this therapy is suggested as being appropriate for the treatment of plantar ulceration, its success will depend on the patient's concordance. The footwear with orthoses needs to be worn for the great majority of the time that the foot is in ground contact. Patients are advised to wear their new footwear for 30 minutes initially, and to then examine their feet for any indicator of pressure from footwear. If any areas of redness, which might be associated with the footwear, are identified, they are asked to stop wearing the boots or shoes, and to inform the clinician of the problem at their next appointment (4 weeks). If there are no problems, they are asked to extend wear time by an additional 1 hour each day and to examine their feet following this period of wear. Once this initial phase has been successfully completed, patients are asked to wear their footwear at all times except when visiting the bathroom at night. Some patients find it difficult to wear their boots or shoes indoors. They may have always worn slippers at home, and breaking the habit of a

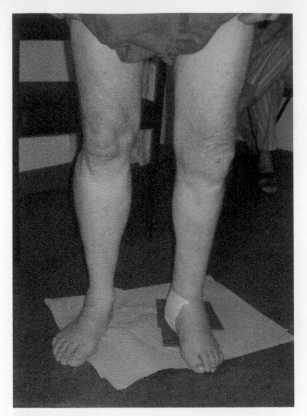

Figure 14.13 Blocks placed under left heel of the patient in case study 5 to evaluate the height of the required raise.

left heel, Mr R was seen to be more symmetrical and indicated that his hip and lower back felt more comfortable (he had not previously complained of pain in these regions). His feet were then measured, drafts were taken and plaster of Paris impressions of both feet were made. Mr R prefers to wear boots because of his ankle problems. The preferred boot quarter height was identified as 130 mm and measurements of leg circumference at the malleolar level and at the top of the boot level were taken. Velcro® fastening was preferred for ease of attachment.

The foot measurements were as shown in Table 14.8.

Because of the ankle fixation, the outer sole unit of the shoes was designed to include only 12 mm of heel height with 12 mm at the tread line (i.e. level from heel to joint) and a rocker to the toes. To give additional stability, a rigid wedged sole and heel unit was requested. Orthoses were prescribed to include

Table 14.8 Case study 5: foot measurements

	Length seated (mm)	Length standing (mm)	MP joint width (mm)	MP joint girth (mm)	Waist girth (mm)	Instep girth (mm)	Long heel (mm)	Short heel (mm)	Heel width (mm)	Malleolar circumference (mm)
Left	260	260	96	258	258	250	350	320	71	255
Right	278	280	105	265	263	250	360	340	65	245

MP, metatarso-phalangeal

lifetime is difficult. They need to understand that the footwear and orthoses prescribed for them are actually a therapy. It may be equated with medication: if they fail to take their medication, it will be ineffective. Similarly if they fail to wear the prescribed footwear, the foot problem will not benefit from it, and the ulceration or other lesion will fail to heal.

Mr R was prescribed boots (Fig. 14.14). He has worn boots for a number of years, having found that shoes irritated the lateral side of his left ankle and heel. Following examination of his foot shape, it was considered wise to continue to use boots. At fitting stage, it is helpful to use a structured approach to check fitting. In Mr R's case, as with all patients, a footwear insole template was compared with the foot to ensure that the width of the footwear made was adequate throughout both boots, to match the length

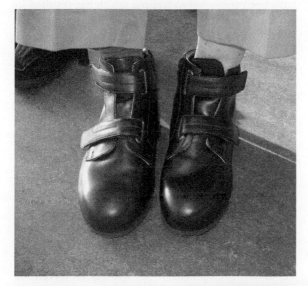

Figure 14.14 Patient in case study 5 wearing boots.

of the boots with the length of the feet and to check that heel-to-ball measurements were satisfactory.

We had asked the shoe manufacturer to allow an additional depth of 1 cm to house orthoses for Mr R; these will not be made until the original dimensions of the inner sole are available, therefore a piece of material equating to the depth of the orthoses is cut and inserted into the boots before fitting. With the mock orthoses in place at fitting stage, it is useful to first evaluate whether the boots can be donned without great effort first by the clinician and then later by the patient himself, as he will need to be able to do this adequately in normal daily wear. Then, with the boots fastened, the height of the quarter was checked to ensure that it matched the prescription, and the fit around the leg circumference at the top of the boot was checked to ensure that it was neither too snug nor too loose, bearing in mind the hosiery worn and the likelihood of any ankle oedema.

The short heel and long heel measurements were then checked, and the match of the facings across the instep and throughout the fastening were checked to ensure that they were not too tight and that the Velcro® straps fastened with adequate length still available to fasten across the entire attachment point. While the length and width measurements had been checked against the insole template, both dimensions plus the girth dimensions were checked again, both visually and by palpation of the foot within the footwear.

The fitting for Mr R was firstly checked semi weight-bearing, next fully weight-bearing and finally walking. In walking, the ability of the boot to retain the heel within the counter was also checked to ensure that the boot did not slip and also that the forepart of the foot was not impacted against the toe box of the boot. In gait, it is also essential to look for fluency to ensure as far as possible that the tread line appears to be in the correct position, that heel strike is normal and that there is no slippage at the back of the shoe or boot or excess creasing across the vamp. On fitting this footwear, each aspect seemed satisfactory and the footwear was returned for finishing.

The finished boots were received and fitted 2 weeks later, by which time the orthoses were made. Wear advice was given. However, Mr R was reluctant to wear his boots indoors and it may be possible to find a house shoe within which we may use an orthotic. In the meantime, he has undertaken to wear his shoes as advised and has been given a return appointment for evaluation in 2 weeks.

The expectation for Mr R is that he will follow the wear advice given, that gradually his ulceration will show signs of improvement and that within a period of about 8 weeks, all other things being equal, his ulceration will have healed. In healing this ulceration, it is also important to ensure that the footwear will not cause any other foot problems. We must remember too that all the factors which led to the development of the heel ulceration, its history of recurrence and failure to heal are still present. The limited joint mobility, the high pressure area on the lateral border of the left heel, the underlying osteomyelitis and a circulatory status concomitant with an age of 82 years are all factors which need consideration. Therapeutic footwear provides the opportunity to break the cycle: it can remove the high pressure on the heel area and, by using materials which insulate, can help improve circulation to the feet. It is also anticipated that the hip and lower back discomfort that Mr R obviously suffered, but did not complain of, will resolve.

It is hoped that the footwear will have a positive impact on Mr R's general health and that it will help him lead a more active lifestyle and reduce the number of hospital visits he has to make – at present about 2 per week – and also reduce the number of calls from the district nurse required to dress his ulceration. The aim is to improve quality of life, to reduce morbidity and minimize the likelihood of amputation.

Case study 6 (bespoke orthopaedic footwear)

Mrs G is a lady born in 1958 who has spina bifida. She has worn surgical footwear with an external calliper on the left leg throughout her life and has a considerable limb length discrepancy of 8 cm. Her left leg is shorter than her right. This discrepancy is so great that she cannot even attempt to visit the bathroom at night without her footwear, and showering is impossible. In her early twenties, she underwent a triple arthrodesis which fused her ankle at 90° to her leg and her midtarsal joint in 15° of plantar flexion. She also had a deformity affecting her left third toe where the proximal interphalangeal joint was in fixed plantarflexion, and the distal interphalangeal joint was also fixed. The resultant toe apex was at a lower level than the other digits. Both her feet also demonstrated a small amount of plantar callous over the plantar surface of the metatarso-phalangeal joints.

Her previous footwear was made to reflect only the fixation of the ankle, and in prescription and manufacture, the plantarflexion of her midtarsal joint appears to have been ignored, as was the toe problem. In consequence, the apex of her plantarflexed left third toe developed first heloma durum and later ulceration. A decision was made to amputate the distal phalanx of that toe. Unfortunately the amputation site proved difficult to heal, and it was at that time that Mrs G was first referred to the specialist footwear service. It was identified that a suture remaining in her toe was contributing to the extended healing time, but also a sequestrum of bone was found on further investigation under epidural. During this procedure, her spinal nerves appear to have been subjected to trauma which has resulted in uncontrollable tremors of her left limb, a progressive loss of motor power and abnormality of sweating. The tremors were most pronounced at rest, particularly in bed at night, but she is still able to walk with the aid of orthopaedic footwear, callipers and arm crutches (Fig. 14.15).

On first meeting Mrs G, biomechanical assessment was carried out. It was identified that her left ankle joint was fixed at 90° and the plantarflexed fixation of her left midtarsal joint was identified and measured. Her limb lengths were measured with the patient supine, and a tape measure held on the zyphoid process and measured to the medial malleolus of both ankles and from the anterior superior iliac crest of both hips to the medial malleolus. The hip measurements were difficult to assess because of the underdevelopment of her left leg. However, we then placed an 8 cm raise under the left leg with the

Figure 14.15 The patient in case study 6.

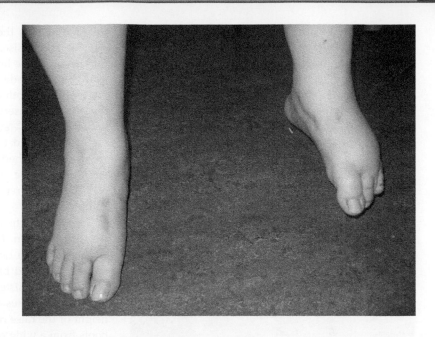

Table 14.9 Case study 6: foot measurements

	Length seated (mm)	Length standing (mm)	MP joint width (mm)	MP joint girth (mm)	Waist girth (mm)	Instep girth (mm)	Long heel (mm)	Short heel (mm)	Heel width (mm)	Malleolar circumference (mm)
Left	215	215	80	223	230	245	330	320	62	250
Right	233	235	98	240	243	250	330	320	60	255

MP, metatarso-phalangeal

patient standing. The pelvic level measure appeared satisfactory when the elevation was assessed. This equated with the previous elevation which the patient identified as comfortable. But while this was adequate at the heel, the identified discrepancy at the midtarsal joint indicated that the forefoot elevation needed to be modified. The limb length discrepancy required an 8 cm heel elevation, a 7 cm tread line elevation, tapering to a toe elevation of 4.5 cm, thus permitting a rock over for toe spring. A calliper entry socket also needed to be included in the raise.

Drafts of both feet were taken with an appropriate elevation under the left foot to hold the draft pad at a suitable height from the ground to allow the foot to make contact with it and rest on it comfortably.

Her foot measurements were as shown in Table 14.9.

A plaster of Paris impression was taken of both feet with a heel elevation of 1 cm from the horizontal under the impression while it set. This represented the 15° plantarflexion at the midtarsal joint and allowed the foot to retain a fully plantargrade position. A vertical line was drawn on the outside of each cast from the lateral malleolus proximally along the leg, and a horizontal line drawn directly beneath that line. The instructions to the manufacturer included the detailed medical history and identified the problematic areas on her feet. Overall, the shape of her feet is relatively normal, but the function is reduced because of the lack of motor power and control as a result of the spina bifida and because of surgical intervention (Fig. 14.16).

In addition to the footwear, we also intended to make total contact orthoses for both her feet. The therapeutic rationale was to aid healing of her left third toe and to ensure that there was optimal weight distribution over the plantar surface of both feet to reduce loading over the metatarso-phalangeal joint area where callous was beginning to form.

The footwear prescribed, which reflected the angulation at the midtarsal joint, was received at fitting stage and returned for finishing without further modification (Fig. 14.17). It is difficult to assess

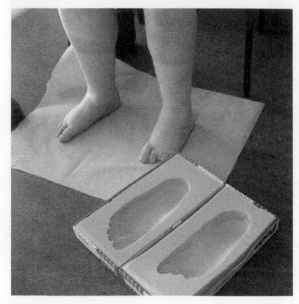

Figure 14.16 Phenolic foam impressions: case study 6.

the fit in gait as the shoes are sent for fitting without the final raise. However, the indicators were that fitting at the heel was excellent, and width and girth appeared adequate when an inner sole reflecting the final depth of the orthotic to be used within the shoe was inserted. Once the dimensions of the boot inner soles were available, work could begin on the orthoses, and these were made while the boots were being finished. They were issued some 3 weeks later, and as the patient has full sensation in her feet, she could report that she found the footwear comfortable.

The apex of the left third toe healed without further complication. The patient was pleased to be able to choose from a range of colours, as previously she had been offered black or brown boots only. While the clinician insisted that she needed boots rather than shoes because of stability problems with the height of the raise needed, she was able to select her boots from a wide range of colours. She chose bright blue. There was one later complication in that the dye from the shoe leached out and stained her hosiery and her feet. This was made worse by the sweating abnormality which developed following surgery. She was unwilling to use her previous footwear and we had to wait for a second pair of boots made to the new prescription before we could address the problems with staining from the leather dye.

Figure 14.17 Note the angulation of the sole of the boot reflecting the angulation of the surgical fixation of the ankle and midtarsal joints: case study 6.

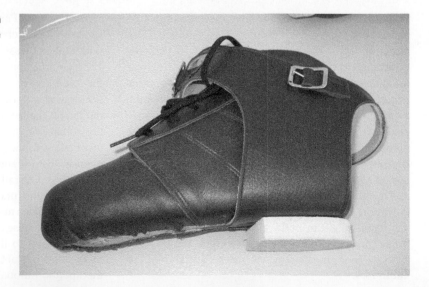

Figure 14.18 The patient in case study 6 in well-worn footwear.

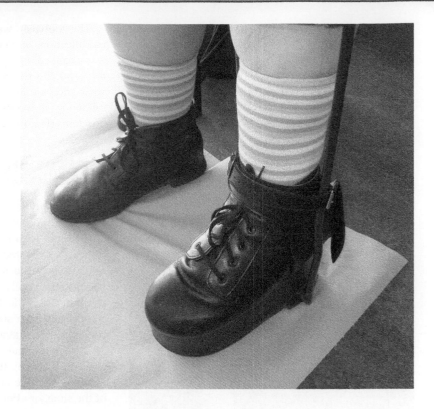

Once her additional boots were ready, the first pair was returned to the manufacturer, who sprayed a compound inside the boot to prevent the staining. This was effective (Fig. 14.18).

The patient remains with feet free of superficial lesions, and while her mobility levels are declining because of the long-term affects of spina bifida, she is still able to walk. She dreads the thought of losing the ability to walk when she might become confined to a wheelchair. She is also undergoing physiotherapy to maximize the muscular capability, and this, accompanied by her determination to remain independent, should ensure that she retains maximum ambulatory capacity for as long as possible.

Case study 7 (bespoke orthopaedic footwear)

Mr K was born in 1936, and at the age of 8 years, he contracted poliomyelitis. He appeared to recover adequately from the condition but retained a 'weakness'

in his right leg. As he has aged, over the past 10–15 years, his foot condition has deteriorated and he demonstrates the typical post polio syndrome. His right leg is shorter than his left, has reduced calf muscle girth and power, and his right foot is inverted and plantarflexed. He also has ankle equinus and footdrop of his right foot (Fig. 14.19).

Despite this, he is quite active. He is retired from his work as a local government officer but walks regularly, has an allotment where he grows his own vegetables and has an active social life and regularly goes on holiday when he travels to various parts of the world.

His feet are of very different sizes. Bespoke footwear was indicated and drafts were taken which indicated the measurements shown in Table 14.10 (Fig. 14.20). Plaster of Paris impressions were taken with the required raise in place beneath the right foot (Fig. 14.21).

Mr K's footwear demands were simple. He wanted to have black shoes. It was suggested that boots might be better because of the raise required for the right leg, which was 34 mm shorter than the left, but he preferred to have shoes. His limb length discrepancy was measured and an elevation prescribed to raise the right heel by 34 mm, the right tread line by 17 mm and the area under the toes by 8.5 mm. A bridged raise was prescribed to gain some symmetry between the left and right shoe. The patient's preference was that both shoes should appear with a distinct heel unit (rather than a through wedged unit).

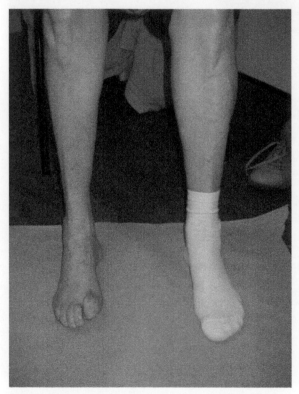

Figure 14.19 Post polio syndrome affecting the right leg: case study 7.

The footwear was received for a fitting and no modifications were required. The completed footwear was received 4 weeks later. The fitting was satisfactory and the shoes were issued to the patient with wear and care instructions. The patient was seen for follow-up 4 weeks later and reported no adverse problems (Fig. 14.22).

Conclusion

The prescription of therapeutic footwear may at first seem daunting, but bear in mind that about 75% of all patients requiring orthopaedic footwear can be satisfactorily fitted from stock ranges. These are returnable to the manufacturer if they don't fit the patient adequately. It is also possible to liaise with some orthopaedic footwear manufacturers to have a supply of each size and fitting held in your clinic, provided you have sufficient secure storage space. This provides the opportunity of trying the shoes, and either issuing them to the patient immediately if the fit is suitable and they like the colour and style of the shoe, or alternatively ordering footwear of the correct size and fitting of the desired style and shade with certainty of fit.

By beginning to work with an available range of stock shoes, clinicians can become familiar with the features of the manufacturer's styling and will be able to evaluate the fitting features and address the way in which each feature may be used to address a patient's therapeutic needs. By becoming familiar, clinicians will develop an understanding of the parts of the shoe which may need modification to best suit particular pathologies and, in this way, gradually progress to prescribing modular footwear.

Table 14.10 Case study 7: foot measurements

	Length seated (mm)	Length standing (mm)	MP joint width (mm)	MP joint girth (mm)	Waist girth (mm)	Instep girth (mm)	Long heel (mm)	Short heel (mm)	Heel width (mm)	Malleolar circumference (mm)
Left	252	255	108	256	256	250	350	325	61	235
Right	222	222	100	268	268	255	325	315	60	205

MP, metatarso-phalangeal

Figure 14.20 Taking drafts for footwear measurements: case study 7.

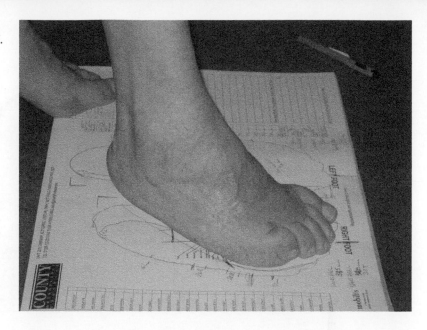

Figure 14.21 Plaster of Paris impressions (case study 7) are taken with the required raise in place. Note that the impression is marked with horizontal and vertical reference points.

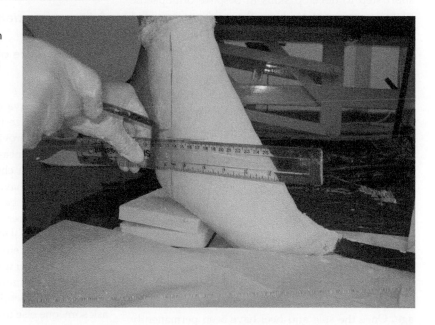

Figure 14.22 Footwear for patient in case study 7 – note raise on right shoe.

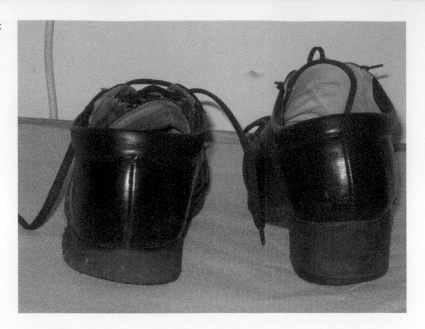

From modular footwear prescription, it is only a short step to develop skills in bespoke orthopaedic footwear prescription. Here the guidance provided by the British Standard is invaluable. The drafting system may seem arduous at first, but is an extremely useful tool which is relatively straightforward to use. In addition, taking a cast of a highly complex foot gives the last maker a clear vision of the patient's problem and is the key to the manufacture of a successful shoe or boot for feet which have been subject to pathological or traumatic changes.

Both modular and bespoke footwear is best made to a fitting stage, where it is received without permanent soles and heels attached, at a point in manufacture when alterations to width, girth and length can easily be made. Where changes are made at fitting stage, it may be worthwhile having subsequent fittings, just to ensure that the shoe fits perfectly. It is better to take time to ensure that a shoe fits well rather than providing a patient with an ill-fitting shoe which may cause them discomfort or damage. Once the sole and heel have been permanently attached, the shoe or boot cannot be altered.

Footwear can be an extremely valuable therapy, providing patients with a means of relieving pain and discomfort, optimizing gait patterns, increasing mobility levels and improving quality of life.

Appendix

Advice to patients with diabetes

Wear and care of special footwear and orthoses

Because you have diabetes, your feet need special care. To minimize the risk of damage to your feet, you have been provided with special shoes. Your feet were carefully measured and the selection of shoes from which you chose has been specially designed for people who have diabetes.

There should be no problem with your footwear. Great care has been taken in fitting it. It should be comfortable and it should be easy to walk in.

However, to ensure that there are no problems, the first time you wear your shoes it should be for no more than 30 minutes. Then, take your shoes off and examine your feet (if you have poor eyesight, please ask someone else to do this for you). If you find:

- any colour change in any part of your foot
- any new pain or throbbing in any part of your foot
- any new swelling in your foot or leg
- any rub

- any blisters
- anything else which concerns you

DO NOT WEAR THE SHOES. If you are concerned, please contact the clinic (the telephone number is on your appointment card).

IT IS ONLY IN VERY RARE CIRCUMSTANCES THAT ANY OF THESE PROBLEMS OCCUR.

If all is well and your feet appear normal after the first 30 minutes of wear, please gradually increase wear time by an additional hour each day. Once you have built up wear to an entire day, please begin to wear your shoes every day. They should become your normal footwear. Please wear them. They should be worn throughout the day, every time your foot touches the ground. You should wear them indoors. Slippers should be worn only for very short periods of time, for example for a visit to the bathroom at night.

You will be given an appointment to attend the footwear clinic again, in about 4 weeks and then again at regular intervals. Please ensure that you keep these appointments.

Your shoes contain orthoses (insoles). Each orthosis has been made specifically for each of your feet and has been fitted to your shoes. Each is made to fit one shoe and should be worn in that shoe and not in any other.

Caring for your shoes

Your shoes are made from soft leather, and creasing of the uppers will occur as you wear them. To prolong the life of your shoes and to help keep their appearance, polish them regularly and wipe away any debris or mud which may become attached to them. If for any reason your shoes or orthoses get wet, allow them to dry away from direct heat.

To clean your orthoses, wipe them with a damp cloth. Do not immerse them in water.

When your shoes need to be repaired, please remove the orthoses and any laces in your shoes and return them to clinic. They will be repaired free of charge.

Index

Index

Printed and bound by CPI Group (UK) Ltd, Croydon, CR0 4YY
03/10/2024
01040366-0012